Transactional Analysis Proper—and Improper

Transactional Analysis Proper—and Improper: Selected and New Papers offers a critical reading of transactional analysis (TA), which analyses, deconstructs, and reconstructs its foundational theory.

Keith Tudor's work is detailed, informative, and critical, and written with deep affection for TA and its founder, Eric Berne. Beginning with its philosophical foundations, Tudor considers TA's ontological assumptions about the essence of human beings, its method and methodology, and its treatment philosophy. A series of chapters then review and advance TA's theory of transactions, ego states, life scripts, and psychological games, and the book concludes with two chapters which both honour TA's traditions and look forward to what TA might do differently.

This book offers a unique 'insider but independent' perspective on transactional analysis. It will be essential reading for students and practitioners of transactional analysis and encourages free, independent, and critical thinking about TA and its place in the world.

Keith Tudor is professor of psychotherapy at Auckland University of Technology, Aotearoa New Zealand where he is also a co-Lead of Moana Nui—Centre for Research in the Psychological Therapies. He has been involved with transactional analysis (TA) for over 40 years and is a Certified and a Teaching and Supervising Transactional Analyst in the field of psychotherapy. He is a well-published author and editor in the field, with over 100 publications about TA, including most recently an edited book: *Claude Steiner, Emotional Activist* (Routledge, 2020). He has a small private practice as a therapist, trainer, and supervisor, based in West Auckland.

'A magisterial summary and reflective critique of transactional analysis and its relationships to the psychodynamics of most of the last century, this latest book by Keith Tudor is truly revolutionary. This is for the serious student, teacher and practitioner of transactional analysis. It covers and evaluates all the developments in the field since Berne and their potentials as practitioners encounter different populations and circumstances. Yet all, as Tudor emphasizes, are rooted in the same philosophical and ethical principles. Notwithstanding its complexity, the book is written in simple and clear language. I especially appreciated the extraordinarily useful tables. They also highlight that transactional analysis is not a one-size fits all approach for true believers with one set of techniques, but a rich and generative background from which, within a contractual framework, to come alongside our clients. For future students, teachers and practitioners, this will be The Book!'

James R. Allen, *MD, MPH, Teaching and Supervising Transactional Analyst, Formerly Professor of Psychiatry and Behavioral Sciences, University of Oklahoma Health Science Center Oklahoma City, USA and Past President of the International Transactional Analysis Association*

'This tour de force is an unfolding exploration of the core ideas of TA from philosophy to theory to methodology to practice. Keith Tudor constructs, critiques and examines the different views of the conceptual roots of transactional analysis, including I'm OK, You're OK, thinking Martian, ego states, scripts, and much more. He explores the implications of concepts philosophically and politically, locating them in space and time within the wider field of psychological thought as well as within society.

It is a challenging book and also a deeply respectful, inclusive and even a gentle one. It is also erudite and stimulating – a wonderful resource for others writing in the field. I found that it was not a quick read. In every chapter there was something to make me stop and have a discussion with the author in my head, to look things up, to make notes, to agree and disagree, and much to muse about!

The collection of papers, some previously published and some new, also tracks the author's own journey from his beginnings as a qualified transactional analyst in the 1990s through to the present day. At its heart, of course, are transactions – or, rather *present-centred relating* – from a deeply relational standpoint. There is a rich elaboration of Keith's thinking about relating as well as his contribution to Stark's (1999) modes of therapeutic action, namely "two-person plus" relating, which invites the reader to embrace a constant higher level of awareness of the wider world, including issues of ecological and intersectional importance on one hand, and on the other, the professional and personal identity of a transactional analyst.'

Professor Charlotte Sills, *Teaching and Supervising Transactional Analyst, Ashridge Hult University, Berkhamsted, and Metanoia Institute, London, UK*

'Beginning with its title, the book *Transactional Analysis Proper – and Improper*, comprises a challenge from the author to transactional analysts to identify TA both in its "proper" form (traditional, classical and transactional) and its less proper form, i.e., one which is more deconstructive, and acknowledging of the incongruent elements of the original theory and methodology of TA.

Drawing on his personal and professional journey as a transactional analyst, and as someone who has worked with, taught, and reflected on TA for some 35 years, Keith Tudor offers this detailed analysis using both scientific method and philosophical analysis. In doing so, he has created an intense book, full of bibliographical references, through which he traces the evolutionary path of thought in TA and its different and sometimes opposing orientations.

In this volume, which comprises some of his previous publications, as well as seven new chapters, the author attempts to give some answers to the contradictions he identifies in TA theory, and, in doing so, poses many questions for the reader to reflect upon, including that of the paradigm of ego states which lies at the heart of TA. The author does this on various levels – conceptual, clinical, phenomenological, and existential level, inviting us to go beyond a "skin-to-skin" schema characteristic of the Western view of personality. The author proposes that we move towards a psychology of "we-ness" in order to replace the top-down anthropocentric and anthropomorphic psychology with one that restores the inseparability of the self from the world. Visible in this new paradigm is the importance of recognising the self, the other, others and the environment in a co-creative relational mode that is oriented towards collective well-being as well as individual autonomy. What this book proposes and demonstrates is that the construction of postmodern identities cannot be reduced to the action of intrapsychic determinants alone.

This important contribution is vital for the future development of TA on both a theoretical and a methodological level. In various chapters, the author attempts to identify a map within which to move in order to review the main theoretical and methodological assumptions of TA, starting from the use of words and their meaning. The text emphasises the importance of the clinical and environmental context and their influence in the construction of theory, a construction that cannot fail to take into account the context in which we live and form our psychological world, a context in which we are in deep and constant relationship. Last but not least, this important volume suggests that the future of TA must be fluid and oriented towards the present and the future, and free from a past (including its contradictions), within which the present cannot be imprisoned.'

Dr Gaetano Sisalli, *Clinical Transactional Analyst,*
Teaching and Supervising Transactional Analyst,
and Psychiatrist, living and working in Catania, Italy

'In many ways reading Keith Tudor's book feels like stepping into a craftsman's workshop and watching him immersed in his work, assessing the weight of various materials, measuring their length, finding out their melting point, or how easily they break if bent. The author takes Berne's pivotal ideas and critically observes them, playfully, but vigorously challenging them at times, turning them on their head and, ultimately, transforming them. His lens regarding the nature and purpose of TA, its practice, or the nature and purpose of transactional theory is often radical; however, it is not subservient to forms of radicalism, but remains (self) reflexive, committed to complexity and dialogue. Throughout the book, some passages convey echoes of either hopefulness, or disappointment in relation to the use or misuse of theory, yet each time the author's relentless curiosity remains in place, unwavering.

The reading of Keith Tudor's book becomes all the more meaningful when considered in relationship to other TA papers and in the broader context provided by philosophical and political writings. It is a reading that equally fosters the freedom to agree, as well to disagree with the content, the courage to exercise the craft of testing out the coherence of our theoretical frameworks. Therefore, it becomes a good companion for the reader's mind and heart alike.'

Diana Deaconu, *Psychologist and Certified*
Transactional Analyst, Bucharest, Romania

'In his aptly titled book, *Transactional Analysis Proper – and Improper*, Keith Tudor has surveyed and updated six decades of transactional analysis (TA) literature. The title points to a clear discussion of, and a careful balance between, the two poles of TA critique – that it is an overly simple "pop" psychology, and that it has tried too hard to become complex, colonising other, particularly psychodynamic models. The book's layout in three, roughly chronological parts, makes it immediately accessible to readers with both beginning and sophisticated sensibilities, and, read in sequence (though they do not have to be), they take the reader on a philosophical journey through TA theory, from foundational ideas to a complex future. The book offers depth and informed perspective to both social studies (and particularly psychotherapy) students and experienced practitioners and academics. It is likely to become a standard text in the field, and deservedly so.'

Seán Manning, *Teaching and Supervising*
Transactional Analyst, Dunedin, Aotearoa New Zealand,
and former President of the New Zealand
Association of Psychotherapists

Transactional Analysis Proper—and Improper

Selected and New Papers

Keith Tudor

Routledge
Taylor & Francis Group

LONDON AND NEW YORK

Designed cover image: The Last Night (2) by Charlotte McLachlan

First published 2025
by Routledge
4 Park Square, Milton Park, Abingdon, Oxon OX14 4RN

and by Routledge
605 Third Avenue, New York, NY 10158

Routledge is an imprint of the Taylor & Francis Group, an informa business

British Library Cataloguing-in-Publication Data
A catalogue record for this book is available from the British Library

Library of Congress Cataloging-in-Publication Data
Names: Tudor, Keith, 1955– author.
Title: Transactional analysis proper-and improper:
selected and new papers / Keith Tudor.
Description: Abingdon, Oxon; New York, NY: Routledge, 2025. |
Includes bibliographical references and index. |
Identifiers: LCCN 2024021184 (print) | LCCN 2024021185 (ebook) |
ISBN 9780367027209 (hardback) | ISBN 9780367027216 (paperback) |
ISBN 9780429398223 (ebook)
Subjects: MESH: Transactional Analysis
Classification: LCC RC489.T7 (print) | LCC RC489.T7 (ebook) |
NLM WM 460.5.T7 | DDC 616.89/145—dc23/eng/20240625
LC record available at https://lccn.loc.gov/2024021184
LC ebook record available at https://lccn.loc.gov/2024021185

ISBN HB: 9780367027209
ISBN PB: 9780367027216
ISBN EB: 9780429398223

DOI: 10.4324/9780429398223

Typeset in Times New Roman
by codeMantra

Contents

Introduction

The best physician is also a philosopher.

(Aelius Galenus)

This book presents and develops a critical and reflexive perspective on transactional analysis (TA), informed by contemporary relational perspectives both within and outside TA. Comprising six previously published papers, and seven new chapters, the volume both represents my existing contribution to TA over some 35 years and offers further developments of TA.

The title of the book plays on a central piece of TA theory, the analysis of transactions, otherwise known as 'transactional analysis proper' or TA Proper, and confronts it, in the Bernean sense of the word, by developing what might be considered as TA 'improper', i.e., that which challenges the language and rhetoric of TA, some of its tradition and received wisdom, its authority and convention, and its claims to objectivity and universalism, as well as the conservatism of much of TA therapeutic practice. My own interest in critical thinking, criticism and critique is long-standing (for the background to which, see Tudor, 2018b), and, alongside some of my other writing in TA (Tudor, 1996, 2008d, 2010d, 2011e, 2016ca, 2016d; Tudor & Widdowson, 2008; Tudor et al., 2022), this book represents such thinking, applied to TA. Moreover, despite his own social conservatism, Berne appreciated independent thinkers—in *Principles of Group Treatment* (Berne, 1966a), he cites Karl Abraham approvingly in this respect—and himself advocates 'the "Martian" approach' (Berne, 1962, p. 32), which represents a way of thinking without preconceived ideas (see Chapter 13). In his commentary on this, Hostie (1982) refers to this as 'that impertinence which prompts extremely pertinent questions' (p. 169). Whilst this was very much part of Berne's own style, and of some of the early discussions in the San Francisco Social Psychiatry Seminars, and, of course, of the radical psychiatry tradition in (and outside) TA, there is, with a couple of notable exceptions, i.e., Deaconu (2020) and Barrow and Marshall (2023b), now comparatively little Martian thinking, speaking, or writing in TA (for discussion of which, see Chapter 13).

I have been inspired by other critical thinkers in TA, and especially those who invite us all to think critically and reflexively about theory. These include Robert

DOI: 10.4324/9780429398223-1

Massey (e.g., 1986), William (Bill) Cornell (e.g., 1988), Marilyn Zalcman (1990), Graham Barnes (1994, 2000, 2004, 2005), James (Jim) Allen (e.g., 2009), Helena Hargaden (2016), Salma Siddique (2017), and, most recently, Victoria Baskerville (2003). I particularly appreciate Zalcman's (1990) critique of the (then) development of TA theory and practice, which she views as slowed down and misdirected, due to four trends:

(1) The rapid generation of new TA concepts and techniques without adequate conceptual integration with what already exists;
(2) The adoption of concepts and techniques from other methods without sufficient critical evaluation or integration into TA theory and practice;
(3) The reframing of TA into psychoanalytic and neo-psychodynamic terms, often to make it 'more respectable', or presenting TA in pop psychology terms, often to make it 'more marketable'; and
(4) More recently, the tendency to quote Berne and to proceed as if his words were gospel and not to be questioned (Zalcman, 1990, p. 5).

Thirty five years on, these trends are still trending. Thinking about this book in relation to Zalcman's observations, I think that, by considering the philosophical basis of TA (in Part I), I offer some clarity with regard to conceptual integration; by exploring and emphasising the frame that is transactional analysis, I present a depth and breadth that can hopefully inspire a renewed confidence in this analysis, rather than psycho-analysis or pop analysis; and, by researching what Berne wrote (throughout, but especially in Chapters 2, 6, 9, and 11), I provide both the old testament, or, at least a critical exegesis of it, as well as some contributions to a new testament. In this sense, I hope that this contribution addresses some of what Zalcman refers to as negative outcomes of such trends, and, in any case, is something on which I reflect in Chapter 13.

I refer to 'therapeutic practice' as, although TA has a number of fields of application (counselling, education, organisations, and psychotherapy), my experience, training, and practice has been predominantly in the field of psychotherapy, although, interestingly, my first article on TA, published in 1990, was an early attempt to understand organisational dynamics, and, nearly 35 years later, and as I am again working in an organisation, this time a university, I find myself returning to the application of TA to and in organisations—and continuing to value the independence, impropriety, and impertinence that gives rise to pertinent questions. Also, as someone who has been teaching—or, rather, facilitating the learning of— TA for 30 years, and as a full-time university lecturer (and now professor), my primary identity is that of an educationalist and academic.

For many, psychotherapy or soul healing is concerned with freeing the soul (or spirit), mind, heart, and body. Psychotherapy, however, is paradoxical; as Casement (2002) puts it: 'It can either free the mind or bind it. It can liberate creativity and spontaneity, but it can [also] foster compliance' (p. 1). This paradox may be expressed in TA terms as one between helping people to become autonomous, that is, aware, spontaneous, and intimate (Berne, 1964/1968a)—and, I would say, homonomous and socially responsible; and, on the other hand, encouraging people to be self-controlled, to settle for symptomatic relief and short-term solutions, and to be compliant. Forty years ago, Lasch (1979) challenged what he analysed as the culture of narcissism. Unfortunately, psychotherapy has, by and large, contributed to a psychological and social/political culture that promotes such a culture of self-obsession and self-delusion based on an individualism which, arguably, is the narcissistic focus of mainstream therapy. As such, conventional and state regulated psychotherapy (see Chapter 10) is as much part of the problem as it is the solution to the psychological and social ills of this world. At worst, such therapy promotes isolation, mystification, and (internalised) oppression, which Claude Steiner and other radical psychiatrists identified as a formula for alienation (see Chapter 12). If we are to maintain and enhance psychotherapy—and other forms of 'psy' healing (clinical social work, clinical psychology, counselling, counselling psychology, psychiatry, shamanism, etc.) as a form of personal *and* social liberation for the interpersonal and interdependent human organism, then we need to address the threats to this project and process, such as dogma and fundamentalism (see Tudor, 2007b, 2018b). Given its origins in criticism of and opposition to psychoanalysis, and the positive influence of radical psychiatry on TA (see Althöfer & Riesenfeld, 2020; Althöfer & Tudor, 2020; Jenkins et al., 2020), TA should be in a good position to do this; yet it has become and is widely viewed as being conservative and conformist (see, for example, Kovel, 1976; Karpman, 1981; Tudor, 2010d). Another tension within TA—and that TA reflects—is that between action and reflection. As Berne (1966a) himself put it:

> Transactional analysis is an actionist form of treatment, where psychoanalysis is to a much greater extent, a contemplative one. The transactional analyst says, 'Get better first, and we can analyse later.' …. Thus the transactional patient and his family benefit from the accomplishments that take place before the deeper analytic phase of his treatment, so that it is of relatively less consequence how long he remains in treatment after that. The psychoanalyst, on the other hand, may imply, 'After you have been analysed, you will get better.
>
> (pp. 303–304)

Me and transactional analysis

I first came across TA in the late 1970s when I was undertaking social work training at the University of Kent at Canterbury in the UK. The social work training was one informed by critical thinking and radical politics (Bailey & Brake, 1975; George & Wilding, 1976; Sayers, 1976), and it was in this context that I came across the literature on radical psychiatry and radical therapy: Wyckoff (1970, 1976b), The Radical Therapist Collective (1971), The Rough Times Staff (1973), and Steiner et al. (1975). During a placement in a community social work agency in South London, I met two inspiring community activists who were part of a TA study group run by Dr Roger Kreitman and Lily Stuart, a group I joined and attended regularly during that placement. I did my first introductory 'TA 101' course in 1985 with Dr Petrūska Clarkson and Dave Gowling at what was then called the Metanoia Group and Training Institute, and another one in 1987 with Susanna Ligabue at il Centro di Eric Berne in Milan when I was living in Italy. On my return to the UK in 1987, I began training at Metanoia and had the good fortune to train with Maria Gilbert and, later, Charlotte Sills, as well as a number of other, visiting trainers, including Frances Bonds-White, Vann Joines, Gisela Kottwitz, Carlo Moiso, Hank Nunn and Jenny Robinson, Alice Stevenson, Ian Stewart, and George Thomson. I also attended conferences where I had the good fortune to meet many luminaries who, indeed, illuminated my thinking about and practice of TA. I also began writing about TA, and, in 1991, had my first article published in the international *Transactional Analysis Journal*, on the subject of children's groups I had run with two TA colleagues.[1] I passed my certifying TA exam in 1994 in Maastricht, and my accrediting exams as a teaching and supervising transactional analyst in 2004 in Rome. In both these journeys I was both supported and challenged by my supervisors: Dr Brian Dobson, Maria Gilbert, Sue Fish, Dr Ian Stewart, Dr Adrienne Lee, and Robin Hobbes. I have also had the good fortune to have made and maintained close collegial relationships in TA and I especially want to acknowledge Dr Helena Hargaden, Professor Charlotte Sills, and Graeme Summers, both individually and collectively, for their personal and professional support, intellectual stimulation, and sustained and sustaining friendship over more than a quarter of a century. For seven years, we met as a peer supervision group, which not only fulfilled its purpose of supervision but which also led to the elaboration of different perspectives on relational TA: firstly, an article Graeme and I wrote about co-creative TA (Summers & Tudor, 2000), which was published in the *Transactional Analysis Journal*, and for which we received the Eric Berne Memorial Award in 2020; secondly, Helena and Charlotte's book *Transactional Analysis: A Relational Perspective* (Hargaden & Sills, 2002), for two chapters of which they received the Eric Berne Memorial Award in 2007; and, thirdly, other work that Graeme and I produced over subsequent years which we later published in *Co-creative Transactional Analysis: Papers, Dialogues, Responses, and Developments* (Tudor & Summers, 2014).

TA has a strong and international community and I count myself fortunate to have many colleagues and close work friends not only here in Aotearoa New Zealand but all over the world and specifically, in the UK, where I have presented many times at conferences and meetings, but where I have also been invited to present (in 2002, 2005, 2006, 2007) and, notably, to give the keynote speech to the Annual Conference of the United Kingdom Association for Transactional Analysis (in 2015), an invitation I was honoured to accept. I have also been invited to present in Lithuania (2000 and 2002), Australia (2006, 2012, 2015, and 2019); Aotearoa New Zealand (2006, before emigrating here in 2009, since when I have taught on several training programmes in this country); in India (2007 and 2019); Italy (2008, 2011, 2018, 2020,[2] and 2023); Spain (2011); Japan (2014); to online international colloquia (2014 and

2015); in Slovenia (2015 and 2023); Singapore (2015 and 2018); Germany (2016); Croatia (2018 and 2023); Brazil (2019); Kyrgyzstan (2019); and Romania (2023). Most recently, and due to travel restrictions as a result of the coronavirus pandemic, I have also presented at workshops and conferences online 'in' Brazil, India, Italy, Japan, the Netherlands, South Africa, the UK, and Ukraine. I have been both honoured and humbled by the interest in my work and ideas about TA from colleagues in these and other countries, especially amongst students/trainees, and it is to this next generation of transactional analysts that I dedicate this book.

I am an enthusiastic researcher, writer, and editor. I tend to write from experience; thus, for instance, my first publication on TA in organisations was as a result of working in a social services department and wanting to understand some of the dynamics I was experiencing and observing in terms of TA, in which I was training at the time (Tudor, 1990). I am also a critical thinker, a perspective that has been informed by education (in the disciplines of philosophy and theology, social work, psychotherapy, and mental health, and at various levels); experience (in the various professions of social work, counselling, psychotherapy, and academia); and politics (for further details of which, see Tudor, 2017a). Thus, when faced with a situation, for instance, with regard to practice, policy, or theory, I have been and still am interested to explore this from a critical perspective, grounded in practice (see Tudor, 2018b). In this, I am inspired by Berne's (1972/1975b) elaboration of 'the map–ground problem' whereby an aviator flies according to a map but doesn't check this against the ground, as a result of which he gets lost. Berne concludes: 'The moral is, look at the ground first, and then at the map, and not vice versa' (p 409).

My areas of interest have been quite diverse and this is no less true within TA: from the personality of organisations (Tudor, 1990) to a transactional group analysis of war (Tudor, 2023).[3] I have also written about different aspects of TA theory, i.e., transactions and the therapeutic relationship (Tudor, 1999b), ego states (Tudor, 2003b, 2010c), and scripts (Tudor, 2001b, 2008d), as well as about TA theory and meta-theory (Tudor, 1996, 2008d, 2009a, 2010e, 2016b, 2016d, 2016e); and several chapters that offer introductions to TA, i.e., Clarkson et al. (1996), Tudor (2000), Tudor and Hobbes (2002, 2007), Summers and Tudor (2007), Tudor and Sills (2006, 2012), and Sills and Tudor (2017, 2023). All of this writing has been done, in a sense, writing forward: that is moving from one interest and subject to another. Sometimes, one article leads directly to another as, for instance, was the case with my article on '"Take It": A Sixth Driver' (Tudor, 2008c), which, in turn, led to a broader critique of the process model and the theory of personality adaptations in an article I co-authored with Mark Widdowson, which was published later in the same year. However, in thinking about and putting this book together, and in applying some of the analysis I offered in my book *Psychotherapy: A Critical Examination* (Tudor, 2018b) to TA, I have had the benefit of time to look back and to see both the themes in my writing as well as new areas on which I want to focus in order to provide a comprehensive critical review of TA. In this sense, the book is both a retrospective as well as a prospective.

Looking back on my writing in TA, I realise that I tend:

- To return to source, usually Berne—I do this partly because I focus on transactions; partly because, as a scholar, I tend to go back to original sources; and partly because I am interested in the history and development of ideas (for which reason and where possible, I tend to note citations in chronological rather than alphabetical order). In this sense, I am quite Classical and I note with interest that in her work on the schools of TA, Lee (2001) associates me with the Classical as well as the Constructivist School.
- To re-read these sources—I am constantly surprised at how much I get from re-reading a book, including what appears 'new'. One example of this for me was with regard to Berne's four requirements for a complete ego state diagnosis, i.e., that it is based on behavioural, social, historical, *and* phenomenological analysis, which he outlined in his book *Transactional Analysis in Psychotherapy* (Berne, 1961/1975a) and which I first read in the mid-1980s. However, it was only in re-reading this book some years later, and partly influenced by my interest and reading in person-centred psychology, that I really 'got' that, while the behavioural and social diagnosis could be made by the clinician, the historical and phenomenological diagnoses could only be made by the client. In this sense, these two requirements do centre on the client and can only be ascertained in dialogue with the client (and could, therefore, be viewed as being client-centred). These requirements reflect Berne's radicalism in the same vein as his insistence on staff–patient staff conferences (Berne, 1968b). Moreover, this theory of diagnosis means that any statement that a client is 'in their Child' (or Parent or Adult) based only on behavioural observation and social reaction is, by definition, an incomplete diagnosis. I'm not saying that I didn't understand this on my first reading of the book; I am saying that I get more of the theory when I re-read it and do so in the context of reading other theory. Elsewhere, I have noted the challenge and the benefit of re-reading this particular book of Berne's with regard to different views of ego state theory in TA (Tudor, 2010b, and Chapter 6).
- To think about TA both philosophically and politically—in an interview Diana Deaconu conducted with me in 2016, she said (with reference to herself and her collaborators) that 'we did catch that edge of philosophy and politics in your writing' and was kind enough to say that I was 'an astute observer of the philosophical and political side of things' (Tudor, 2018a). This is related to my background, having studied philosophy (and theology), and having been a political activist (and now being an activist scholar). This includes an interest in and attention to language (rhetoric) and the philosophical basis of theory, concepts, models, and practice, which involves referring to certain philosophical concepts. In the Preface to *What Do You Say After You Say Hello?*, Berne (1972/1975b) suggests that conventional psychotherapy uses different dialects, i.e., therapist–therapist, therapist–patient, and patient–patient, and states that he

favours the *lingua franca* of basic English [as it] increases the "communication" which many therapists… court' (p. xv).[4] He then goes on to justify his choice of openness and simplicity (with which I agree) by saying in a somewhat cynical vein (with which I don't agree):

I have thrown in with the 'people,' tossing in a big word now and then as a sort of hamburger to distract the watchdogs of the academies, while I slip through the basement doors and say Hello to my friends.

(p. xvi)

While retaining Berne's challenge to be open (see Chapter 2) and straightforward (see Chapter 13), I think there are times when we need to engage with 'big' words and concepts, which reflect the complexity of life,[5] and, with regard to psychotherapy, as, globally, this is predominantly a post-graduate activity and discipline, we should be able to do so. In this sense, I think it is important to develop other dialects, such as educator/trainer–educator/trainer, theorist–theorist, philosopher–philosopher, researcher–researcher, theorist–educator/trainer, and the multiple variations thereof, not least so that we develop the theorist-practitioner (see International Transactional Analysis Association [ITAA] International Board of Certification [IBoC], 2022),[6] the therapist-philosopher (see Tudor & Worrall, 2006), the critical thinker-therapist (see Tudor, 2018b),[7] and the researcher-practitioner (see Tudor & Francis, 2022).

- To be critical and reflexive (as noted above) and meta[8]—which, in this book, is reflected in two ways: (a) my use of TA to assess theory, for instance, applying Berne's (1964/1968b) taxonomy of the advantages of games to assessing the advantages of theory (in Chapter 2); and (b) to reflex theory on itself, thus, to consider the life script of scripts (in Chapter 9), and the possible game invitation in the conflicting definitions of games (in Chapter 11). This reflexivity also extends to thinking about the education and training of transactional analysts. Originally, I had planned that another part of this book would comprise chapters on the philosophy of education, and its application to training and supervision (see Tudor, 2002, 2009). However, as this book became more substantial, I had to make some choices about the scope of this book, and those chapters will now form part of another book. Nevertheless, I have retained a strong thread in this book that links the ideas presented and critiqued to the training requirements for transactional analysts for certification in counselling, education, organisations, and psychotherapy. These are laid out in two handbooks: the *Teaching/Certification and Examinations Handbook* published by the International Transactional Analysis Association's International Board of Certification (IBoC) (2022) and the *Teaching and Examinations Handbook* published by the European Association for Transactional Analysis' (EATA) Professional Training Standards Committee (PTSC) (2022).[9]

The book

The book is arranged in three parts, each of which I preface with a brief introduction that offers an overview of the constituent chapters, both old and new. The first part comprises three chapters that discuss the **basic assumptions** of TA, which explore the ontological, epistemological, and methodological basis of TA theory and practice. The second part, entitled **new wine from old roots**, comprises two chapters (one original and one new) on each of the four fundamental pillars of TA, i.e., transactions, ego states, scripts, and games, which gives me an opportunity to revisit some of my earlier thinking about these fundamentals of TA, and to offer my latest thinking about them. The third part of the book **looking back, looking forwards** comprises two chapters, the first of which considers the various schools/traditions/approaches/sensibilities that are found within TA, and the second of which, based on a playful reference to Berne's independent, 'Martian view' of human interactions and life, offers a 'Vulcan view' of the future of TA.

Over the years, in my writing and editing, as well as my practice, I have sought to collaborate and, as a result, have appreciated and enjoyed both the co-creative process involved as well as the final outcome or output.[10] In TA, this has been mostly with my friend and colleague, Graeme Summers, to whom I owe profound thanks for his part in the development of my thinking and practice. However, in choosing the six previously published contributions for this book, I have focused on my own sole-authored work, whilst acknowledging, of course, that this has been profoundly influenced by such collaborations. With regard to the book as a whole, the original papers have been reproduced as originally written and edited only to make them consistent with the house style of this book, i.e., predominantly using the present tense, first person rather than third person language, gender-sensitive language, and British/New Zealand English rather than US English (with regard to spelling and punctuation). I have taken the opportunity of editing them into the book as a whole adding to these chapters citations to work published since the original publication (noted in square brackets), and endnotes in order to address or reference more contemporary theory, to connect points to other chapters in the book, and to offer some reflections. Some repetition has been retained in order to facilitate the flow of a particular argument. Finally, in order to avoid undue repetition, and to promote the coherence of the book as a whole, the references of the original contributions and those of the new chapters have been combined in a single list.

Acknowledgements

Finally, as it takes a whole village to raise a book, I'd like to acknowledge and thank those colleagues, friends, and family who have formed the village for this particular book, notably:

- Dr Helena Hargaden, Professor Charlotte Sills, and Graeme Summers, my closest TA colleagues and friends, from and with whom I have learned so much over the years—ngā mihi nui ki a koutou katoa | my regards and thanks to you all.

- Colleagues who acted as peer-reviewers for the new chapters, namely Dr Giles Barrow (Chapter 9), Victoria Baskerville (the Introduction, Chapters 7 and 13), Dr.ssa Antonella Fornaro (Chapter 12), Tatjana Gjurković (the Introduction, and Chapters 2 and 12), Jan Grant (Chapter 12), Hayley Marshall (Chapter 7), Chitra Ravi (Chapter 5), Paul Robinson (Chapters 9, and 11), Dr Brian Rodgers (Chapter 13), D.ssa Anna Rotondo (Chapter 2), Graeme Summers (Chapter 11), and Gregor Žvelc (Chapter 5)—ngā mihi nui ki a koutou katoa.[11]
- Colleagues who were involved in the publication of the original chapters, namely the peer-reviewers of the original articles for the *Transactional Analysis Journal* in which the papers that form Chapters 1, 3, and 6 first appeared; Colin Feltham, who was the editor of the book in which Chapter 4 first appeared; Francesca Hannah, who was the editor of the *ITA News* in which the article which forms Chapter 8 first appeared; and Katrina (Kate) Jacobson, who was the editor of the *TAttler* magazine in which Chapter 10 first appeared—ngā mihi nui ki a koutou katoa.
- Shirley Rivers (Ngāi Takoto, Ngāpuhi, Te Kawerau-a-Maki, Te Waiohua, Waikato-Tainui) for her interest in both Western traditions I inhabit (i.e., person-centred psychology and TA), and her wisdom and guidance in relation to te Ao Māori (the Māori world)—tēnā koe, whaea | thank you.
- James (Jim) Allen, Diana Deaconu, Seán Manning, Charlotte Sills, and Dr Gaetano Sisalli for their generous endorsements—I very much appreciate your interest in and your support for my work—ngā mihi nui hoki ki a koutou katoa | thank you all, too.
- Dr Elizabeth Day, my colleague and friend at Auckland University of Technology, who, for four years was also Head of the Department of Psychotherapy & Counselling, during which time she was not only an excellent leader and manager but also incredibly supportive to me, not least, in facilitating me to take overdue and much needed research and study leave, which has enabled me to finish this book—tēnā koe, rangatira | thank you.
- Angie Strachan, my editorial assistant, with whom I have worked closely on a number of projects, especially over the last three years, from whose skill and sensibility with regard to language and good sense I have benefitted enormously—tēnā koe e hoa | thank you.
- Susannah Frearson, Saloni Singhania, Priya Sharma and Sophie Dixon-Dash at Routledge—tēnā koutou katoa | thank you.
- Rebecca Wise for her fine copy-editing—tēnā koe āno e hoa | thank you again.
- Charlotte McLachlan, a local (New Zealand) TA colleague and artist for giving me permission to use her beautiful artwork as the cover image for the book—tēnā koe e hoa | thank you.
- Louise Embleton Tudor, my friend, colleague, partner, and wife, the longevity of my relationship with whom almost exactly parallels that of my relationship with TA, and who, during that time, has always been supportive of both my engagement and struggles with it—kei te mihi nui ahau ki a koe, hoa rangatira, mō tō tautoko tonu | my deep appreciation for your continued support.

Notes

1 Interestingly, when I came to submit this article, a number of colleagues, including some supervisors and trainers, said that I couldn't (and shouldn't) be published in the *TAJ* as I wasn't (then) yet qualified (as a transactional analyst). This was presented as a fact rather than a prejudice which, fortunately, was not part of the journal's submission criteria. While the article was peer-reviewed, published, and well-received, these responses were one of the first times I had experienced this Parental prejudice and discounting of adult—and Adult—experience in TA, though sadly it was not to be the last (for discussion of which, see Tudor, 2008/2017d).

2 Which, sadly, was first postponed and then cancelled, due to the outbreak and spread of the coronavirus pandemic (see Tudor, 2024/in press).

3 In between which, I have published on: working with children (Tudor, 1991, 2008a) and Gjurković and Tudor (2018); ending psychotherapy (Tudor, 1995b); shame (Tudor, 1995a, a paper which forms Chapter 8); integration (Tudor, 1996; Tudor & Widdowson, 2002); contracts (Tudor, 1997b, 1997d, 2006); groups (Tudor, 1999a, 2013a); brief therapy (Tudor, 2002c); citizenship (Tudor & Hargaden, 2002); supervision (Tudor, 2002b); creativity (Tudor, 2003a, 2014a); culture and identity (Naughton & Tudor, 2006; Minikin & Tudor, 2016; Tudor et al., 2022); ethics (Cornell et al., 2006); change (Tudor, 2007a, 2011a); teaching (Tudor, 2009); statutory regulation and state registration (Tudor, 2010b, 2011e); empathy (Tudor, 2011b, 2011g); research (Tudor, 2013b); politics (Tudor, 2009a, 2016c, Tudor, 2020g); treatment planning (Gjurković & Tudor, 2018; Tudor & Widdowson, 2002); religion, faith, and spirituality (Tudor, 2019); courage (Tudor, 2022a); and ecotherapy (Clare & Tudor, 2023).

4 The irony of Berne using a French phrase (which he doesn't translate) to justify using 'basic English' is not lost on this reader and commentator.

5 When I first use such words (big or otherwise), I tend to offer a translation of them, thus: ontology (the essence of things).

6 One of the two aspects of the purpose of the certified transactional analysis (CTA) written exam is that the candidate 'works effectively and ethically as a theoretically based transactional analyst' (ITAA IBoC, 2022, Section 8.1.2). Moreover, when it comes to the oral exam, one of the criteria refers to the capacity to conceptualise the particular application or field of TA (i.e., counselling, education, organisational, or psychotherapy) in terms of different TA theoretical concepts/models, and with reference to 'different trends and approaches as well as recent developments' (ITAA IBoC, 2022, Section 12.7.9).

7 In my inaugural professorial lecture, I extended this to include the argumentative therapist (Tudor, 2016a).

8 In epistemology, the prefix meta- is used to mean about. In its definition of the word meta, the Urban Dictionary (2017) puts it well as being 'about the thing itself', explaining it as 'seeing the thing from a higher perspective, like being self-aware' (para. 1). It also offers some useful clarification of the incorrect use of meta. Thus, making a film about the film industry isn't meta; making a film about making films is. This highlights the reflexive sense of meta-activity, thus, in TA, offering a transactional analysis of transactional analysis; an ego state analysis of ego states; a script analysis of script theory; and a game analysis of games. Having a meta-perspective is one of the assessment criteria for the certification of transactional analysts (see ITAA IBoC, 2022, Section 12, Form 12.7.7; and Chapter 11).

9 The two handbooks overlap considerably, though there are some differences. They are also updated regularly and publicly available at: https://www.itaaworld.org/iboc-certification-examinations-handbook (ITAA IBoC, 2022) and https://eatanews.org/ta-training-2/ (EATA PTSC, 2022). In this book, I tend to refer to the one published by the ITAA IBoC.

10 In TA, 20 out of my 68 peer-reviewed publications in TA to date (i.e., 30%) have been co-authored.

11 I note this not only to acknowledge my colleagues in this respect, but also because, in some academic and administrative circles, books are not rated as highly as peer-reviewed articles in high-impact journals. Whilst I and many other colleagues disagree with this (see Harley, 2019, Tudor, 2021e), I now make a point of noting how books I write are peer-reviewed (e.g., Tudor, 2021b)—and more so than many journal articles. Also, I have included a number of points my colleagues raised in reviewing these chapters and am grateful to them for allowing me to do so as I consider that it supports and, indeed, enhances the reflexive perspective and flavour of the book.

Part I

Basic assumptions

The three chapters in this first part of the book discuss the basic assumptions of transactional analysis (TA) and explore the methodological basis of TA theory and practice, that is the 'ology' or study of method. This includes its assumptions about ontology (the essence of things); epistemology (the knowledge of things); and, specifically, how we know what we know; and axiology (or the value of things), which generally refers to ethics. Not many writers directly address the philosophy of TA. The principal exceptions to this are Oden (1974) who discusses the theology of transactions; Weinhold (1977) who offers a philosophical analysis of various TA treatment styles; Brady (1980a, 1980b) who discusses both Kant and Hegel with regard to the Adult ego state; Grant (2004) who discusses how the philosophical assumptions of TA complement the theory of adult education; and Rotondo (2020) who offers a philosophical context to Berne's theory of bilateral contracts. Novellino (2012) refers to TA literature as 'a series of themes expressed by Berne [which are] half-way between methodology and philosophy' (p. 103), but does not elaborate either the methodology or the philosophy of the themes he (Novellino) identifies, and, indeed, equates methodology with method, i.e., techniques and tactics, decontamination and deconfusion.

From an early age I was interested in philosophy (see Tudor, 2018b), and had the good fortune to study philosophy and theology as the subjects of my first degree. This education and intellectual training has given me an interest in ideas, where they come from, how they are or may be organised, and how different ideas may be understood in relation to each other—and, as noted in the Introduction, my interest in philosophy and politics has been acknowledged and commented on by others, notably, Bill Cornell about *Conscience and Critic* (Tudor, 2017a), Diana Deaconu (in Tudor, 2018a), Donna Orange about *Psychotherapy: A Critical Examination* (Tudor, 2018b), and Richard House (in Tudor & House, 2019). This interest in ideas and their organisation, as well as meta-theoretical analysis informed an article I wrote on integration—or, as I referred to it, *intra*gration—in TA (Tudor, 1996), in which I offered a paradigm analysis of different aspects of TA theory. Since then, in undertaking further research for this book, I came across Weinhold's (1977) analysis of metaphysical theories underpinning different TA treatment styles, on which I have drawn in Chapter 2.

DOI: 10.4324/9780429398223-2

Taking my starting point as ontology or the essence of things, in Chapter 1, I advance an interdependent, pluralistic, 'we' perspective as a starting point for human beings and, indeed, being human, as distinct from one that is based on 'I', 'I'm OK', and, more broadly, a 'me' psychology. Margaret Thatcher (British Prime Minister, 1979–1990) (in)famously said about society 'There is no such thing!' (Thatcher, 1987/2022). I am more with Donald Winnicott (1947/1957), the British psychiatrist and psychoanalyst, who said that 'there is no such thing as a baby' (p. 137). This chapter provides a different ontological basis for thinking about the essence or existence of things and, especially, of human beings, than the predominant individualistic and anthropocentric one found in the Western—and Northern—intellectual tradition. The original article, '"We are": the fundamental life position', was originally published in the *Transactional Analysis Journal* (*TAJ*), 46(2), April 2016, pp. 164–176, © International Transactional Analysis Association (ITAA), and is reprinted with permission.

Transactional analysis is based on the contractual method, i.e., 'an explicit, bilateral commitment to a well-defined course of action' (Berne, 1966a, p. 362). Whilst this is clear, what is less clear is the methodological and epistemological basis of this method—and, indeed, the 'course of action' or process of the contract or, more accurately, contract*ing*. Moreover, there is confusion and, often, elision between method and methodology. In an attempt to clarify some of this confusion, in Chapter 2, I elaborate the theory of knowledge (epistemology) that underlies the contractual method of TA. The reason I focus on this area of TA is that Berne asserted that transactional analysis is based on the 'contractual method', i.e., a mutually agreed statement of change, as well as on 'open communication' (also see Chapter 4).

In Chapter 3, I (re)turn to method, i.e., what transactional analysts *do*, and discuss what transactional analysts refer to as the three 'Ps' of TA treatment philosophy, that is, permission and protection (from Crossman, 1966), and potency (from Steiner, 1968). In the chapter, I discuss the history of these three concepts, identify what I refer to as four groups of permission, and, from a perspective of 'two-person psychology' (Stark, 1999), critique and reconsider all three. My aim in doing so is to enhance the praxis of therapeutic—and other—relationships that emphasise engagement in relationship and, as such, sets the scene for the rest of the book. The original article, 'Permission, protection, and potency—The 3 Ps, reconsidered', was originally published in the *TAJ*, 46(1), January 2016, pp. 50–64, © ITAA, and is also reprinted with permission.[1]

Note

1 I have a particular fondness for this article, and, in reviewing it for this book, was delighted to see that, according to the statistics available on Taylor & Francis Online, it is currently the fourth most read article in the *TAJ*, with, to date (July 2024) 5,471 views.

Chapter 1

'We are'

The fundamental life position (2016)

This chapter argues that the existential statement 'We are' most accurately describes the fundamental life position of human beings and identifies some ontological, epistemological, methodological, and practical implications of this. Taking the phrase 'I'm OK, You're OK' and its variants as its theme, the chapter critically examines the three elements of this central aspect of transactional analysis theory and philosophy, that is, in terms of the person, OKness, and existential life positions. In doing so, it offers some clarification regarding Melanie Klein's influence on Berne and some variations that are informed by and advance 'we psychology'.

The chapter takes the view that the individual can only be understood in the context of society, the group or groups, and the other, and that, developmentally, socially/politically, and philosophically, 'I' comes from and comes after 'we'. Rather than working from the individual outward, which implicitly privileges the individual, many—arguably most—cultures in the world conceptualise human beings from the outside or wider context inward (see also Chapter 7). This perspective resonates across cultures, societies, and time as encapsulated in the following words, phrases, and statements:

- 'Man is a naturally a political animal' (Aristotle, 350BCE/2004, section 1253a).
- Ubuntu (from the mid-19th century), which Eze (2010) interprets as meaning 'a person is a person through other people' (pp. 190–191).
- 'It takes a village to raise a child' (African proverb).
- 'There is no such thing as a baby... A baby cannot exist alone but is essentially part of a relationship' (Winnicott, 1947/1957, p. 137).
- 'No organism is self-sufficient... There is always inter-dependency of the organism and its environment' (Perls, 1947/1969, p. 38).

The person

In his original article on the 'Classification of Positions', Berne (1962b) states that 'the subjects of all positions are particulars of the polarity I–Others' (p. 23), formulating 'I' as including 'we' and 'you' as including 'they'. Some ten years later, in *What Do You Say After You Say Hello?*, Berne (1972/1975b) shifted this somewhat

DOI: 10.4324/9780429398223-3

by extrapolating 'they' as a third-person position distinct from the second-person other 'you'. As a result, he identifies eight life positions, which he summarises as follows (pp. 90–91) (+ meaning 'OK'; – meaning 'not OK'):

I + You + They + which represents the position of a democratic community

I + You + They - the prejudiced snob- or gang-position of a demagogue

I + You - They + the position of the agitator or malcontent and sometimes missionaries

I + You - They - the solitary, self-righteous critic position

I - You + They + the self-punishing saint or masochist, the melancholic position

I - You + They - the servile position

I - You - They + the position of servile envy and sometimes of political action

I - You - They - the pessimistic position of cynics or those who believe in predestination or original sin.

Berne (1972/1975b) justifies this expansion by using the metaphor of an accordion 'which can expand enough to include a vast assortment of attitudes besides the basic four' (p. 90). I have always thought that the third-handed (i.e., third-person) life position represented Berne's social psychiatry and that, as an aspect of transactional analysis (TA) theory, it has been somewhat overlooked and underrated both in the literature and in practice.[1] Although Berne himself does not view the personal pronoun 'we' as describing anything more than the plural 'I' and does not use the phrase or concept 'We're OK', a number of others writing in transactional analysis have done so.

In an editorial for a special issue of the *Transactional Analysis Journal*, Zechnich (1975) uses the phrase to acknowledge that TA does not have all the answers and that other theories and clinicians have much to teach us, hence, 'We're OK and They're OK' (p. 105). To Berne's 'They', Groder (1977b) adds 'We' and 'It', arguing that 'to be really, really OK, one must pass the test of an "I'm OK, You're OK, We're OK, They're OK, It's OK" analysis' (p. 162). He continues: 'This 5-OK analysis can be very chastening, especially for OK therapists who don't care what effect they have on the world at large' (p. 162). Citing Groder's extension of the basic life positions, Barnes (1981) clarifies that 'even the child who decides that "I'm not-OK, You're not-OK" can make exceptions and make the "We" OK' (p. 24).

In an article about protection and what they name *nutritional nervosa*, Karpman and Callaghan (1985) refer to health fanatics as operating from a 'We're OK, They're Not OK' position. Micholt (1992) uses the phrase in the context of elaborating three-cornered contracts, a use Fischer (1993) picks up in addressing the changing organisational Parent. Clarkson (1993) uses the phrase 'We're OK—They're not OK' to describe the position confirmed by one of 12 Bystander games she identifies as 'I'm Just Keeping My Own Counsel' (or 'I'm All Right, Jack!'). In an article on facilitating OKness-based groups, Steele and Porter-Steele (2003) refer to 'We're OK', stating that 'sitting calmly and quietly is a powerful nonverbal assurance' of these life positions. (They also referred to 'It's OK'.) Drego (2009) uses the term in the context of describing an ecopsychology and ecotherapy that models 'an attitude cum praxis of "I'm OK, You're OK, We're OK, They're OK, [and] planet Earth and its ecosystems are OK"' (p. 205). Following Berne, all of these authors use the pronoun 'we' to represent the first-person plural, that is, 'I' and another 'I'.

Other writers within transactional analysis, however, have used 'we' to represent something more than this. In his article on autocratic power, Jacobs (1987) places 'We're OK' at the heart of his master-follower projection system and, significantly, separate from 'I'm OK, You're OK'. Although he does not explain this directly, he indicates that he views this kind of 'we' as symbiotic: 'The effort then, is to forcibly repress the "Not OK" feelings while simultaneously creating the illusion of being rid of them. It is at this moment that the crowd forms; when I and You become WE' (pp. 66–67). In a rare use of 'we' in a four-handed position, involving 'I', 'you', 'we', and 'they', and in the context of discussing gay and straight sexual identities, Kellet (2004) refers to the existential position of 'I'm OK, You're OK/Not OK, We're OK, They're Not OK':

> For a straight man, this position may be part of a defence against homoerotic desire by keeping threatening aspects of the self split off and located in the other-group imago. For a gay man, this position may (additionally) represent a defense against heterosexism whereby persecutory cultural values are more properly located as individual-other and group-other. Either way, the individual maintains a 'clean' sense of sexual identity.
>
> (p. 186)

In an article on the application of transactional analysis in South Africa, Salters (2006) uses the word 'we' to represent 'our common humanity' (p. 152) and, adapting Ernst's (1971b) OK Corral, presents a group version of what she referred to as 'The OK Kraal'. This usefully and visually distinguishes the positive 'We're OK, You (plural) are OK' and the 'we/they' of the other positions, commenting that, 'in my experience, the word "they" is used to convey a sense of troublesome otherness rather than just out-group difference' (pp. 153–154).

In his formulations of 'I'm OK, You're OK, They're OK', Berne used the personal pronouns in the role of subject ('I', 'you', and 'they'), to which I add 'we'. This accords with W. James' (1890/1981) concept of the personal self. James also identifies the social self, the respective pronouns of which are 'me', 'you', 'they', and 'us'. This is significant because, in human development, the sense of the social self and specifically 'me' (as in when a child says 'me do, me do') comes before the sense of the personal self. We may represent the development of personal and social identity as follows: We (i.e., mother–infant merged subject) → You (mother object) → You (mother subject) → Me (social self) → We (autonomous and homonomous plural subjects) → I (personal self) → Them (object) → They (subject).

We psychology

This sense and use of 'we' draws on we psychology, that is, a psychology that focuses on and, indeed, derives from a perspective that considers 'we' before 'I' or, as G. S. Klein (1976) puts it, 'we-ego' before ego. In Western psychology, this perspective has its origins in the social psychology of Mead (1934) and Vygotsky (1962), the organismic psychology of Goldstein (1934/1995) and Angyal (1941), and has become the focus of research among developmental psychologists such as Stern (1998). As a term, we psychology is attributed to Fritz Künkel (1889–1956), who drew on the work of Freud, Adler, and Jung in synthesising an explicitly religious psychology (see Künkel, 1984).

The ontological assumption of we psychology is characterised by Winnicott's (1947/1957) famous phrase, 'there is no such thing as a baby' (p. 137). The most extreme example of this of which I am aware is reported by Alford (1994), who writes about the Wolini, a now-extinct tribe who lived in the Amazon rain forest on the border between Venezuela and Brazil. They were distinguished in the anthropological literature by the absence in their language of the first-person singular pronoun 'I'. The Wolini were known to each other by a combination of birth order and family name. Thus, 'Lowan' would be the third (Lo) child of the Wan family. The person's name thereby designated not an individual (as conceived) but a member's place in the tribal group. Thus, when Lowan said, 'Lowan did this and thinks that', it did not translate as 'I did this and think that' but, rather, was more akin to the statement 'the part of the group that is located here in Lowan did this and thinks that'.

It follows that the epistemological focus of we psychology is on the knowledge that derives from and is found in relationship. In a later version of his phrase, Winnicott (1960/1965) wrote, 'There is no such thing as an infant... without maternal care one would find no infant' (p. 39, note 1). Interestingly, he wrote this in an article entitled 'The Theory of the Parent–Infant Relationship'. This is significant because we psychology is interested in the theory of relationship(s)— parent–infant, individual–family, family–family, family–couple, and so on—and in drawing on and developing knowledge about knowledge from relationship(s). Taking this further, and paraphrasing Winnicott, we might say that there is no such thing as a relationship, only relationships-in-context. Thus, we psychology acknowledges context and, therefore, social and political worlds as well as personal and interpersonal worlds.

An example of the kind of inquiry that reflects this psychology is understanding how people, including a particular individual, might be alienated from a sense of themselves, others, and the(ir) world (as distinct from focusing on what is wrong with an individual, for instance, in terms of their psychopathology). In this sense, much radical psychiatry (The Radical Therapist Collective, 1971; Roy & Steiner, 1988; Steiner, 1975a; Wyckoff, 1976b) reflects a we psychology. The epistemological focus given to *me psychology* is perhaps most apparent when working with couples. For instance, in therapy, a couple was arguing. Abe was telling his partner, Bea, that she did not understand him. Bea responded by saying, 'But, actually, you...' The therapist interrupted, saying to both of them, 'It sounds like you're fighting about who's right and who knows what about the other. How about you talk with each other about how you know what you know and feel?' Abe and Bea were quiet for a while. Gradually, both began to speak about how they felt and when they felt that the other did not listen to or understand them. This illustrates a common dynamic in couples therapy whereby each person separately argues what he or she knows and talks at the other with a view to convincing the other—and the therapist—of their case. The couple's willingness to move from this to a space in which they talk with each other not only about how each of them feels but, importantly, how they co-create meaning, represents a move from an individual(istic) basis of knowledge to a shared one and, thus, an epistemological shift.

The methodology of we psychology—that is, the philosophical underpinnings of the method—is reflected in theories of relationship. Various philosophers, such as Martin Buber (1878–1965) and John Macmurray (1891–1976) have contributed to our thinking about the centrality of relationship. In his work, Macmurray (1957/1969) challenges the assumptions of a theoretical and ego-centric view of the (reified) self:

> Against the assumption that the self is an isolated individual, I have set the view that the Self is a person, and that personal existence is constituted by the relation of persons.... The idea of an isolated agent is self-contradictory. Any agent is necessarily in relation to the Other. Apart from this essential relation he does not exist. But, further, the Other in this constitutive relation must itself be personal. Persons, therefore, are constituted by their mutual relation to one another. 'I' exist only as one element in the complex 'You and I'.
>
> (p. 12)[2]

As early as 1942, Rogers referred to his then newer psychotherapy as 'relationship therapy', a term he credits to Taft (1933/1973) and that prefigures the more recent relational turn in psychotherapy. Noel and DeChenne (1974) write about a we dimension in therapy that 'involves discussion of processes occurring between the client and the therapist, processes which are co-owned and must be dealt with collaboratively' (p. 253). Saner (1989) names the 'we'ness of the therapeutic relationship itself as the medium for human development and change, and more recently, Summers and I discuss 'we'ness as one of the principles that underpins co-creative transactional analysis and the practice of exploring and expanding new relational possibilities (Summers & Tudor, 2000).

The method or practice of we psychology that follows from this relational methodology focuses on working with and within relationships. As Schmid (2006) puts it:

> Dialogue is an irreversible principle and condition of being human. Humans do not only substantially rely on dialogue, they are dialogue. [Moreover,] dialogue is the authentic realization and acknowledgement of the underlying We.... The restoration of the underlying We is the therapy in psychotherapy.
>
> (p. 251)

Although it is possible to do this with an individual in individual therapy, it is more consistent with the approach to do this with different relational forms or complexes such as a couple, a family, a group, a class, a community, an organisation, and so on. Indeed, we psychology questions the assumption that individual therapy is the form of therapy of choice (see Tudor, 1999b) and, indeed, recommends and priori-tises working with groups.

To reflect this perspective and the reality of the third, relational element to any 'I–You' dyad or complex, I propose the addition to Berne's two-handed life posi-tions of 'we', thus giving us, for instance, 'I'm OK, You're OK, We're OK'.

OKness

Together with the propositions that everyone has the capacity to think and that people decide their own destiny (and that they can redecide it), the idea that people are 'OK' forms part of the basic philosophy of transactional analysis. As a con-cept, OKness has been widely discussed in the literature, notably by Harris (1967), Harris and Dusay (1967), Erskine (1995), English (1995), Hine (1995), Jacobs (1997a), White (1994, 1995a, 1995b), and Harley (2006). These authors and others have described OKness in a number of ways, which I have organised here into four categories.

The nature of OKness

Interestingly, there is little if anything in the transactional analysis literature about the general meaning of 'OK', which, in common usage, denotes approval, accept-ance, agreement, assent, or acknowledgment. In other words, 'OK' (okay, okeh, 'kay, okie dokie, etc.) is more often used to mean that something is adequate and even mediocre (as in 'The food was OK') rather than exceptional or wonderful, and is, thus, a far cry from existential well-being. Indeed, used with a certain tone of voice, 'OK' can indicate doubt or disparagement. Berne's (1966a) hypothesis was that we fix on one life position that represents a pervasive attitude and on which we base our life scripts. Harris (1967) also views OKness as a decision but argues that the first one is 'I'm Not OK, You're OK' and that the three positions 'I'm Not OK, You're OK', 'I'm OK, You're Not OK', and 'I'm Not OK, You're Not OK' are unconscious early decisions, with 'I'm OK, You're OK' being a later, conscious, verbal decision.

By contrast, Ernst (1971b) argues that OKness shifts from moment to moment. Kahler (1979) identifies three positions (I+U-, U+I-, I-U-) as behavioural, whereas White (1994) uses the sign '?' to alter one of Berne's original positions and added three others to propose a total of seven life positions: 'I'm OK, You're Irrelevant' (I+U?), 'I'm Not OK, You're Irrelevant' (I-U?), 'I'm Not OK, You're Not OK' (I-U-), 'I'm Not OK, But You're Worse' (I-U--), 'I'm a Bit More OK Than You Are' (I++U+), 'I'm OK, You're OK' (I+U+), and 'I'm Not OK, You're OK' (I-U+). He argues that all positions are both a surface, minute-by-minute position and a character position. Linking OKness to Klein's positions or states of psychic or-ganisation (see next section), Harley (2006) argues that the not-OK positions are important developmentally and must be worked through and integrated in order for the fourth 'I'm OK, You're OK' position to be more than superficial and conditional.

The scope of OKness

In transactional analysis, OKness encompasses a number of psychological positions (M. James & Jongeward, 1971; Steiner, 1974); a total life direction or destiny (Berne, 1972/1975b); a conviction and 'faith in human nature' (Steiner, 1974, p. 2); and, beyond that, planetary OKness (Drego, 2006).

OKness as existential

The positions or life positions are frequently referred to as existential life positions, which, according to Steiner (1974), are 'feelings about oneself and others' (p. 2). Kahler (1979) argues that only the I+U+ position is existential. By contrast, Barnes (1981) views all four positions as an attitude or existential stance and not an emotional or psychological state. He also contends that the three positions (I+U-, U+I-, I-U-) are existential 'in that they describe the social order that in the best of families is far from the ideal or the reality of the existential position of OKness' (p. 24). I suggest that the existential statement, encapsulated in the use of the verb *to be*, is simply 'I am', 'You are', 'She is', 'He is', 'We are', and 'They are'. The attribution of OKness and not OKness is, in effect, a value judgment about these existential statements. Sills puts this succinctly when she said (personal communication, 6 May 2001) that OKness is a humanistic influence on the existential position 'I am, You are'.

One of the problems with OKness is that it is binary: a person is—or, rather, is viewed as—either OK or not OK, a polarity that does not account for the more subtle, ambiguous, or ambivalent evaluations of ourselves and our behaviour(s) by ourselves or others. Some of these subtleties are captured in White's (1994) use of the '?' and the double positive (+ +) and double negative (- -). In both therapy and training groups, I have seen and experienced OKness and the evaluation of OKness used, wittingly or unwittingly, as an avoidance of the existential, face-to-face encounter 'I am, You are'—or not: the philosophical version, as it were, of the intimacy experiment (Berne, 1964/1968a). For example, in a training group, in response to one member who consistently arrived late, several other members had been very understanding ('It's OK', 'We understand you're looking after yourself', etc.). Eventually, another member of the group said, 'No, it's not OK. I miss you. I want you to be here, with us, on time'. In debriefing this exchange, the person who had been coming late said that what had impacted him was when his colleague said, 'I miss you'. It was an 'I–You' moment in which the parties were, in effect, naming an 'I am, you're not (here)' relationship. In my experience, using or implying the verb *to be*, which, grammatically, shows the existence or condition of the subject, focuses people more directly on their existential relationship(s) with each other.

OKness as essentialist

There is a second set of definitions of OKness in transactional analysis that derives from and represents a different philosophical tradition, that of *essentialism*. This tradition, which, in Western thinking, dates back to the Greek philosophers Plato and Aristotle, posits that for any entity (animal, group of people, object, or concept) there are attributes that are intrinsic and necessary to its identity and function. An example of this with regard to OKness is Barnes' (1981) description of the position 'I'm OK, You're OK' as 'a statement of essence that affirms the humanity, worth, dignity and the right each person has to live and grow by virtue of the fact that he or she exists' (p. 24). Similarly, Stewart and Joines (1987) define OKness in terms of the 'essential value' that one perceives in oneself and others (p. 117). Salters (2006) writes about OKness as a 'way of experiencing oneself and others in the world... and a statement of belief about the intrinsic value of human beings that is shared by many cultures' (p. 153). Also, when people describe OKness in terms of qualities such as strength, power, and dependency, as Harris and Harris (1985/1986) do; or as having the three aspects of thinking, feeling, and doing, as White (1995a) does; or as meaning that 'I am fair with myself and fair with others, I see myself and others as equal, that is, with equal rights. It is a moral position', as Jacobs (1997a, p. 198) does, they are describing something essential or that they consider to be essential about the concept.

Positions

It has been argued that Berne derived his terms *positions* and *life positions* from the work of Melanie Klein on psychic positions and that his four life positions reflect Klein's as follows: 'I'm OK, You're Not OK' (I+U-) (paranoid); 'I'm Not OK, You're Not OK' (I-U-) (schizoid); and 'I'm Not OK, You're OK' (I-U+) (depressive). To these Berne adds a fourth—'I+U+'—which might be viewed as the healthy, integrated, or integrating position (see Clarkson, 1992; Stewart, 1992).

In his book on *Eric Berne*, Stewart (1992) was specific that '[Berne] adopted both the term and the concept of "positions", with acknowledgement, from the child psychoanalyst Melanie Klein' (p. 49). However, reading Berne's (1966a) work, it is clear that this is a more general reference to the psychodynamics of early childhood pathology and not a specific reference to positions. Indeed, Klein's and Berne's own definitions of the term *position* reveal significant differences. In her preface to the third edition of her book *The Psycho-Analysis of Children* (which was originally published in 1936), Klein (1936/1949) explains that 'the term "position" was chosen... [to] represent specific groupings of anxieties and defences which appear and re-appear during the first years of childhood' (p. xiii), a definition she had first given in an article published in 1935. In contrast, Berne (1962) offers a more general view of position as 'the fundamental variable of human living' (p. 23) and later, that it 'involves a view of the whole world and all the people in it' (Berne, 1972/1975b, p. 85). He specifically distinguishes between this general view (e.g., futility) and its clinical manifestations (e.g., schizoid and schizophrenic).

Another difference between Klein and Berne in this area is in the ages when these positions are adopted. For Klein, the paranoid (later paranoid-schizoid) position extends from birth until age three, four, or even five months of age; the depressive position that follows is established about the middle of the first year of life. Although Berne (1972/1975b) also suggests that 'the first script programming takes place during the nursing period, in the form of short protocols which can be later worked into complicated dramas' (p. 83), he does not distinguish epigenetically between the different positions, though others have (see, for instance, Harris, 1967; and Harley, 2006). For Berne, any life position justifies the decision the child has made on the basis of their programming, from birth onward. Another way of putting the distinction is that Klein's is a developmental model, whereas Berne's is a conceptual model.

In her book *Transactional Analysis in Psychotherapy*, Clarkson (1992) also writes of the direct influence of Klein on Berne: 'The three not-OK basic positions Berne identifies are paranoid, depressive and schizoid. These terms are taken directly from Klein (1949)' (p. 248). In fact, they appeared in Klein's earlier work—in 1935 when she introduced the framework of positions and contrasted the depressive position with the earlier paranoic phase and in 1946 when she introduced the paranoid-schizoid position—and are only referred to briefly in Klein's 1949 preface.

I suggest that the claim of a connection between Berne and Klein further breaks down when we consider that Klein postulates two (not three) psychic positions: the (unseparated) paranoid-schizoid position, which she described as the state of mind of children from birth to four to six months of age, and the depressive position, which refers to a capacity to bring together the nearness or proximity of what is experienced as good and bad and thus describes an integration of the ego. In other words, Klein's depressive position is not the same as the experience of being depressed (and a one-down view of oneself) and, in Bernean terms, would arguably be an aspect of I+U+.

Berne cites Klein in three of his works: *Transactional Analysis in Psychotherapy* (Berne, 1961/1975a), *Principles of Group Treatment* (Berne, 1966a), and *What Do You Say After You Say Hello?* (Berne, 1972/1975b). And all of the citations are to the same book: *The Psycho-Analysis of Children* (Klein, 1936/1949). Although Berne had clearly read the third edition of that book, there is no evidence that he had read anything else of Klein's, and it is just as likely that he derived his understanding of Klein through the work of Ronald Fairbairn, whom Berne also references:

> The fairy godmother and witch-mother, 'electrode-like' introjects, derived from transaction and introspective observations, will be easily recognized as allied to the good and bad introjected objects of Melanie Klein postulated on psychoanalytic grounds, and to the elaborations of her concepts by Fairbairn. *In fact, Fairbairn is one of the best heuristic bridges between transactional analysis and psycho-analysis* [emphasis added].
>
> (Berne, 1972/1975b, p. 134, note 2)

Jacobs (1997a) offers a different view, that 'life position is relative and variable' (p. 198), and proposes a significant addition to Ernst's OK Corral: calibrations for both axes whereby the plotting of points creates multiple locations within the quadrants and, thus, relative or degrees of OKness.

In addition to the people or persons, as represented by personal pronouns, and the OKness and not OKness, as designated by + and – signs, one or two other notations have been introduced. In his book *I'm OK, You're OK*, Harris (1967) described four other positions: 'You Can Be OK If', 'I'm Not OK And I'm Not Sure About You', 'I Can Be OK If', and 'I Am OK As Long As'. In his last book, Berne (1972/1975b) introduces the use of the question mark to describe insecurity and flexibility, for example, 'I + You + They?', which he describes as an evangelistic position, and 'I + You? They –', which he describes as an aristocratic class position. On the basis that all four original positions establish our character, which is in some way adapted, English (1975a) describes an individuated and autonomous fifth position: 'I'm OK, You're OK (Adult)'.

In keeping with the we psychology perspective of this chapter, incorporating 'we' into Berne's (1972/1975b) three-handed positions results in 16 basic life positions.[3] I suggest that these variations more explicitly describe a relational perspective on what are, in effect, individual, group, and social life positions. I outline them here and include three examples.

I + You + We + They +

This represents the position of democratic communities or groups getting along with each other.

I + You + We + They –

This describes a position and a series of relationships whereby a person, with others, colludes with and justifies negative attitudes toward and actions against another or others, usually referred to as 'Them' (over there). This, in terms of language, objectifies and distances the object and makes 'them' and their troublesome otherness not OK. J. James (1983a) writes about this dynamic with reference to dominant and nondominant cultures and the challenge to transactional analysis of cultural consciousness in this regard. In an article on therapy, thought reform, and cults, Singer (1996) refers to the three-handed position 'I'm OK, You're OK, They're Not OK' as describing the therapist/Master, client/Follower dynamic of cults. Adding the fourth hand of 'We'—or 'We?'—to this example adds something of the collective collusive quality of the projections from 'Us' onto 'Them'. There are numerous historical examples of this particular four-handed position in practice that describe forms of oppression, war, and, ultimately, genocide. We may analyse, for instance, the attitude of the United Kingdom and United States governments to the war in Iraq (2003–2011) whereby both the enemy and other countries who did not support the war were 'They' and 'Not OK'.[4] With regard to other countries who did not join the coalition, the position was represented by 'I + You – We + They –'. In the context of psychotherapy groups, I notice the change when people stop referring to 'them' as objects, even when referring to other people in the group (e.g., 'men… them') and begin to use the word 'they'. Although this represents the third-person plural, it is a subject rather than an object pronoun. The final shift is from this abstraction to the more direct use of 'You': a personal, subjective other. In my experience, these changes in language often mark the beginning of less certainty, rigidity, and fixity and the development of more uncertainty, ambivalence, and fluidity as well as dialogue on the basis of intersubjective experience. In this sense, the movement to 'we' is through the more intimate appreciation of 'you'. This may be represented as: 'I + Them (generalised object) → I + They (plural subject) → I + You (subjects) → Us (social self) → We (personal self).

I + You + We – They +

This represents the position of internalised oppression when the split-off aspects of self are located in the identified group (see also the I – You + We – They + position below).

I + You + We – They –

This describes a prejudiced position (as described earlier) with the addition of this being justified with a cause.

I + You – We + They +

This represents the position of the agitator, malcontent, and sometimes missionaries, also often justified with a cause. Berne (1972/1975b) illustrates the position 'I + You – They +' as 'You people here are no good compared to the ones over there.' (p. 90)

I + You – We + They –

This describes the position of the self-righteous and collusive critics.

I + You – We – They +

This is the position of the (self-righteous) agitator or malcontent who actually despises the cause.

I + You – We – They –

This is a position that Groder (1977b) says that Berne describes as that of 'I'm going to make the world pay' (p. 163).[5]

I – You + We + They +

This represents the position of the self-punishing saint or masochist or the melancholic.

I – You + We + They –

This is the servile position with the additional complexity of some identification with the other that makes 'We' or 'Us' in some way OK.

I – You + We – They +

This represents another position in the experience and process of internalised oppression (see earlier) when the subject is both internalising the form of alienation against herself or himself and, at the same time, externalising it by projecting the positive norm onto the dominant other.

I – You + We – They –

This position describes a person (a real but anonymised client) who was socially phobic and who joined a therapy group out of some desperation. He did not much like himself, others, or human beings as such. He was in considerable internal distress and felt out of sync(hrony) with the world. He described that when he mixed socially, he often ended up in trouble because of his sarcasm, cynicism, and overall rejecting manner. He was an example of what Bion (1961/1968, p. 131) describes as 'the individual [as] a group animal at war, not simply with the group, but with himself for being a group animal and with those aspects of his personality that constitute his "groupishness"' (p. 131). This particular client idealised the group therapist ('You') as the fount of all wisdom, someone to whom he looked for how to do it, for answers and solutions to the meaning and dilemmas of life. This is consistent with Berne's (1972/1975b) reference to the three-handed version of this position as servile. Drawing on the four-handed perspective, the group therapist initially encouraged the client's positive 'You're OK' position and worked with him to apply this to other individuals in the group. At the same time, other group members recognised both the individual's difficulty in joining the group as well as his contribution to them as individuals. Gradually, the client was able to accept that, for others, he too was OK and began to internalise this as 'I'm OK'. The next phase of his therapy in the group focused on his development of a we perspective through a series of transactions and interactions in which the therapist highlighted their co-constructed nature. Following this, the client became an enthusiastic member of, and advocate for, the group. He talked about the group as a refuge in an uncaring and alien world and, at that time, made several proposals that the group should meet socially. The group was clearly important and, at this stage, the client was idealising it and setting it ('Us') against the world ('Them'). The final phase of this client's group therapy involved confronting his idealisation of the group and his discounting of others and other groups, which was important with regard to describing and analysing intergroup relations. Apart from the usefulness of the four-handed positions in describing the client's development, this brief example also highlights the necessity of the group context for therapy because it provides otherness and difference.

I – You – We + They +

This is the position of servile envy and sometimes of political action often justified by a certain righteousness.

I – You – We + They –

This is the pessimistic position of cynics who seek to justify their pessimism and most accurately describes the terrorist and/or suicide bomber. Berne (1972/1975b) describes the three-handed version (I – U – They –) as the pessimistic position of cynics. However, this in itself does not adequately explain the vision of the terror-ist, however distorted, and their sense of belonging to a movement or cause that is justified and supported by others. It is arguable that such ideology generates more of an (object) 'Us' rather than 'We' because terrorism is ultimately an 'Us versus Them' dynamic.

I – You – We – They +

This is the pessimistic position of cynics who know that they are misguided or wrong.

I – You – We – They –

This is the pessimistic and critical position of cynics who are also self-critical.

Conclusion

Having a key formulation of theory that uses the verb *to be* offers a linguistic link to existentialism. Using the first- and second-person singular pronouns 'I' and 'you' reflects a singular—that is, individualistic—psychology. Extending Berne's three-handed position to include 'we' offers a conceptual link to we psychology based on an ontological view of the person-in-relationship in-context and a more context-oriented psychology and transactional analysis both in theory and practice in its various fields of application. The application of this perspective supports groups and group work as well as individuals who view themselves primarily as members of groups (families, tribes, communities, etc.). Although I have made a strong case here for we psychology, I am aware that some people may need to find the 'I' before or from the 'we', developmentally and/or socially. There is further work to be done in elaborating the different identified life positions; in considering the implications for the different needs of clients, students, and trainees; in relation to other aspects of transactional analysis theory and practice, such as assessment, diagnosis, stages or phases of cure, and so on; and, not least, with regard to different therapists and their preferred ways of working.

Notes

1 During a workshop in which I commented favourably about this addition to the two life positions, Claude Steiner said that he didn't think it was a significant part of Berne's theory (in Steiner & Tudor, 2014, 27:15f).
2 Tony Blair, (Prime Minister of the United Kingdom, 1997–2007) said that John Macmurray was his favourite philosopher. He had been introduced to Macmurray's ideas when he was studying Jurisprudence at the University of Oxford in the 1970s (Hunt, 1988/2022). In a speech in 2006, Blair said that Macmurray's ideas help confront 'what will be the critical political question of the 21st century: the relationship between individual and society'. Blair's answer to that question was an acceptance of our social nature and that 'human life is inherently a common life' (Blair, 2006).
3 Accounting for the use of the '?', as well as the '+' and '−', in all four 'persons' yields a total of 64 life positions.
4 President George W. Bush's famous statement (2001): 'Every nation, in every region, now has a decision to make. Either you are with us, or you are with the terrorists' is an example of a statement that splits and polarises 'You' or 'They' (every nation) so that those who choose not to be 'with us', or who choose not to make that choice or not to accept that form of speech act (which creates a false dilemma) is positioned as You – and/ or They –.
5 Though Groder doesn't cite where Berne writes or said this.

Chapter 2

There's methodology in the contractual method

Philosophy in practice

Working on the basis of a contract with the client or clients initially distinguished transactional analysis (TA) from many other therapies and other applications of psychology to the fields of education, and work in and with organisations—and, at best, our focused, engaged, co-operative, and egalitarian way of working with clients still distinguishes TA practitioners from those of many other schools and methods of therapy (see Gellert & Wilson, 1977; Stummer, 2002). Moreover, the centrality of the contract in TA has influenced thinking across modalities about the terms and conditions of therapy and how this is understood by the various parties to therapy, and, by extension, to supervision, education/training, service delivery, and professional organisations. Nowadays, most codes of ethics and frameworks for professional practice contain some reference to a contract with clients (and others), though generally this concerns the administrative aspect of engagement with therapy. Whilst acknowledging the administrative or business contract, Berne (1966a) also identifies two other types of contract: the professional (or treatment) contract, and the psychological contract. I suggest that this tripartite taxonomy is significant because, if contracts about and in therapy remain entirely administrative, they contribute to a more mechanistic than therapeutic or relational view of that therapy. However, despite identifying these various types of contract, and, at one point, proposing a contractual method, in his writing about contracts, Berne (1947/1971, 1963, 1966a, 1972/1975b) does not identify the philosophical basis or assumptions of this central element of his method. In keeping with the other chapters in this part of the book in which I explore the methodology, and epistemology, ontology, and ethics of TA practice, in this chapter, I do so with regard to contracts and the basis of TA practice: the contractual method. Although Berne himself does not discuss methodology, 'TA methodology' is a required component of the TA 101 introductory course (International Transactional Analysis Association [ITAA] International Board of Certification [IBoC], 2022, Section 12, Form 12.11.1).[1]

The title of this chapter is inspired by the line from Shakespeare's *Hamlet*, spoken by Polonius: 'Though this be madness, yet there is method in't' (Shakespeare, 1602/1985, Act II, scene 2, line 195). In effect, this chapter explores the statement: 'Though this be method, there's methodology in't.' In order to elucidate the largely unexamined methodology of the contractual method of TA, in the first part of this

DOI: 10.4324/9780429398223-4

chapter I discuss what Berne and other transactional analysts write about contracts. In the second part of the chapter, I apply the difference between method and methodology to the subject of contracts, contracting, and the contractual method; and in the third part of the chapter, I discuss methodology and philosophy and outline the importance and advantages of having both method and methodology.

Contracts in transactional analysis

As Stewart (1992) points out, Berne's interest in and commitment to the contract dates back at least to 1947 (see Concannon, 1971), though, given its centrality in his thinking about the practice of transactional analysis, it is surprisingly absent in his first major book on the subject: *Transactional Analysis in Psychotherapy* (Berne, 1961/1975a). In his book *A Layman's Guide to Psychiatry and Psychoanalysis* ('*Layman's Guide*') Berne (1947/1971) clearly links the treatment contract to the importance of results, arguing that 'making an Adult type of contract which will consider objectively the patient's individual needs' (p. 316) avoids patients being dependent on the therapist (Child ego state) and/or the therapist responding with prejudices (about what they think the patient needs) (Parent ego state). Berne's interest in 'hooking' the Adult of the client or patient is epitomised in his approach to staff–patient staff conferences (Berne, 1968c). Table 2.1 summarises Berne's writing on contracts.

From this, a number of points emerge regarding Berne's thinking about contracts:

1. That it is primarily and predominantly confined to the context of working with groups and in organisations.
2. That it is focused more on goals than process (for further discussion of which, see Stewart, 1996).
3. That the most widely quoted of Berne's definitions of a contract in TA—that it is 'An explicit bilateral commitment to a well-defined course of action' (Berne, 1966a, p. 362)—appears in the glossary of *Principles of Group Treatment*, and is not discussed in the text.[3]
4. That, in his last book, *What Do You Say After You Say Hello?*, Berne (1972/1975b) changed this definition in a way that refocused attention to the *goal* of treatment rather than the course of action.

Berne's own descriptions of the qualities or requirements of a therapeutic or treatment contract are that it should be clear, operational, and bilateral (Berne, 1966a); and Adult-to-Adult, and stated simply and in well-defined words (Berne, 1947/1971). Clarkson (1992) suggests that this Adult-to-Adult contract 'emphasise[s] the responsibility of both client and psychotherapist to be clear about the changes that the client wishes to make and how the psychotherapist will effect this' (p. 20). Moreover, according to Berne (1947/1971), 'If the patient is unable to form an Adult contract, this inability becomes the chief concern in the treatment' (p. 316).

Table 2.1. A summary of Berne's ideas on contracts (in chronological order)

Contract	Purpose	Note/definition
Social contract (Berne, 1963)	To support the social etiquette of the group—which, in turn, enforces the contract	'The most important influence in the group culture' (Berne, 1963, p. 109) 'You respect my persona, and I'll respect yours.' (Berne, 1963, p. 109) 'An unspoken contract of etiquette which requires the members to respect each other's personas as presented in the individual structure.' (Berne, 1963, p. 239)
Constitutional contract (Berne, 1963)	To maintain roles in an organisational structure	'I promise to support the constitution of this group.' (Berne, 1963, p. 109) 'The contract entered into by a member [of a group] to respect the roles of the organizational structure on the terms stated in the constitution.' (Berne, 1963, p. 239)
Administrative contract (Berne, 1966a)	To understand the occasion for and purpose of a particular project and any organisational goals involved	'The statement between the administration and the therapist concerning the occasions, purposes, and goals of treatment group, usually in sociological language.' (Berne, 1966a, p. 362)
Professional contract (Berne, 1966a)	To identify the goal of therapy	'The professional goal of the therapy' (Berne, 1966a, p. 16), such as social control, symptomatic cure, personality reorganisation, etc. 'A statement of the technical goals of the treatment group, usually in psychiatric language.' (Berne, 1966a, p. 362)
Psychological contract (Berne, 1966a)	In an organisational context, to clarify the personal needs of various relevant colleagues	As Berne describes it in the organisational context, this is akin to the 'valid consideration' of a contract as described by Steiner and Cassidy (1969), i.e., 'The therapist's assessment of the ulterior motives of the administration that will influence the fate of his treatment group in the organization.' (Berne, 1966a, p. 362) As Berne describes it with regard to the therapist–patient relationship, it is 'the psychological aspects of the contract which become part of the therapeutic struggle.' (Berne, 1966a, p. 20)

(Continued)

Table 2.1. (Continued)

Contract	Purpose	Note/definition
Therapist–patient contract (Berne, 1966a)	To clarify the relationship between the therapist and the patient	Has the same aspects as the organisational contract, i.e., administrative, professional, and psychological—in which context Berne refers to these as 'levels'. 'Administratively, this concerns the relationships between therapist, the patients, and the organisation. Professionally, it states the goals of the therapy. Psychologically, the therapist (inwardly) tries to anticipate which games the patients are likely to play in the group.' (Berne, 1966a, p. 362)
Contractual treatment (Berne, 1966a)	To identify the goal of treatment	Defined as 'bilateral rather than unilateral' (Berne, 1966a, p. 88)
Transactional contract (Berne, 1966a)	To distinguish between getting better and analysis	
Psychoanalytic contract (Berne, 1966a)	To distinguish between the procedure (long-term analysis) and cure	
Contract (Berne, 1966a, 1972/1975b)	To define the process, and goal of treatment/therapy (and other applications of TA)	'An explicit bilateral commitment to a well-defined course of action.' (Berne, 1966, p. 362); 'An explicit agreement between a patient and a therapist which states the goal of the treatment during each phase.' (Berne, 1972/1975b, p. 442)
Organisational contract (Berne, 1966a)	To clarify the relationship between the therapist and the organisation	'The agreement concerning group treatment between the therapist and his organisation.' (Berne, 1966, p. 362)
Treatment contract (Berne, 1947/1971)[2]	To consider objectively the patient's individual needs	Adult-to-Adult Based on four requirements (see Steiner & Cassidy, 1969) 'An explicit agreement between a patient and a therapist which states the goal of the treatment during each phase.' (Berne, 1972/1975b, p. 442)

Also, in *A Layman's Guide* Berne notes four requirements for a contract, which, drawing on the basic requirements for contracts to be legally valid (in the United States, at the time), Steiner and Cassidy (1969) had identified as:

- Mutual consent—which, in the therapeutic context, implies a clear and understandable offer on the part of the therapist of what they will give, in return for some act or promise on the part of the client.
- Valid consideration—which refers to the benefit conferred both by the therapist (amelioration, cure, etc.) and by the client (in the form of payment and/or attendance, active participation, etc.).
- Competency—which refers to the ability of the parties to enter into a contract and is, therefore, mediated in the case of legal minors, and certain levels of dysfunction and intoxication (see also Steiner, 1971a, 1979).
- Lawful object—which refers to the broader consideration that, as Steiner and Cassidy put it: 'The contract must not be in violation of law or against public policy or morals' (p. 31).

Writing in the context of UK law, Jenkins (1997) identifies similar requirements or conditions, i.e., legal capacity; firm offer and unequivocal acceptance; clear intention of the parties to create a legally binding agreement; and consideration of exchange. However, whilst Steiner and Cassidy's basic requirements provide a useful set of criteria for the practitioner at least to think about, they are also problematic for a number of reasons:

1. That they are highly contextual and relative
   The question of what defines a contract varies significantly between jurisdictions, for example, in Scots' law, there is no need for consideration. Thus, any proposed principles have to reflect this fact, which means that practitioners need to be familiar with the law regarding contracts and contracting in the jurisdictions in which they work, and that consequent practice—as well as the theory that supports such practice—is context-dependent.
2. That these particular requirements are contested
   The question of capacity/competency is a contestable issue, particularly under the United Nations (2008) *Convention on the Rights of Persons with Disabilities* because it can lead to adults with intellectual or other impairments being infantilised. As Gledhill (personal communication, 27 September 2018) put it: 'What to do in this context is a cutting edge issue, which is going to affect all sorts of areas—e.g., banks, utility service providers, accommodation providers, given that everything turns on a contract.'
3. That using the metaphor of 'legal requirements' restricts free thinking
   Given Steiner's radicalism as far as radical psychiatry was concerned, it appears somewhat strange that he put his name to promoting a criterion of lawful object that was defined in terms of (United States) law, public policy, and, especially, morals. This is not only because they are relative, but also because

they are precisely subjects which transactional analysts and their clients analyse transactionally—and should be able to do so freely (Younger, 2017/2020) and, not least, by thinking Martian (see Chapter 13). Moreover, the use of a legal framework to define the requirements of the therapeutic contract supports the managerial, audit culture in psychotherapy and other applications of TA (for a critique of which see King & Moutsou, 2010).

There may be ways in which drawing on criteria for legal contracts is useful, but only in context, i.e., with reference to specific and relevant national and international law, and, I would say at a meta-level. For instance, as Gledhill (personal communication, 27 September 2018) notes:

> there have been major developments in relation to concepts such as undue influence as a basis for setting aside, and [thus] some might argue that some form of parity in bargaining power could be seen as an important element of contracts.[4]

This raises an important point about the 'parity in bargaining power' that a client has—and/or experiences—with regard to what are viewed as certain norms of therapy (regarding frequency, length of sessions, payment, etc.). One client with whom I worked appeared somewhat frustrated about what he experienced as the short length of the 50-minute session and, quite early on in the course of the therapy, asked to book sessions of a session and a half (i.e., 75 minutes). I gave this some thought and agreed, following which we experimented with sessions of an hour, and sessions of either an hour or 50 minutes. From some perspectives such flexibility would be viewed as compromising the therapeutic frame (Milner, 1952); for me it was important firstly, to respond openly and positively to this client's request, and secondly, to analyse his frustration, a response which, it transpired, was in itself therapeutic and reparative or expansive.

Both during Berne's lifetime and since his death, transactional analysts have developed the concept of the contract, i.e., the goal or outcome of TA intervention; and the concept of contracting, i.e., the process of making the contract and defining treatment/intervention, as a result of which TA has a number of different models of both contract and contracting. Table 2.2 summarises these models in the context of the different approaches within TA (see Tudor & Hobbes, 2002; and Chapter 12).

From this, it is clear that there are a number of concepts in TA about the contract and about the process of contracting. It is also clear that, in some cases, the two terms—contracts and contracting—are used interchangeably, and also that both are covered by the term 'the contractual method'.

The contractual method in transactional analysis

While Berne did write about contracts predominantly in terms of goals, he did also define the contract in terms of process, i.e., 'An explicit bilateral commitment to a well-defined *course of action* [emphasis added].' (Berne, 1966a, p. 362) This short,

Table 2.2. Contracts and contracting in different approaches in TA

Approach	Contracts	Contracting
Classical (psychodynamic)	(Contract) for cure (Berne, 1961/1975a) Social contract and constitutional contract (Berne, 1963) Contract completion (Drye, 1980)	With regard to the dynamics of script, and, specifically, compound script beliefs (Stewart, 1989)
Classical (cognitive behavioural)	Levels of contracts: administrative, professional, and psychological (Berne, 1966a) Four requirements for an effective contract: mutual consent, valid consideration, competency, and lawful object (Steiner & Cassidy, 1969; Steiner, 1974) Autonomy contract (relating to script), and the social change contract (relating to ego states) (Holloway & Holloway, 1973) Escape hatch closure (Holloway, 1973); no psychosis contract (M. M. Goulding & R. L. Goulding, 1979; White, 1999) Three-cornered contract (English, 1975c) The contract card (Moiso, 1976) The transactions of a 'mutually-informed-consent relationship', i.e., the request, an offer, and an acceptance (Steiner, 1979, p. 124) Classroom contracts (Rovics, 1981) Effective contracts, i.e., phrased positively: specifying the positive (for the Child); achievable; with specific and observable goals (phrased in eight-year-old language); made from Adult (with Free Child co-operation); including with an assessment of the cost (Stewart & Joines, 1987); marking a movement out of script (Stewart, 1989); and finishable (Stewart, 1996) Sensory-based (Stewart, 1996) Contact contract (White, 2001)	Six steps for effective contracting (M. James, 1971) Closing escape hatches (Holloway, 1973); see also Boyd and Cowles-Boyd (1980), M. M. Goulding and R. L. Goulding (1979), and Mellor (1980) Process contracting (Lee, 1997)
Radical psychiatry	Social contracts (Tudor, 1997d)	Co-operative contracts (i.e., contracting): be honest; no lies, no power plays, no rescues (Steiner, 1974)[5]

(Continued)

Table 2.2. (Continued)

Approach	Contracts	Contracting
Cathexis	Initial 'soft' contracts[6] and specific mini contracts (as patients in the initial stages of treatment are 'sufficiently dysfunctional' (Schiff et al., 1975, p. 101) Reparenting contracts (Mellor, 1980)	
Redecision	Levels of contract, i.e., care, social control, relationship, and structural change (Loomis, 1982) Contract for change (de Saint-Pierre, 2004)	Contracting (R. L. Goulding, 1972; M. M. Goulding & R. L. Goulding, 1979)
Integrative	Viewed as implicit in Erskine's work—see Stummer (2002)	Contracting emphasises mutual and respect between the two parties and responsibility on the part of the client (Clarkson, 1992) Process contracting (R. Erskine, 2002, personal communication, cited in Stummer, 2002)
Constructivist		Co-creative contracting, based on principles of 'we-ness', shared responsibility, and present-centred development (Summers & Tudor, 2000)
Relational	Therapist–patient contract (Berne, 1966a) That 'the therapist and client have a shared idea of why there in the consulting room together... Any change that can be named is part of the imaginable assumptive world of the client.' (Hargaden & Sills, 2002, p. 32)	
Systemic	Social contract and constitutional contract (Berne, 1963) Types of contracts: administrative, professional, and psychological (Berne, 1966a) Three-cornered contract (English, 1975); and multi-handed contracts (Tudor, 1997a) Five levels of contract (Sills, 2006)	Contracting matrix (Sills, 2006)

ten-word sentence contains four key elements of the definition of the term contract in TA:

- That it is explicit...
- ... rather than implicit, and, therefore, clearly stated.

Example

Client: I have a problem with sleeping.
Therapist: So, what would you like to talk about?
Client: My problem with sleeping.
Therapist: What do you want to achieve by talking about your problem?
Client: Well, I'd like to get to sleep more easily, and to stay asleep at night longer.

While, at first blush, such explicitness may appear straightforward, obvious, and desirable, in cultures in which subtlety, ambiguity, and indirectness are valued, the unfolding, openness and clarity demanded by this Bernean (and Western) view of a contract is problematic. In such contexts, the following definition of a contract may be more widely acceptable and applicable: an explicit or implicit, bilateral or multi-lateral sense of what's wanted or needed in a given situation.

- That it is bilateral

    This means that there are two sides to the agreement, or, in the case of a multi-lateral contract, more than two sides or parties to the agreement. In this way, contracts are distinguished from rules (which are unilateral) and working agreements (which may come from any ego state) (see Woollams & Brown, 1978; Tudor 1999).[7] In his article on staff–patient staff conferences, Berne (1968c) emphasises the need for staff members who are observing the staff conference to say something, which he asserts 'makes the situation bilateral' (p. 43). Thus, it is clear that bilaterality requires engagement and openness. In her excellent article on 'Rethinking contracts', Rotondo (2020) emphasises the bilateral nature of the contract and the 'specific, innovative, relational quality of reciprocity' (p. 2) this represents between the therapist and the patient. Citing Berne, she writes: 'just as the therapist analyzes the patient, it is appropriate for the patient to analyze the therapist and to ask what the therapist can offer' (p. 2). Yet, despite this emphasis on the bilateral nature of contracts, in the context of reading TA case studies and examining candidates presenting at certifying TA oral examinations over nearly 30 years, I rarely see an acknowledgement of the therapist's side of or engagement with(in) the agreement. In her discussion of bilaterality, Rotondo (2020) highlights two aspects to this. The first is the importance and significance of the equality of the partners to the contract and their respective OKness, as well as the 'intersubjective vision between the two individuals involved in the relationship, both with their own competence and both worthy of respect and attention' (p. 8). The second is the qualities of the relationship. Quoting the Holloways' vision of the clinician as 'an equal and mutual participant in the process of change (Holloway & Holloway, 1973, p. 36), Rotondo (2020) considers this as acknowledging the 'specific potential and influencing capacity' (p. 8) of both partners to and in the contract 'both with their own responsibility for the process of change' (p. 8).

Example (continued):

Therapist: So, it sounds like you want to talk as much about some solutions to the problem as the problem itself.

Client: … I guess so, but I'd still like to tell you the problems I have in getting to sleep and in waking up during the night.

Therapist: OK…. So, in talking about the problem and in finding solutions, what do you want from me?

Client: Well… to listen… maybe to give me some advice.

Therapist: OK: you want me to listen and to offer you any advice I may have about getting to sleep and sleeping through the night. Would you also be interested in me offering any thoughts about connections I see between this problem about sleep and other things you talk about?

The fact that this contract is bilateral also suggests that it is or might be the subject of some discussion and negotiation, not merely an acceptance of what the client wants (which is discussed in the literature), or of what the therapist is offering—or an absence of what the therapist is or could be offering (reference to or comments on which are largely absence in the literature).

- That it is – and represents – a commitment
  Berne's use of the word commitment suggests a certain engagement and investment on the part of both or all parties to the contract. Berne (1966a) himself defines commitment as 'An operationally ratified decision to follow certain principles of action in order to achieve a certain goal' (p. 362). Following on from the previous point about the negotiability of the contract, this might mean that the therapist offers something to the client – which is consistent both with Steiner's (1979) transactional analysis of a contract, and with the co-creative principle of shared responsibility (Summers & Tudor, 2000).

Example (continued):

Client: What do you mean?

Therapist: Well, I'm aware that you've already told me something about yourself and your family history and I'm wanting to check whether it's OK with you that I offer any observations or reflections about connections I see.

Client: Yeah, that's fine. Thanks.

- That it is well-defined

    Writing about the professional contract, Berne (1966a) suggests that this should be phrased as 'a clear statement in operational form' (p. 88). This is particularly important when a therapeutic goal might be an internal one, such as 'to feel good'; a comparative one, such as to feel 'less' anxious or to have a 'better' relationship, or, as in the above example, what constitutes getting to sleep 'more easily', and sleeping 'longer'; or a vague one, such as for the family 'to be working well together'. From a TA perspective, all of these goals would need further clarification.

However, that this definition refers to the contract as a course of action suggests that the focus of the contract—and, indeed, the purpose of its explicitness, its bilateral nature, the agreement of the parties concerned, and the clarity of its definition, and of the parties' commitment to it—is on a process, i.e., the course of therapy. This perspective on the contract as method is close to what Rawls (1971) describes as a 'method of discovery' (p. 159). While it is relatively easy to see and hear the word 'contracting' (the gerund of the verb 'to contract'), as a noun that indicates process, it is perhaps harder to understand the noun 'contract' as referring to a course of action and, in that sense, a process. Nevertheless, I suggest that thinking about the contract in TA as a *method* is helpful, especially in distinguishing it from the concepts of goal(s) and outcome(s).

    The strength of Berne's approach to contracts is precisely its explicitness, definition, and engagement. However, this is also its weakness, as not all human experience can—or should—be so defined. While the concern of Berne and other transactional analysts to be open in and about their communication is very client-centred and egalitarian, the over-concern, even obsession to define everything makes it problematic. We can't control ourselves, others, or the world simply by defining things; people don't necessarily know what they want, let alone what they want to feel or achieve in 50 minutes, and even if they do, by defining what they know they want and, therefore, what's 'in', they implicitly discount or disavow what's more unknown and, thereby, what's 'out'—and what might emerge through the process of therapy. Writing about therapy as bringing new dimensions to the client's life, Hargaden and Sills (2002) put this well: 'Having a detailed goal can be restricting in itself and preclude a journey of discovery', one which can open the client to 'ways of seeing the world that are outside his present consciousness' (p. 32).

    Having reviewed various ideas about the contract and contracting in TA, I now discuss the difference between method and methodology in order to explicate the methodology of the contractual method.

Method and methodology

According to the online *Oxford English Dictionary* (2023a), method, from the Latin *methodus*, refers to 'a procedure for attaining an object' and, more generally, 'a way of doing anything, esp. according to a defined and regular plan'; 'a mode of procedure in any activity'; 'a scheme, a plan of action'; 'a set of rules and procedures proper to a particular practical art'; and, in philosophy, '[a]ny of various principles or canons of inductive reasoning'; and systematic arrangement and order. According to the same *Dictionary*, the word methodology (as it was formed in English), refers to

> the branch of knowledge that deals with method generally or with the methods of a particular discipline or field of study... [and] the study of the direction implications of empirical research, or of the suitability of techniques employed in it; [and] (more generally) a method or body of methods used in a particular field of study or activity.
>
> (*Oxford English Dictionary*, 2023b)

From this we can see that methodology refers to the thinking behind the method, the method of method(s), the meta-method, or meta-theory. One way of summarising the difference between method and methodology is that method refers to practice, i.e., what we do, while methodology refers to the philosophy underpinning practice, i.e., what and how we think about what we do. For example, historical materialism is the sociological analysis (the method) of Marxism (the methodology). In TA, Berne's only formal reference to methodology is to be found in his book *The Structure and Dynamics of Organizations and Groups* (Berne, 1963), in which he refers to 'general methodology' (p. 297) and quotes approvingly the British mathematician and historian Jacob Bronowski (1953) who writes: 'we must look for the evidence for the laws in the cross-connections between them. What we must adduce, I think, is the amount of simplification or order the laws bring into the wilderness of natural facts' (p. 142). Apart from revealing Berne's antipathy to wilderness, this also suggests his interest in cross-connection, which is not only reflected in his interest in transcultural psychiatry (see Berne, 1949, 1956, 1959a, 1959b, 1960a, 1960b; Bernstein, 1939) but also supports Rotondo's analysis of the influence of the intersubjective vision that characterises humanistic psychology and its therapies, including TA.

Berne addresses the issue or problem of cross-connection in his last book, *What Do You Say After You Say Hello* (Berne, 1972/1975b), when he reports a discussion at the San Francisco Transactional Analysis Seminar in which people were talking at cross purposes, that is they were using (four) different theories or frameworks and different terms to those different theories and frameworks. Berne offers the following explanation of this:

> The first framework was structural and transactional, with four key ego state terms: states, transactions, games, and scripts. The second was validating, again with four key terms. They could talk about her behavior, which offered operational criteria; her mental processes..., her developmental history..., and the kind of social responses she elicited by her behaviour. The third language dealt with naming her ego states. They could be named according to psychobiological

principles: the Parent in her Child, the Adult in her Child, etc, or described functionally by adjectives: Adapted Child, Natural Child, etc. [Fourthly,] the arguments themselves could be termed logical on the one hand, or empirical on the other.

(pp. 410–411)

Table 2.3 offers a summary of this analysis of terminology.

With his usual interest in logic and maths, Berne noted that this analysis accounts for 64 possible paths for discussion! Moreover, if we then extend any of these—and I would certainly argue for a greater range of methodologies as the basis for argument in TA, i.e., existential, humanistic, and phenomenological (see Chapter 12)—then matters become more complex and the paths more than double to 160! The point here is that it is useful to know the basis on which we are analysing, validating, and modifying transactions, ego states, scripts, and games, as well as the philosophical basis on which we do things, for example, changing the order of these fundamental pillars—or pillows[8]—of transactional analysis, as Graeme Summers and I did in our article published in 2000, which I tend to follow (see Part II).

Elsewhere, in furthering the practice of co-creative transactional analysis (Tudor, 2011d), I have written about empathy and co-creative transactional relating as methods which derive from phenomenological methodology, both hermeneutic and heuristic, which, in turn, is based on an epistemology that views knowledge as based in relationship, which, in turn, is based on a view of human nature as organismic, which, therefore, describes the ontology or essence of things in terms of the integrating Adult ego state—at least for the time being (see Chapter 7)! These derivations are represented visually in Table 2.4 which may be read from top to

Table 2.3. A terminological grid for the analysis of transactional analysis

Transactional	Validating	Modifying	Methodology
Ego states	Operational Phenomenological Historical Social	Structural (biological) Functional (descriptive)	Logical Empirical
Transactions	Operational Phenomenological Historical Social	Structural (biological) Functional (descriptive)	Logical Empirical
Games	Operational Phenomenological Historical Social	Structural (biological) Functional (descriptive)	Logical Empirical
Scripts	Operational Phenomenological Historical Social	Structural (biological) Functional (descriptive)	Logical Empirical

Table 2.4. Assumptions about the nature of social science applied to the development of co-creative TA

Empathic and co-creative transactional relating (Tudor, 2011b, 2011g)
Method
Phenomenological—hermeneutic and heuristic
Methodology
(the philosophy of method)
That knowledge is created and co-created in relationship
As embodied in 'Co-creative transactional analysis' (Summers & Tudor, 2000) and 'Empathy: A cocreative perspective' (Tudor, 2011b)
Epistemology
(the knowledge of knowledge)
Based on the nature of the organism (Tudor, 2003b; Tudor & Worrall, 2006)
Human nature
Understood in terms of the neopsyche or integrating Adult ego state (Tudor, 2003b) as well as the archeopsyche and exteropsyche
Ontology
(the essence of things)
Based on Burrell and Morgan (1979), and developed from Tudor (2011d).

bottom (as described in this paragraph) or from bottom to top (in working from fundamental principles or categories to practice).

In terms of principles and categories, I now tend to include human nature (which Burrell and Morgan had as a distinct category) as part of ontology, as I regard human 'nature' as part of the essence of things or the consideration of what constitutes the essence of things. Also, this Table doesn't explicitly account for ethics, which Levinas (1961/1969) considers 'first philosophy' and, therefore, prior to ontology, a point I pick up later in this chapter in a brief discussion about transactional ethics.

So, let's see how this works with regard to TA theory, taking the example of the permission transaction (see Figure 2.1).

Here, the method is the permission transaction, while the methodology is as follows:

- Regarding epistemology (the knowledge of knowledge)—that the therapist knows what the client needs, and, therefore, knows more than the client. This is represented in the classical or traditional diagram of this TA transaction as stimulated by the client (in Child) (in this case an ulterior transaction though it could equally be a social level transaction) which elicits a response from the therapist (in Parent). The fact that the therapist is represented on the left-hand side of the page (in Western script) also reinforces the priority given to the therapist and to their authority and power over that of the client. Inspired by Bob and Mary Gouldings' (1975/1978) perspective and slogan, 'The power is in the patient', I tend to diagram transactions beginning with the client and with the client on the left-hand side of the page (see, for example, Tudor, 2011g).

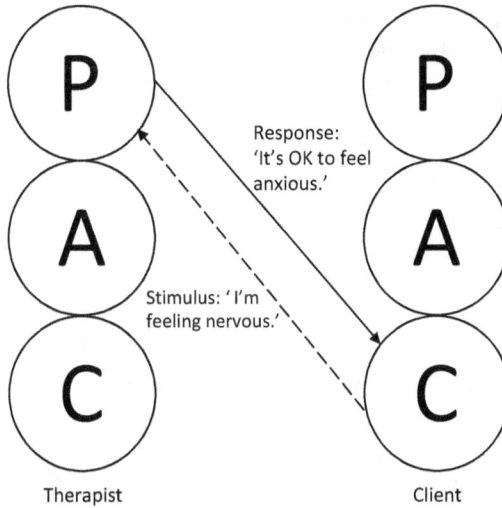

Figure 2.1. The permission transaction

- Regarding human nature—bearing in mind that 'every transaction has political consequences, every message has a meta-communication, a message about the message' (Steiner, 1981, p. 171), I suggest that the message that this transaction conveys about human nature is that you (over there) are a separate individual, and in some ways less than or under me as I have power over you to give you the permission (I think) you need, and, therefore, that human nature and society is hierarchical.
- Regarding ontology (the essence of being)—that the client is nervous or anxious, and that this is a problem, and that the therapist knows the 'essence' of the client. There are a number of implied assumptions with this:

  1. The first is the view that the 'fact' that the client is nervous or anxious is a problem, when it may not be the case. From a person-centred perspective, a client's declaration that they are feeling nervous might demonstrate that they are being congruent or authentic; from an existential perspective, it may be that, given their circumstances and the state of the(ir) world, the client could or should be *more* anxious.
  2. The second assumption is that is it OK for the particular client not to feel anxious, when this also may not be the case. For instance, from a holistic perspective of the person, I don't know what role anxiety plays in maintaining the client's homeostasis and, as Berne (1964/1968a) argues, stabilising homeostatic functions is the general advantage of a game (see Chapter 11). Considering the implications of this for practice, Novellino (2012) writes:

     This states that the therapist should maintain a sense of balance, so as not to confront the game either too soon or too late. If he does it too soon, that is,

---

before establishing a therapeutic alliance and before having reinforced the Adult of the patient, he takes away from the latter some of his 'known' strokes. If the game is confronted too late, when the 'escalation' is beginning to move towards abandonment of the therapy and, therefore, becoming a repetition of the previous therapeutic relationships, the therapist is experienced as a 'Victim' ('I have trapped him as well'), and the Child of the patient enters into a situation in which he no longer expects the therapist to be a different parent.

(p. 104)

Thus, like Novellino, I am generally cautious about confronting a game until I know more about the context of the client's stable and unstable functioning.

3. The third is that this transaction implies a particular ontology of the person, in this case a three ego state model of personality and a three ego state model of health (Figure 2.2), in which one of the aims is to acknowledge the Child ego state as (conceptual) place of nervousness and anxiety and to grow or develop it as the place of either feeling OK about this or no longer feeling or having to feel those particular feelings or emotions. A different view of the essence of the person is offered by the integrating Adult, which, while still based on a three state model of personality, proposes a one ego state model of health (Figure 2.3).

The completeness of the three ego state model of personality is emphasised by Berne in his last book in which he puts a skin around all three ego states (for discussion of which, see Chapter 7).

Using the example of the permission transaction to illustrate my argument about the importance of method and the methodology 'in't', I am arguing that as—or,

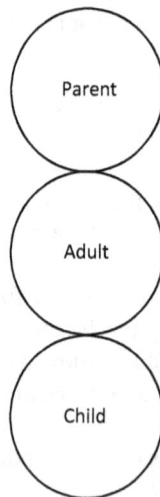

Figure 2.2. The three ego state model of health

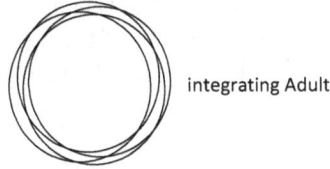

integrating Adult

Figure 2.3. The integrating Adult model of health
(Summers & Tudor, 2021).

preferably, before—we do something, we need to have a view about the nature of human beings and, indeed, about the nature of nature—and that consideration of this would include whether there is a 'nature' or essence of things. To a large extent this is about making explicit what is more often implicit. As Rogers (1957b) puts it: 'One cannot engage in psychotherapy without giving operational evidence of an underlying value orientation and view of human nature' (p. 199) and goes on to state his preference—with which I agree—'that such underlying views be open and explicit, rather than covert and implicit' (p. 199). Given Berne's preference for being open and explicit, Rogers' point stands well for transactional analysts, too.

Applying the distinction between method and methodology to the subject of the contract and contracting, we can say that a contract is a statement (about a process or an outcome) which is elicited through a method of contracting (asking questions, etc.) which, in turn, is based on a methodology or philosophy. In this sense, the contract is linked to what is generally viewed as Berne's other therapeutic method, that of open communication.

Open communication

In his discussion of Berne's approach to therapy, Stewart (1992) refers to open communication as 'a *sine qua non* of the therapeutic relationship' (p. 78), citing in support of this Berne's actions as a psychiatrist:

a) When he abolished the practice of having observers hidden behind a one-way mirror during sessions of his out-patient groups (see Callaghan in Levaggi et al., 1971); and

b) When he introduced staff–patient staff conferences, whereby, following their observation of a psychotherapy group therapy session, staff who had sat outside the group for the session, then formed an inner group to discuss the session they had just observed (see Berne, 1968c).

To this, I would add:

c) That he also introduced in these conferences a blackboard on which he drew explanatory diagrams for both staff and patients (also reported by Callaghan in Levaggi et al., 1971).

These methods, which were seen as radical and challenging at the time, were based on Berne's critique of the so-called 'purity' of the therapeutic and especially the transferential relationship, and of intellectualisation on the part of psychiatric staff.

However, despite the fact that 'open communication' is commonly referred to as one of Berne's two therapeutic methods, it has not been discussed or elaborated in TA, at least in the literature; and is, I suggest, viewed as more a principle (philosophical or otherwise) by Stewart (1992), Newton and Wong (2003), and Cox (2007); a basic assumption by Napper (2009); and a philosophy and a method by Bestazza and Ranci (2015). Describing the work of a therapeutic community based on TA, Robinson (2003) notes the importance of open communication, which is required by the group structure and contained by and within the confidentiality boundary that surrounds the community as a whole: 'This degree of contact and openness makes it hard for someone to initiate and engage others in a serious game without someone else recognizing what is happening' (p. 316). Writing about those executive coaches who are also TA practitioners, Krausz (2005) refers to the establishment of 'open communication channels' (p. 369) especially in working with issues of trust. In a rare article that links the concept of open communication to a broader context, van Tol (2017) reminds us that members of the United Kingdom's Association of Transactional Analysis (UKATA) are, by virtue of their *Code of Ethics* (UKATA, 2008) directed to work with—and, presumably, also by means of—open communication.

In terms of the focus of this chapter, I view the practice of open communication, as exemplified in Berne's staff–patient staff conferences, as a method which implies a methodology, thus:

- Regarding method—for example, that 'the staff is trained and expected to say everything worth saying while the patients are listening' (Berne, 1968c, p. 44), a method that, along with the discipline of having no other staff conferences or meetings without patients present (and, therefore, no post-conference conferences), implies and embodies openness, what Berne refers to as 'talking "straight"' (p. 44), and with 'frankness' (p. 45), and respect.
- Regarding epistemology—that what is communicated is or can be known, not only in terms of what the client communicates, both explicitly and implicitly, but also what is or can be analysed between the client and the therapist, which, of course, is the basis of TA, that is, the analysis of transactions. Furthermore, thinking about this in terms of epistemology invites us to think about the assumptions about knowledge that are contained in transactions such as 'I don't know what I'm feeling' (which negates self-knowledge), 'Others know best' (which gives away knowledge), and 'The world's a scary place' (which externalises knowledge). These statements are poignant examples of Steiner's (1981) point about the meta-communication of the message, and, of the political—and, I would add, philosophical—consequences of that. Fundamentally, open communication is based on phenomenology, a philosophical tradition that acknowledges subjective experience and thus, in the therapeutic context, questions the emphasis on the clinician's knowledge based on the categorisation of symptoms

and labelling; as Berne (1968c) puts it: 'As a logical product of this "equality", categorization of patients has been abolished' (p. 45; see also Rotondo, 2020) This suggests that transactional analysts could and should focus on TA ways of understanding patients and their pathology and not rely on psychiatric diagnosis and manuals. It also suggests that that Berne comes close to Rogers' (1951) view of diagnosis: 'In a very meaningful and accurate sense, therapy is diagnosis, and this diagnosis is a process which goes on in the experience of the client, rather than the intellect of the clinician' (p. 224).

• Regarding ontology—that human beings are naturally open and/or have the capacity to be open, and are communicators (*homo communicans*); and that people are equal. As Berne (1968c) himself puts it: 'The staff–patient staff conference first attacks the comfortable and well-established sociological roles of "therapist" and "patient" and substitutes a "bilateral contract"... Everyone is treated as a 'person' with equal rights on his own merits' (p. 45).

Having discussed methodology as implying philosophy, I now turn to the relationship between the two.

Methodology and philosophy

As methodology is viewed as the philosophy underpinning method or practice, it is worth examining what the philosophical roots of TA are. However, before doing so, and in the spirit of the contractual method and open communication, I first offer some justification for why I think it is important to have a method and methodology and for them to be coherent and consistent, and I do so, appropriately enough, with reference to TA theory.

The importance and advantages of method and methodology

Writing about games, Berne (1964/1968a) states that 'The general advantages of a game consist in its stabilizing (homeostatic) functions' (p. 56), a view that finds echoes in contemporary ideas about regulation. Here, I consider Berne's six categories of advantages of games (or, from a co-creative perspective, confirmations), together with the addition offered by Bary and Hufford (1997), with regard to the importance and 'advantages' of having a methodology that underlies method and practice—and of knowing it.

1. The *biological advantage*, which, for Berne, is 'stated in tactile terms' (1964/1968a, p. 56)—is, in this context, I suggest, the physical sense of belonging to a community with a shared view of method and methodology, a physicality which is often manifested in the exchange of physical strokes when people meet and greet each other at TA (and other) events by shaking hands, hugging, and kissing. Moreover, the fact that colleagues greet each other with different

degrees and intensity of affection—and animosity—is based in no small part on theoretical and methodological differences.

2. The *existential advantage*, which Berne defined as 'a demonstration of the co-herent structure which underlies all games' (p. 56)—is, in this case, the co-herent structure and consistency of one's thinking, and being and living that thinking.

3. The *internal psychological advantage*, which Berne describes as the 'direct ef-fect on the psychic economy (libido)' (p. 57)—is reflected in feeling good and excited about oneself as a theoretical, philosophical, and thinking being.

4. The *external psychological advantage*, which Berne describes as 'the avoidance of a feared situation' (p. 57)—is represented by the protection that theoretical and philosophical coherence and consistency provides, for instance, when an-swering questions about one's practice, whether in the context of taking exams or making presentations, or from colleagues who work on the basis of other theoretical orientations.

5. The *internal social advantage*, which 'is designated by the name of the game as it is played in the individual's intimate circle' (p. 57)—is represented in how people identify themselves as a transactional analyst, a relational transactional analyst, an eco transactional analyst, etc.

6. The *external social advantage*, which 'is designated by the use made of the situation in outside social contacts' (p. 57)—is reflected in the ways people rep-resent that identity both within and outside the TA community.

7. The *physiological* advantage, the restrictive game version of which Bary and Hufford (1997) describe in terms of body armouring, and the freedom from which as a softening—which is reflected in the idea that theory is and needs to be open and flexible (see Rogers, 1959; Tudor, 2018b), even pliable and cer-tainly adaptable (Berne, 1972/1975b; see also Chapter 12).

Considering that a part of the stated purpose of the written examination for cer-tification as a transactional analyst is that the candidate 'works effectively and ethically as a theoretically based transactional analyst' (ITAA IBoC, 2022, Section 8.1.2), I suggest that the greater the alignment of these biological, existential, psy-chological, and social aspects and advantages, the more the candidate is likely to experience themselves as an integrated transactional analyst.

TA and philosophy

Berne himself was widely read and was interested in ideas and their derivation, and made quite extensive study of anthropology, and cross-cultural psychiatry and psychology. However, in his writing, he tended to reference such ideas in footnotes or at the end of his books, rather than declare or elaborate them 'up front'. Indeed, in his foreword to *A Layman's Guide* he is explicit about this:

> In order to help in preventing misunderstanding on the part of professional read-ers of what I am trying to say, notes are added at the end of each chapter, in

which qualifications and reservations are made, and the more technical aspects of the matters dealt with are discussed.

(Berne, 1971, pp. 19–20).

However, although he named these 'Footnotes for Philosophers', Berne uses the term very loosely and in his *Layman's Guide* refers to only one book on philosophy: *The Philosophy of as If* by Hans Vaihainger, published in 1966. Indeed, in *The Mind in Action*, Berne defines a philosopher as 'anyone who likes to think about what he reads' (p. xvi). Table 2.5 summarises the references to philosophical and/or philosophical traditions in Berne's books.

Berne's preference for working from practice to theory to philosophy (if at all) is most explicit in his discussion of group treatment in which he proposes that the therapist should decide on the goals of such treatment, and have a contract with each patent, following which 'the therapist must then choose the method best adapted to the attainment of each one [goal]' (Berne, 1966a, p. 8). He identifies three kinds of method or techniques: borrowed, opportunistic, and indigenous. Borrowed methods are those derived from training, while opportunistic methods refer to those that the more experienced therapist tries and integrates, at which point Berne suggests that the group therapist may 'relinquish his clinical orientation in favour of a sociological or even metaphysical interest in the group as a whole' (p. 9). Interestingly, for our current discussion, Berne defines indigenous methods as those that make 'specific use of the inherent richness of the group situation' (p. 9); in other words, the methods—of group analysis and of transactional analysis—derive from the essence or ontology of the group. As we are social—and, following Aristotle, political—animals, so we transact, and as we transact, we analyse transactions. Thus, according to Berne's logic—and, I would argue, his philosophy—transactional analysis as a method derives from our indigeneity as *homo sapiens*, or what we might term *homo transagiens*.

In what little Berne did write about philosophy, he focuses predominantly on existentialism, and, indeed, in its discussion of ethical principles, the International Transactional Analysis Association's (ITAA) International Board of Certification's *Certification and Examinations Handbook* refers to 'Our primary existential philosophical perspective' (ITAA IBoC, 2022, Section 3.1.2, p. 2). In a short passage on the ratification of a contract in the context of group treatment, Berne (1966a) refers to rare cases in which the therapist makes a unilateral amendment to a commitment. In a passing comment about this, he writes that the fact that this amendment may have to be unilateral 'is unfortunate both clinically and existentially' (p. 96), which suggests that his commitment to the bilateral nature of the contract was existential. This suggestion is confirmed later in the book (*Principles of Group Treatment*) when he writes about TA and existential analysis:

In so far as actual living in the world is concerned, transactional analysis shares with existential analysis are high esteem for, and a keen interest in, the personal qualities of honesty, integrity, autonomy, and authenticity, and their most poignant social manifestations in encounter and intimacy.

(p. 305)

Table 2.5. Books by Eric Berne and their reference to philosophy and/or philosophical traditions

Book	Reference
The Mind in Action (1947)	In which Berne states that the term 'Philosopher is used to mean anyone who likes to think about what he reads.' (p. xvi) In which Berne cites Zeno the Semite who talks about physis; writes that 'The idea of Physis was not originated by Zeno, but he did much of the thinking about it in connection with the growth and development of living things' (Berne, 1947, p. 68); and acknowledges that his own conception of physis derives from Murray (1915). In which Berne cites Schopenhauer on creative evolution; and Halliday on the general philosophy of etiology.
Transactional Analysis in Psychotherapy: A Systematic Individual and Social Psychiatry (1961/1975a)	In which Chapter 20 comprises 'Theoretical and technical considerations' in which Berne refers briefly to number theory and psychodynamics.
Sex in Human Loving (1970/1973)	None.
The Structure and Dynamics of Organizations and Groups (1963)	In which Appendix 1 comprises 'Suggested reading' which encompasses texts from the Ancient world (India, China, Greece, and Rome), the Middle Ages, the Renaissance, and the 19th and 20th centuries (including Bion, Burrow, Ezriel, Foulkes, and Moreno).
Games People Play: The Psychology of Human Relationships (1964/1968a)	In which Berne refers to the existential advantage of games.
Principles of Group Treatment (1966a)	In which (in Chapter 13) Berne discusses the relationship between TA and existential analysis in some detail, with reference to personality structure, dynamics, games, the script, and the therapeutic problem.
The Happy Valley (1968b)	Not applicable.
A Layman's Guide to Psychiatry and Psychoanalysis (1969/1971)	None.
What Do You Say After You Say Hello? The Psychology of Human Destiny (1972/1975b)	In which, in a brief passage (in Chapter 21), Berne addresses philosophical objections to script theory which he identifies as transcendental and existential.
Intuition and Ego States (Berne, 1977e) (comprising papers originally published by Berne between 1949 and 1962)[9]	Restricts his consideration of the nature of intuition to 'clinical intuition... [to] avoid the dangers run by those who try to scale the walls of philosophy' (p. 4)
A Montreal Childhood (2010)	None (though Berne does refer to the influence of his Jewish upbringing).

Berne illustrates his existential leanings with reference to his favourite game, poker:

> Poker is one of the few really existential situations left in the world. Now here's what I mean by existential: Everybody's on their own. Nobody's going to feel sorry for you. You're fully responsible for everything you do. Once you put the money in the pot, you've put it in the pot. You can't blame anybody else. You have to take the consequences of that. There's no copping out.
>
> (Berne, 1947/1971, p. 8)

From this, it is clear that what Berne meant by existentialism was a very individual-istic kind of existentialism, one that emphasises aloneness, personal responsibility, and self-sufficiency—and which is more associated with American existentialism (and the work of Rollo May, and Irvin Yalom) as distinct from European existen-tialism (and the work of Søren Kierkegaard, and Jean-Paul Sartre).[10]

In her commentary about contracts and contracting, Clarkson (1992) makes the link between Berne's Adult-to-Adult contract and existentialism: 'Working contractually maximises individual responsibility for the outcome of the psycho-therapy and thus combines the existential principle of individual freedom with a behavioural practice of goal setting and feedback' (p. 20). In his analysis of Berne's work as representing 'a profoundly existential–phenomenological attitude in his approach to psychotherapy' (p. 214), Nuttall (2006) suggests that 'transactions con-stitute intersubjectivity, ego states and life positions represent Being-in-the-world, games manifest inauthentic Being or bad faith, and script denotes the existential project and possibilities for-Being-in-the-world' (p. 214). In their excellent chapter, Heiller and Sills (2010) recover the existential perspective on life scripts which was originally in Berne's writing but which 'has been all but lost' (p. 240). They do so by suggesting that 'the children of each generation are asked to struggle with the existential questions that their parents could not accept' (p. 24), and that, while the various script mechanisms represent ways of managing this, 'these important ele-ments of script... [rest] on a subtle but inexorable foundation of existential realities' (p. 240).

Some writers have identified other philosophical influences in TA, including empiricism (Stewart, 1992; Tudor & Hobbes, 2002, 2007; Weinhold, 1977), and some have written specifically about such influences with regard to TA theory and practice, i.e., humanism (Clarkson, 1993), phenomenology (Nuttall, 2006), and constructivism (Allen, 2009; Hine, 1993; Kenny, 1997; Kreyenberg, 2005; Stapleton & Stapleton, 1998; Steinfeld, 1998). In an early article that offered a philosophical analysis of various TA treatment styles based on metaphysical theo-ries of the sources of knowledge and the nature of reality, and putting these together as axes, Weinhold (1977) identifies a number of philosophical traditions as well as their expression in the work of some early transactional analysts (see Table 2.6, into which I have inserted relevant quotations from different authors).

Table 2.6. Metaphysical theories of the sources of knowledge in TA

The nature of 'man'—a posteriori

Nature of reality—subject (inner world)

Experimentalism
Logical empiricism

Claude Steiner and other radical therapists

Writing about the treatment for depression, Steiner describes it as 'to teach the person how to obtain strokes in the outside world [emphasis added] where the rules of stroke economy are usually in force.' (Steiner, 1974, p. 276)

Existentialism
Existential phenomenology

The Schiffs

'Underpinning our interventions is a consciously formulated and experientially supported philosophy. Two major components are that patients know cognitively and/or viscerally what they need to do to get well, and that they can take responsibility for their functioning during treatment if they have a supportive environment while they develop new internal structures and options for behavior.' (Schiff et al. 1975, p. 98)

Logical positivism
Scientific realism

Eric Berne

'The objective of transactional analysis in group therapy is to carry each patient through the progressive stages of structural analysis, transactional analysis proper, game analysis, and script analysis, until he attains social control The attainment of this goal can be validated by observing changes [emphasis added] not only in his own responses, but in resultant, independently observed changes in the behavior of intimates, who have not been exposed to psychotherapy' (Berne, 1961/1975a, p. 165)

Phenomenology
Idealism

Bob and Mary Goulding

As seen in their redecision approach to dream work in which the client plays all the parts of the dream, which, according to the Gouldings, 'enables the dreamer to get into his various ego states very quickly. He experiences his Child, his Adult, his Parent phenomenologically [emphasis added]' (R. Goulding & M. Goulding, 1976, p. 47)

The nature of 'man'—a priori structures

Nature of reality—object (outer world)

Based on Weinhold (1977).

A note on TA and ethics

Earlier in the chapter, I referred to ethics and where this subject might sit in a framework of assumptions about the nature of social science, and, specifically, whether ethics is a part of methodological assumptions or whether it underpins ontology.

In TA, the main codes of ethics—of the ITAA IBoC (2022) and the European Association of Transactional Analysis Professional Training and Standards Committee (2022)—draw on the idea that such codes are based on ethical principles which, in turn, derive from values. The ITAA's 'Ethics and professional practice guidelines' (Section 3 of its *Handbook*) explicitly references the United Nations' *Declaration of Human Rights* (1948) from which it extrapolates the guiding principles of responsibility, protection, respect, commitment, and fidelity in relationship, and empowerment (ITAA IBoC, 2022). While these are well-recognised and widely accepted principles, the issue is how they are understood and actioned and, specifically with regard to TA, whether they are understood and embodied as Parent or Adult. As the ITAA IBoC (2022) puts it:

> Global challenges to preserve human rights to dignity and autonomy require trainers and trainees to employ what Berne was describing when he considered the finer structure of the Adult ego state (1961 [/1975a], p. 195): an inclusive, 'world-wide ethos', defined as moral qualities, rules, values, principles; ethical decision-making that engages in logical reasoning, [and] critical thinking.
>
> (Section 3, p. 4)

Both in TA and the wider therapeutic literature, there has been a turn away from prescriptive 'codes' of ethics with their detailed (and usually increasing number of) proscribed behaviours, in favour of frameworks and guidelines that challenge and require practitioners to think about, reflect on, and resolve complex issues, including multiple relationships, in an increasingly complex and global world. Thus,

> Multiple relationships and boundary crossings should be evaluated in the context of the theoretical and philosophical tenets of transactional analysis, the above ethical principles, and the context of the individual situation through informed, persistent, and comprehensive questioning.
>
> (ITAA IBoC, 2022, Section 3, p. 6)

In 2022, the ITAA identified 'New ethical values of responsivity, diversity awareness, relational ethics of care, and responsibility [which] will fortify the capacity of transactional analysis instructors and students to meet these challenges' (ITAA IBoC, 2022, Section 3, p. 3). Whilst I don't disagree with such sensitivities and extensions to the previous ethical codes and guidelines, I think the real challenge—and one that is consistent with my present concern about methodology—is to engage with both the method, i.e., ethical practice, and the methodology, i.e., the philosophy of values or morals. If we do this in a global context, then we need to engage, for instance, with Eastern philosophy—as Suriyaprakash (2011) does when he describes how his ethics are influenced by the Indian philosophy of dharma and karma, describing them as 'two sides of the same coin and exemplify the power of our choices as human beings to determine our own destiny' (p. 133), which, as he acknowledges, is central to transactional analysis philosophy (see Berne, 1972/1975b). In Aotearoa New Zealand, there is much discussion, at least in some quarters, about indigenous-based knowledge (referred to as mātauranga Māori) and theory (kaupapa Māori), which is based on other principles, such as:

- Tino rangatiratanga—the principle of self-determination (which relates to sovereignty, autonomy, control, self-determination, and independence).
- Ngā taonga tuku iho—the principle of cultural aspiration (which, amongst other things, asserts the centrality and legitimacy of te reo Māori, the Māori language).
- Ako Māori—the principle of culturally preferred pedagogy or ways of learning.
- Kia piki ake i ngā raruraru o te kainga—the principle of socio-economic mediation.
- Whānau—the principle of extended family structure (which acknowledges the relationships that Māori have to one another and to the world around them).
- Kaupapa—the principle of collective philosophy (the collective vision, aspiration, and purpose of Māori communities) (from Smith, 1997).

Since then, others have added:

- Te Tiriti o Waitangi—the principle of the Treaty of Waitangi (which is commonly referred to as the founding document of the New Zealand nation, which defines the relationship between Māori and the Crown in New Zealand).
- Ata—the principle of growing respectful relationships (as developed by Pohatu, 2005/2013, primarily as a transformative approach within the area of social services, and acts as a guide to the understanding of relationships and wellbeing when engaging with Māori).

Such knowledge provides the ontological basis for a virtue ethics, that is an ethics of being as distinct from an ethics of doing (for a discussion of which with regard to Māori ethics, see Perrett & Patterson, 1991) and, therefore, a relational ethics.

The point here is that different principles inform different practice(s); thus, if TA practice in different countries and contexts is to respect new—and, for that matter, old—ethical values, then we need to engage with and across different communities, to understand their values and principles, and to be open to dialogue about them. I suggest that, in this way, we can further develop the ethics of relational TA (see Cornell et al., 2006) to a genuine transactional and relational ethics that reflects TA as a culturally-informed social psychiatry/psychology.

Conclusion

While Berne did write and talk about goals and outcomes and many other transactional analysts have followed him in this, it is important to note that what we might think of as Berne's high- or meta-level definition of a contract essentially points to a *process*, and, therefore, I would argue, to a greater focus on contract*ing*, i.e., the process of negotiating, making, and changing a contract, than on the contract itself, i.e., the stated outcome or goal of therapy.

Furthermore, this chapter has argued the need for transactional analysts to pay more attention to the philosophy and the philosophical assumptions of TA, i.e., the methodology underlying or 'in't' method. Making such assumptions and views open and explicit makes it easier for practitioners to embody a 'philosophical congruence' (Tudor & Worrall, 2006) between TA and their own views and, to paraphrase the purpose of the CTA written exam (as noted above), to work effectively and ethically as a philosophically based transactional analyst.

Notes

1 Although this is a requirement, there is very little written about TA methodology—the phrase appears in only five articles in the *Transactional Analysis Journal* (1971–2023)—in most of which, it is simply named as such, or used synonymously with method.

2 Although this appears in *A Layman's Guide* which was a revised version of Berne's first book *The Mind in Action* (originally published in 1947), in his comments about the treatment contract Berne refers to Steiner and Cassidy's work (which was published in 1969), so this passage must have been part of his later revisions for the *Layman's Guide* (which was first published also in 1969).

3 So, those of us who like and use this quotation to support more of a focus in contracting on process, are skating on thin ice—or rather flimsy paper!

4 I am grateful to Kris Gledhill, Professor of Law at Auckland University of Technology for his input on contract law.

5 There are various versions of this contract, for an analysis of which, see Tudor (2020a).

6 It should be noted that the concept of a soft contract was developed specifically in the context of working with patients who were 'dysfunctional'. There is no reference to the concept in any of the 36 issues of the *Transactional Analysis Bulletin* (1962–1970). In her discussion of soft contracts—not insignificantly, in the context of working with clients with eating disorders, with whom hard contracts can be counter-therapeutic—Solomon (1986) reports that, according to a personal communication from Jack Dusday (in September 1980), Berne 'differentiated between hard contracts and soft contracts (hard contracts are linked to specific, observable behavioral change, while the changes implied in soft contracts are not quantifiable)' (p. 226). In a brief summary of some research he conducted in his own private practice, Dusay himself (in Dusay & Levin, 1971) distinguishes between hard and soft contracts thus: 'the "hard" types represented major life changes, for example: "... graduate from college", "... not get fired for one year". The "soft" varieties included: "... know my different ego-states", "... learn how I come on with people", and so forth. These "soft" contracts did not require definite life commitments or change' (p. 63). Boyd and Cowles-Boyd (1980) put it clearly: 'When a practitioner allows patients to be in therapy without first deliberately and specifically closing escape hatches with that patient, he or she is limiting the course of treatment for the

patient to soft contracts and/or awareness contracts' (p. 227). Similarly, Giusti (2002) distinguishes between soft contracts and contracts for change. I offer this brief review as, in recent years, recently, the term 'soft contract'—unfortunately in my view—seems to be used in a generalised rather than specific way, and, in some instances, to window dress the fact that the work is not subject to a clear, transactional contract.

7 Table 2.7 Comparison of contracts, rules, and working agreements in group therapy (developed from Tudor, 1999a)

Table 2.7. Contracts, rules, and working agreements in transactional analysis.

	Contracts	Rules	Working agreements
Definition	'An explicit bilateral commitment to a well-defined course of action' (Berne, 1966a, p. 362)	A non-negotiable requirement set by the therapist prior to and as a pre-requisite for working with the client/s	'Stated intention of behaviors... to provide short-term protection' (Woollams and Brown, 1978, p. 255)
Initiated by	Therapist or client/s	Therapist	Therapist or client/s
Agreed by	Therapist and client/s	Therapist to client/s	Therapist and client/s
	Client/s and therapist		Client/s and therapist
	Client/s and client/s		Client/s and client/s
Laterality	Bilateral	Unilateral (multilateral acceptance)	Bilateral or multilateral
Ego state	Made in Integrated Adult/ integrating Adult	Made from therapist's Integrated Adult/ integrating Adult	Made from any ego state
Negotiability	Renegotiable	Not negotiable	Negotiable in the session
Timescale	Made at any time	Made at the beginning of counselling	Made at any time Performed between meetings

8 During a workshop I facilitated in Zagreb, Croatia, in June 2018, someone heard the word 'pillows' instead of 'pillars' and, while we clarified the misunderstanding, I rather like the substitution as offering a softer and more flexible and pliable view of theory (on which, see also Rogers, 1959; and Chapter 13).

9 That is, Berne (1949/1977f, 1952/1977b, 1953/1977a, 1955/1977g, 1957a/1977c, 1957b/1977d, 1958/1977i, 1962/1977h).

10 Also, in a critical appraisal of Berne's work, Langguth (1966) questions Berne's 'glorification of poker'.

Chapter 3

Permission, protection, and potency—the three Ps reconsidered (2016)

This chapter offers a historical and critical review of the transactional analysis (TA) concepts of permission, protection, and potency. Taking account of permissions that are given and taken, verbal and nonverbal, direct and indirect, I extend the classification of two to four types or groups of permissions. The three Ps are reconsidered not only as qualities and skills of the transactional analyst but also, and rather, as principles that reflect a two-person, relational psychology and psychotherapy.

Background

In TA, the three Ps (or '3Ps') refer to the concepts of permission and protection as outlined by Crossman (1966) (although Steiner had referred to permission as an element of cure in an article published earlier in 1966) and potency as described by Steiner in 1968. Steiner (personal communication, 20 September 2015) recalled a conversation with Berne early in 1966 about the role of permission in curing alcoholics in which Berne talked about the importance of the permission not to drink. Together, the three Ps describe certain attitudes and attributes of the therapist as well as specific transactions and form part of what Steiner (1968) refers to as the treatment philosophy of transactional analysis.

In 1976, Crossman was awarded the Eric Berne Memorial Scientific Award for her 1966 article, although in 1979 she returned the award on the grounds that the original paper was not scientific. She later clarified that point (Crossman, 2002), writing that, because the article was 'pure speculation [it was] potentially dangerous' (p. 5).[1] Whether scientific or speculative, the three Ps have, nevertheless, been hugely influential in the practice of TA for the last 40 years.

Although the concepts of permission, protection, and potency are generally considered together, there is some debate about the similarities, differences, and overlap among them. Woollams and Brown (1978), for instance, argue that permission differs from protection in that 'it never carries an expectation or obligation' (p. 241). On the other hand, in referring to setting limits, J. Allen (in Allen et al., 1996) suggests that 'in these cases, [permission] may slide over into protection, for example, in permission to think clearly about danger' (p. 197). He concludes that 'permission and protection may not be nearly so distinct as we thought 20 years ago' (p. 197).

DOI: 10.4324/9780429398223-5

That the concepts are different is reflected in some of the debates in the literature as to which concept comes—or should be considered—first. As Brook (1996) observes, 'There is consistency in the transactional analysis literature around the idea that protection needs to be present for permission to take hold. What is not consistent is whether the protection should occur before or after the permission' (p. 163). She goes on to summarise the position of various authors as follows: Crossman (1966) notes that permission implies protection, Steiner (1971a) that protection follows logically from permission, and Erskine (1993) that permission comes only after protection. Brook (1996) herself appears to prioritise potency: 'If the therapeutic relationship is potent, the relationship will provide for protection against intrapsychic punishment' (pp. 162–163). Erskine's (1993) position follows Woollams and Brown's (1978), and both draw on M. James's (1977) work in which she conceptualises both permission and protection as qualities and skills of potent TA therapists. In his summary of the concepts, Berne (1972/1975b) discusses them in the order: permission, potency, and protection. However, when describing his version of the permission transaction, he puts potency before permission and protection. M. James (1977) emphasises their interrelationship as 'particular qualities and skills a TA therapist needs to have' (p. 39). She also writes that 'people with authenticity, integrity, creativity, and training are effective. They are able to be *potent* when faced with treatment challenges. They give people *permission* to get well, and they *protect* them psychologically during the process' (p. 39).

The three Ps appear together in the descriptor for the criterion of 'Relationship' in the oral examination for certification in TA counselling (International Transactional Analysis Association [ITAA] International Board of Certification [IBoC], 2022, Section 12, Form 12.7.9, scale 2) and in one of the score descriptors (for the score of 3) for the oral examination in TA psychotherapy under the criterion 'Establishment and maintenance of an I'm OK—You're OK relationship' (Form 12.7.12, scale 2). Protection and permission (but not potency) form one of the criteria of the Teaching and Supervising Transactional Analyst (TSTA) teaching examination (Form 12.11.8, scale 8).

In terms of what has been written about these concepts in the *Transactional Analysis Journal* (*TAJ*) between 1971 and 2015, there have been 16 articles about permission, of which ten were written in the 1970s and 1980s, three were written in the 1990s, and three in the 2000s; six articles on protection were written in the 1970s and two in the 1980s; and only three articles on potency, all of which were written in the 1970s. There are references to the concepts in the wider TA literature, although, again, fewer in more recent publications. The paucity of articles about protection is particularly surprising given its presence in both *Teaching and Examinations Handbooks* (European Association for Transactional Analysis [EATA], 2022; ITAA IBoC, 2022):

- Regarding the protection of clients in the psychotherapy written examination (ITAA IBoC, 2022, Section 8.5.1.3).
- Regarding the protection of candidates:

- In the Certified Transactional Analyst (CTA) written examination (Section 8.1.6).
- In the CTA oral examinations (Sections 9.3.3.3 and 9.5).
- Regarding the protection of candidates in the Training Endorsement Workshop—in the EATA (2022) *Handbook* (Section 10.9), but not in the ITAA IBoC's (2022) *Handbook*.
- As a criterion of the TSTA supervision examination—again, in the EATA *Handbook* (Section 13, Form 12.12.8, scale 5: 'Protection Issues [regarding both Supervisee and Supervisee's client']), but not in the ITAA IBoC's *Handbook*, and, therefore, exam.

Most of what has been written about the three Ps has been from a one-person or one-and-a-half-person psychology (Stark, 1999), that is, they are viewed as something in or about the client (i.e., something absent or needed) or they are used as a therapeutic intervention by the therapist (i.e., something corrective or reparative). Given the relational turn in TA in recent years (see Cornell & Hargaden, 2005) and the increased interest in working relationally, it is timely to reconsider these concepts as both transactional and relational.

Permission

Crossman (1966) identifies permission as

> a particular transaction that occurs between therapist and patient at a particular point in therapy, whereby the therapist effects a change in the direction of the patient's behavior or attitude which before that time would have seemed either impossible or untenable.
>
> (p. 152)

The patient or client needs permission to change or give up their script. Crossman argues that the therapist can give the necessary permission but only after he or she has understood something about the client's script. Otherwise, the client may seduce the therapist into playing into that script. This issue and potential for a game is discussed by Ingram (1980), although his contention that the client can programme the therapist into giving permission lays all the responsibility for this transaction on the client.

With regard to permission, Crossman (1966) makes three points about the therapist:

- They must hook the patient's 'young Professor' (p. 152) by supplying more data, a point that connected to Berne's (1966a) therapeutic operations of specification and confirmation.
- They must be stronger than the patient's original (internalised) Parent.

- They are 'giving permission to the patient's Child to disobey the instructions of his Parent' (p. 153), a point that provides a link between Steiner's (1981) ideas about the importance of disobedience and the concept of permission.

Crossman's reference to parenting has been echoed in the subsequent literature. Woollams (1977) refers to giving a permission as 'like giving a small dose of parenting' (p. 364). Bolten and de Jong (1984) reflect on the fact that the permission to regress was essential to the regressive therapy of Schiffian reparenting. Drego (1994a) describes permission as 'an act of empowerment and nurturing which is at the core of parenting' (p. 4). J. Allen (in Allen et al., 1996) writes in terms of parents providing an environment that gives permission to children.

In his summary of permission, Steiner (1968) defines it as 'a transaction in which the Parent of the therapist directs the patient to perform a certain behavior' (p. 59). Later, in *Games Alcoholics Play*, he describes permission as 'a transaction in which the therapist attempts to align the patient with his original script-free, natural Child ego state' (Steiner, 1971a, p. 175), and describes and diagrammed the permission transaction as

> a combination of a Parent-to-Child command, as described above—'Stop drinking'—and a rational, logical explanation, Adult-to-Adult, in which the rational or logical reason for the command is explained ('You will not regain your job unless you stop drinking', etc.).
>
> (p. 175)

In these two contributions, Steiner (1968, 1971a) makes a number of points about permission and the permission transaction:

- 'This transaction occurs in treatment at a moment when the patient has arrived at an impasse beyond which he cannot or will not move' (1968, pp. 62–63).
- 'The situation is seen as one in which a patient and a therapist who have previously agreed to work on a certain condition of the therapist are confronted' (p. 63). Thus, permission is—or should be—clearly linked to the treatment contract.
- Permission requires the involvement of the patient's Adult because otherwise 'permission simply becomes a Command that can be resisted by the patient' (1971a, p. 175).
- 'The Parent giving Permission should be the grownup Parent (P_2)', which argues that it is only this ego state that has 'the potency required to countermand parental injunctions' (p. 177).
- The timing of permissions is important, that is, they should be given 'only when both the therapist and patient feel that Protection is possible' (p. 178).

Also in 1971, M. James wrote about potency permissions (in contrast to original impotency scripting). Then in *Born to Win,* she and Jongeward (1971) wrote about destructive permissions (e.g., 'Go play on the freeway'), which act as and support injunctions, and giving permission (instead of an authoritarian restriction) to foil a game.

In his own summary of permission, Berne (1972/1975b) defines it as 'a license to give up behaviour which the Adult wants to give up, or a release from negative behaviour' (p. 375). He develops the metaphor of the license when he writes that 'true permissions are merely permits, like a fishing license' (p. 123). Just as a license does not compel one to fish, a permission does not compel one to challenge the injunction or resolve the impasse. Berne also adds three ideas to the concept of permission. Firstly, there are negative permissions: whereas the positive permission cuts off the injunction, the negative permission (e.g., 'Stop pushing him into it') cuts off the provocation. Secondly, permission is, or can be, the cure (e.g., 'The cure for the scriptless aged is permission'). Thirdly, in a section on the dynamics of permission, he suggested a more complex permission diagram.

Also in 1972, Allen and Allen published an article on the role of permission in which they linked it to other factors such as the child's existential position, limited life experience, and level of cognitive development. From infant and child observation and their clinical experience, Allen and Allen hypothesised a series of permissions: to exist, to experience one's own sensations, to be one's self as an individual of appropriate age and sex, to be emotionally close to others, to be aware of one's own basic existential position and to change that position, to succeed in sex and work, and to find life meaningful. These are consistent with Erikson's (1950) assumptions about human psychosocial development. Revisiting the subject nearly 25 years later, Allen and Allen (in Allen et al., 1996) emphasise a number of points, including that there are two groups of permissions, nonverbal and verbal; that they would put more emphasis (than originally) on conditional permissions (i.e., a permission 'provided that...'); that the verbal permission 'not to...' involves setting limits; that nonverbal permissions may be conceptualised as the converse of the injunctions as delineated by R. L. Goulding and M. M. Goulding (1978); and that the original permissions have several different meanings, that is, they are 'cognitively and linguistically ambiguous and slippery' (p. 198).

M. James (1977) acknowledges that permissions may be given indirectly (e.g., 'Winners learn to think for themselves') and emphasised that 'permission can be given from any ego state' (p. 41). In their book *Transactional Analysis,* Woollams and Brown (1978) suggest that 'a permission transaction occurs when the therapist states directly or indirectly to a client who is ready to receive it that "It's OK to..."' (pp. 240–241). They also make a number of points:

- 'Permissions may be given from any ego state', 'permissions delivered from the Child usually have the greatest impact', and 'the most effective permissions are simultaneously communicated from all three ego states' (p. 202). However, in an earlier chapter, Woollams (1977) makes the point that no matter which of the three ego states the therapist sends the permission from, it will be received, if effective, as though from a parent and so will be recorded in the client's Parent while being reacted to in her Child.

(p. 364)

- It is important for the therapist to follow the contract and give only those per-missions that fit with the contract; Woollams adds that 'extraneous permissions are distracting and may be provocative' (p. 202).
- 'Permission is actually something which is taken by the client rather than given by the therapist' (p. 241); this perspective is reflected in the work of a number of authors.
- Consequently, 'it is essential that the client's Free Child and/or Adult ego state be available to take Permission and make the redecision' (p. 241).

The concept of permission has been applied widely in TA practice, particularly with regard to the treatment of sexual problems (e.g., M. James, 1971; Janssens, 1984; Parkin, 2002) as well as to groups (e.g., Steiner, 1974; Woollams & Brown, 1978), parenting through family rituals (Drego, 1994a), and work with young peo-ple (Drego, 1994b). More recently, Hawkes (2007) describes a permission wheel diagram developed by Gysa Jaoui (1988) that offers a useful way of representing the main limits of a person's life script.

Four groups of permissions

Despite the fact that Woollams and Brown (1978) write about permission as some-thing that is taken by the client rather than given by the therapist, both they and the majority of authors writing about this concept in TA practice describe giving permissions, although some authors argue for both perspectives. J. Allen (in Allen et al., 1996) acknowledges that 'if a patient believes the therapist is the solution to their predicament, it can lead to a rapid freeing of Child inhibitions. Ultimately, however, such permission is usually something the patient must give himself or her-self' (p. 196). This difference can be conceptualised as being between transference cure and script cure. Discussing therapeutic work with individuals who make little connection between their somatic complaints and internal psychological states, and helping them to develop skills such as self-regulation, Allen et al. (2004) suggest that 'this can be conceptualized as helping them give themselves the permission they need to be aware of their own experiences' (p. 6). Two subsets of these permissions, as identified by M. James (1977), are those that are direct and those that are indirect.

Another distinction in the literature is between nonverbal and verbal permis-sions, which J. Allen (in Allen et al., 1996), in effect, correlates with permissions that are taken and given, respectively. I think these distinctions are useful because taking permission suggests the more active involvement of the client. Furthermore, in the case of nonverbal permissions, it is important to recognise the significance of the environment of the therapeutic or facilitative relationship and/or group: 'The healing aspects of relationship—for example, potency, permission, protection, support, and challenge—are co-created and co-maintained by active contributions from both therapist and client' (Tudor & Summers, 2014, p. 4). This is very different from the therapist's permission transaction, as Steiner (in Allen et al., 1996) notes: It is important 'to distinguish permission, a specific therapeutic transaction, from permissiveness. A permissive attitude or environment is quite different from a permission transaction' (p. 203). Commenting on the relationship between the two, Hawkes (2007) is explicit: 'Although we have the permission transaction... most of this work is done through the therapeutic relationship' (p. 215). The shift here is from viewing permission as a transaction generated by the therapist to appreciating that permission and permissiveness (as in freedom or liberation) are aspects of the therapeutic relationship and environment, an appreciation that represents the different methodological or philosophical stance of the two-person approach to psychology. We also know, from communication studies, that as much as 90% of communication between people is nonverbal (see Fromkin & Rodman, 1983).

From my research and reading of the literature, there is, I suggest, another category: clients giving themselves verbal permission. This distinction produces four forms or groups of permissions: verbal (direct), verbal (indirect), verbal (given to self), and nonverbal (taken). The underlying differences between these forms, and especially between giving permission and taking or deriving permission, are more than technical. They are philosophical because, in effect, they reflect different views of responsibility, that is, they place different emphasis on the therapist's role and the client's responsibility, respectively.

Critiques of permission

Firstly, one of the problems with the concept of permission is that it derives from a parental relationship and metaphor, neither of which necessarily translates well into therapy or other applications (for a critique of this, see Lomas, 1987/2001). If practitioners wish to use either the relationship or the metaphor (or both), it seems to me that, in the spirit of the contractual method and open communication, the method—and methodology—should be made explicit (see Chapter 2). Similarly, one of the problems of the permission transaction, at least from an integrative and/ or integrating perspective, is that it assumes a Parental position, and, as M. James (1977) acknowledges, clients may interpret direct permissions ('You can...') as paternalistic. Moreover, it is no accident that the early definitions of permission and diagrams of the permission transaction were based on the theory of a three ego state model of health, that is, that both a healthy personality and the goal of therapy were based on all three ego states (for clarification, see Tudor, 2010c [Chapter 6]). Interestingly, an aspect of Steiner's (1971a) definition is that 'the Parent of the therapist directs the patient to perform certain behavior, *which the patient's Adult already recognizes as necessary*' [emphasis added] (p. 191). The issue with this is that if the patient's Adult already recognises or knows something, the therapist directing him or her to this same end is at best repetitive (and, therefore, inefficient) and at worst patronising. The integrating approach focuses on expanding the Adult or neopsyche rather than 'growing' the Child or Parent.

Secondly, a number of authors who have written about permission (and other subjects) have used the word modelling to describe how the therapist (or teacher or consultant) is in a relationship. In her article on permissions, on the basis of acknowledging the importance of role models in human development, Ford (1987) specifically promotes the idea that therapists should take the opportunity to act as role models. The problem with this (and many other references to modelling in the psychological literature) is that it (and they) do not acknowledge that, as a concept, modelling has its origins in behaviourism, specifically, operant conditioning (Bandura, 1969). As such, it is a deliberate modelling on the part of the person doing it (parent, teacher, educator) of a specific behaviour that the person wishes the observer to introject (see Wood, 1995). Drawing on Wood's criticism of modelling as antithetical to the person-centred approach—and, I would argue, many forms and applications of humanistic psychology—I distinguish between *modelling* a behaviour so that the observer introjects it (i.e., Parental behavioural modelling designed to elicit a Child response) and *demonstrating* something with which a person can engage, to which they can relate critically, and that, if they find it useful, they may integrate (i.e., Adult behaviour that encourages an Adult response).

Thirdly, in his article 'Beyond Permission', Holloway (1974) argues that '"cure" by Permission is a limited achievement' (p. 15). He distinguishes—usefully, in my view—between social control contracts, which 'completed through the Permission transaction may result in the patient no longer following an injunction' (p. 16), and autonomy contracts whereby the patient or client achieves individuation, which, among other capacities, 'implies that the person is capable of the full use of options in attaining strokes from multitudinous others' (p. 15). Woollams (1977) argues that the client's autonomy is not reduced if permission giving is used within the framework of a contract. Holloway also raises the issue that giving permissions may contribute to a sense of omnipotence in the therapist, which Holloway viewed as antitherapeutic and limiting of change in the client. Woollams acknowledges this danger but viewed the solution as the therapist ensuring that they have their needs met outside the therapy situation. Although some transactional analysts view permission as reflecting a stage of cure (i.e., transference cure), the danger is that it may create dependency on the therapist. Pirnie (1976) represents this when she reports and reflects on a five-day TA workshop in which all the permissions she received had been given in a safe and supportive environment and the euphoria of the workshop: 'With this realization and subsequent Adult acceptance of the responsibility for what was to follow from the week's experience, I knew that I had to develop a specific plan to serve as my guide for continued growth' (p. 88).

Reconsidering permission

In her book *Modes of Therapeutic Action*, Stark (1999) distinguishes between three different, although mutually enhancing modes: one-person psychology, in which the therapist is an 'objective observer of the patient' (p. xvi); one-and-a-half-person psychology, which is characterised by the therapist offering the client what

Alexander and French (1946) refer to as a 'corrective emotional experience'; and two-person psychology, in which, because therapy is conceptualised as 'interactive engagement with an authentic other' (p. xix), the therapist focuses more on working in and with the relationship (see Chapter 2). Using Stark's taxonomy, it is clear that most of the TA literature on permission and, specifically, the direct and indirect verbal permissions, reflects a one-and-a-half-person psychology whereby the transactional analyst gives permission(s) to the client in order that the client 'corrects' or repairs a previous and/or early experience. Clients themselves taking permission from the therapist or the therapy could reflect any of the three modes of therapeutic action. For example, near the end of four years of psychoanalytic psychotherapy, my therapist, who had operated primarily in a one-person mode, asked me what, in particular, I was taking away from our work together. After some consideration, I replied, 'What you said to me about acceptance'. My therapist responded, 'That's interesting, because I never said that—you did!' The shift from the giving and receiving of permission(s)—or, in my case, the perceived receiving of a permission—to what I had taken from a permissive and, indeed, liberating therapeutic relationship and environment is, I suggest, more reflective of a two-person psychology approach to permission. It is also a shift from conceptualising permission as a skill (intervention or operation) to being a principle or value that informs therapy.

Protection

In her original article, Crossman (1966) identifies protection as part of the mother's (or a mother substitute's) nurturing role and function, in response to which the child develops 'its growing Adult to explore and find out [about] the world around it with the certainty that it is right and safe to do so' (p. 152). When Crossman introduced the idea of permission, she considered that protection was necessary for behaviour change: it needs 'to be alright to disobey mother, or father, [and] that the Child will not be deserted, die, or be punished for disobedience' (p. 153).

Arguing that protection follows logically from permission, Steiner (1968) writes: 'A patient, having taken a therapist's permission to disobey his parents' injunction, finds himself in a state of panic and [an] existential vacuum and needs temporary protection from the therapist' (p. 63). Commenting on the concept three years later, he acknowledges that 'because the patient has to rely on the therapist's Protection, the timing of Permissions is important' (Steiner, 1971a, p. 178), providing examples of giving protection over the phone. In later work, Steiner (1974) clarifies that protection is temporary: 'Ordinarily, a person does not require Protection for more than three months following abandonment of a script injunction' (p. 263). He adds that, if the client's need for the therapist has not subsided by this time, 'the therapist is probably playing a Rescue game' (p. 263). Steiner also asserted that 'protection is the function of the Nurturing Parent' (p. 263).

Writing about protection, Berne (1972/1975b) clearly links it to potency: The therapist should feel potent enough to deal with the patient's Parent and 'the patient's Child must believe he [the therapist] is potent enough, to offer protection from the Parental wrath' (p. 374). Berne also wrote that the therapist's protective power 'resides as much in the timbre of his voice as in what he says' (p. 375) and diagrammed it as a Parent–Child transaction in the context of the overall permission transaction.

Compared with the concept of permission, protection has been used less often in TA, although there are examples of it being applied in a social context (Haimowitz, 1975); to family therapy (J. James, 1977), parenting (Vago & Knapp, 1977), and eating disorders (Karpman & Callaghan, 1985); and in script prevention work with children (Campos, 1988).

Critiques of protection

As with permission, the concept of protection as presented in the majority of the TA literature assumes a Parental position and a three ego state model of personality and health. In the case of Vago and Knapp's (1978) article, it also assumes a particular model of ego state development, which is that the Parent (P_2) ego state does not fully develop until 18 years of age or even later. (For a summary of the different models of ego state development, see Tudor, 2010c [Chapter 6].)

The argument for protection appears to be based on the view that the transactional analyst can— and should—make it safe for clients to make the changes they need, both intrapsychically (e.g., with regard to their internal Critical Parent and script backlash) and interpersonally (e.g., with regard to other members of a group). An alternative view is that it is more useful and therapeutic to explore the client's fantasies—and phantasies—about safety and to help them work through their anxieties about going against their scripting, being disobedient, and being unsafe. In the context of groups, the desire for safety is often expressed in terms of a concern about confidentiality. For example, six weeks into one psychotherapy group I facilitated, and by way of an introduction to what he was going to say, one group member leaned forward and said, somewhat conspiratorially, 'Now this is really confidential'. After he had finished and other members of the group had commented on both the content and his process, another group member looked at me somewhat accusingly and said, 'We haven't discussed confidentiality'. I acknowledged that we had not, and the whole group then engaged in a lively debate about the basic assumptions of the group, including what had been said and shared up to that point. They also discussed the responsibilities of the leader and the participants, the nature and purpose of confidentiality, and what was meant by 'really confidential'. In deciding not to introduce confidentiality as a ground rule during the first group meeting, I was influenced by the bilateral nature of contracts, co-constructivism, emergent learning, and, specifically, Shohet's (2007) advocacy of goodwill as underlying any agreement to observe confidentiality—and hence the more fundamental concept of goodwill contracts.

Another critique of protection as conceptualised in TA is that it is, in fact, over-protection. In a rare critique of this concept from within TA, Schiff and Schiff

(1971) argue that overprotection is an example of a disturbance in the normal or healthy symbiotic relationship between mother and child and, specifically, a disturbance in the differentiation of the child from the mother. Also, English (1972) views overprotectiveness as an example of racket or inauthentic behaviour and feelings, often expressed as excessive helpfulness, sweetness, and devotion. To these, Douglas and Tudor (2007) add the overprotectiveness of rigid and often legalistic health-and-safety responses to the complexities of life, representative of the 'Nanny state'. In some jurisdictions, the protection of the public has been used as an argument for the state registration of psychotherapists, despite the fact that there is no research evidence that supports this. The fact that proponents of such registration, and the statutory regulation that often goes with it, still pursue this reflects a psychology and politics of overregulation and protectionism (see Smith, 2011; Tudor, 2011e; and Chapter 10). In this sense, and like permission, protection may also be patronising and infantilising, and, at worst, an example of the phoney insurance policy that gave rise to the original concept of the protection racket (Berne, 1964/1968a).

Reconsidering protection

If protection transactions are a Parent ego state response and/or initiative from the therapist and temporary or pseudo protectiveness is a Child ego state defence, then any reconsideration of protection needs to promote an Adult sense of the concept. Etymologically, the English word protect comes from the Latin word *protegere*, which means to protect or to cover in front. Associating to this, I have the image of a client seated in a chair with their back supported but needing protection or cover as they face, front, and encounter the world with, in this case, me as their therapist. Here I find Schmid's (1999) reflections on encounter useful in highlighting that the concept contains a sense of being against (counter from the Latin contra) as well as being face-to-face. Thus protection, or the lack of it, becomes a relational dynamic and issue. For example, following a brief break from work, a trusted colleague told me that, in response to an incident while I was away, another colleague had been criticising me behind my back. On my return, I took this up with the colleague in question, who assured me that she had not done so. I told her what I had heard and said that if she wanted (as it were) to stab me, I would prefer to see it coming, that is, to be stabbed from the front! She agreed to this, following which we enjoyed a better working relationship. A two-person psychological perspective on protection is one in which protection, trust, and mistrust are confronted face-to-face in genuine encounter.

In Aotearoa New Zealand, protection is generally accepted as one of the principles of the Treaty of Waitangi, a treaty signed by Māori Rangatira (chiefs) and representatives of the British Crown in 1840 (see Royal Commission on Social Policy, 1988; Waitangi Tribunal, 2015). Under this principle, the Crown (i.e., the New Zealand government) has a duty to protect Māori interests, resources, and treasures, including intangible cultural assets such as mountains, rivers, and the foreshore.[2] This is a rare example of protection as a principle being applied in the social/political world. It is also a principle that is being used to inform ethical practice (see New Zealand Association of Counsellors, 2020) and therapeutic practice, for instance, in ecotherapy.

Potency

Steiner (1968) describes potency in the context of permission and protection: 'Potency is expressed in permission by the emphasis with which permission is given, and is exemplified in protection by the willingness of the therapist temporarily to carry the burden of the patient's panic when in an existential vacuum' (p. 63). He asserts that 'it is an attribute which transactional analysts seek in their work' (p. 63) and involves a commitment to curing patients, with valid consideration (one of Steiner and Cassidy's (1969) four criteria for contracts [see Chapter 2]), and a willingness to confront the patient at the impasse. In *Games Alcoholics Play*, Steiner (1971a) summarises therapeutic potency as 'the therapist's capacity to bring about a speedy cure' (p. 181), asserting that 'the Potency of the therapist has to be commensurate with the potency of the injunction laid down by the parents of the patient' (p. 181). This point is echoed by Berne (1972/1975b) and by Woollams et al. (1977). Berne also writes succinctly that 'potency means power to confront' (p. 375) and diagrams it as an Adult—Adult transaction.

M. James (1977) defines potency as a quality and skill entailing 'a personal sense of authenticity, credibility, trustworthiness, and responsiveness' (p. 39). It is demonstrated by a certain knowledge and understanding and a commitment to a continuing learning process, self-awareness, and self-care, in part through self-analysis and an ability to change. Potent therapists, James argues, 'know that an informed, experienced Adult will be more potent than an uninformed, inexperienced one' (p. 39).

English (1978) discusses potency specifically with regard to female therapists and, in a poignant and poetic passage, argues that

> a potent female therapist is in a particularly good position to validate a client's heroic trip through life, as does an enthusiastic mother who cheers her child onwards at each stage of development. Women can do much more than nurture. When they give birth, they catapult their infants from out of the dark enclosures of their wombs into the excitement of life.
>
> (p. 299)

Finally, and most recently, Erskine and Trautmann (1993/1997) define potency as 'the result of engagement that communicates to the client that the therapist is fully invested in his or her welfare' (p. 92). This reframes it as a product and a quality of the relationship (see also Tudor & Summers, 2014).

Compared with the concepts of permission and protection, potency is applied less in TA practice, and in an electronic search of the *TAJ* and a hand search of some

30 books on TA analysis, I could find only one article on the application of the concept. It is an article on groups in which, in discussing group boundaries, Gurowitz (1975) puts forward the view that the strength of the external boundary is largely a function of the group leader's potency.

Critiques of potency

More so than permission and protection, potency is an attribute of the therapist. Whereas the transactional analyst may give, offer, or even co-create permission and protection, they are, or are not, potent. With regard to the other two Ps, the equivalent is that the transactional analyst is permissive and/or protective. This clarification acknowledges that potency is about the self of the therapist rather than the relationship, a point reflected in the quotation from Tudor and Summers (2014) cited earlier. In this sense, potency reflects a one-and-a-half-person psychology that offers the client a corrective or reparative emotional experience of power, but, in this mode, it is still power to, or power over, rather than power with. Whereas some therapists may take too much power and even abuse it, others may too readily give it away. Reflecting on Berne's use of permission classes, Cornell (2013) comments on the therapist's loss of potency in referring clients on, concluding that 'the therapist's or counselor's potency is better served by the capacity to reflect on his or her own anxiety and uncertainty in making an intervention rather than referring out to a specialist' (p. 8).

Another critique of potency is that it represents a masculine and, at least implicitly, phallocentric language of experience. As if anticipating this gender critique of potency, both Berne (1972/1975b) and Steiner (1974) make the point that it can be manifested equally by women and men, and Steiner specifically notes that 'potency is often, but mistakenly, mixed up with machismo' (p. 318).

Reconsidering potency

Of the three Ps, potency is the least discussed in the literature, a lacuna that reflects a wider absence of discussion about power (for exceptions to which, see Friedlander, 1987; Guggenbühl-Craig, 1971/1996; Proctor, 2002).

A two-person psychology approach to potency understands it in terms of the therapeutic relationship or relating. In the context of a discussion of some of the differences between integrative and co-creative TA, Tudor and Summers (2014) argue that

> whilst both approaches view empathy as the principal method, the integrative approach tends to rely on the potency of the therapist and the therapist's empathy, whereas in the co-creative model, the therapist's empathic resonance and responsiveness is a stimulus for both client and therapist to engage in a search for further understanding of the client's experiencing process and internal frame of reference. Whilst the power is still in the patient (see [R. L.] Goulding &

[M. M.] Goulding, 1978), from a co-creative perspective, it is more accurate to say that the power or potency of the therapeutic encounter lies in the co-created relational field.

(p. 135)

Again, this represents a shift from potency as a skill or intervention to a principle of a relationship, the ultimate purpose of which is to help the client be the potent person they are and aspire to be.

Conclusion

As well as describing specific transactions, permission, protection, and potency have been viewed in TA as naming certain desirable, even necessary, attitudes and attributes of the therapist. As such, the original conceptualisations of the three Ps reflect a one-and-a-half-person psychology and, within that, the primary use and provision of a corrective or reparative emotional experience and/or a developmentally needed relationship. This chapter suggests that by shifting our perspective from one that is therapist-centred to one that is relationship-centred, these concepts may be reconsidered as principles of therapeutic—and other—relationships that reflect a two-person psychology emphasising engagement in relationship and one that is appropriately permissive, protective, and potent.

Notes

1 This perspective, of course, represents only one view of science and research; for other views about research in psychotherapy, see Leuzinger-Bohleber and Fischmann (2006), Bager-Charleson & McBeath (2020, 2022), and Tudor and Wyatt (2023).
2 Whilst this analysis has its merits, there is more interest in honouring Te Tiriti o Waitangi 1840 and its original Articles (which are concerned with co-governance, Māori sovereignty, equitable outcomes, and spiritual/religious freedom), which is the version of the Treaty of Waitangi that was written in te reo Māori (the Māori language) and signed by rangatira (Māori chiefs). This is line with the principle in international law of contra proferentem (against the drafter), which privileges the Indigenous version of such treaties. For an application of these Articles to TA, see Tudor (2021d).

Part II

New wine from old roots

I have been writing about different aspects of transactional analysis (TA) since 1990 when my first article on TA, on using different ideas about personality to understand organisations, was published in the *ITA News*, the magazine of the UK Institute of Transactional Analysis (Tudor, 1990). Thinking about my contributions since then in terms of what are generally viewed as the four fundamental pillars of TA, that is, ego states, transactions, (life) scripts, and (psychological) games, I realised that I had written about each of these four areas. In the light of this, I decided to reproduce one contribution that addressed something of each of these areas, and to take the opportunity to pair this with four new chapters on the same area of TA theory. Inevitably, this has led to new chapters (the new wine) that draw on, reflect back on, and develop the previously published work and, indeed, critique the original theory (the old roots), and hence the title of the part, which is inspired by and taken from the theme of the conference of the same name, which was held in 1995 in San Francisco.[1]

Chapter 4 "'I'm OK, you're OK—and they're OK": therapeutic relationships in transactional analysis' was originally published in 1999 as a chapter in the book, *Understanding the Therapeutic Relationship* (Sage, 1999), edited by Colin Feltham © Sage Publications, and is reproduced with permission. Colin, who I knew when I lived in Sheffield, in the UK, invited me to contribute this chapter and, in doing so, I took the opportunity to explore the therapeutic relationship in TA highlighting their different ideas about transference. I considered TA with regard to three Schools in TA, which had been the main way of understanding different theories within TA, certainly during my training (1987–1994). For a more comprehensive and contemporary view, see Chapter 12. As I had also experienced and witnessed dual relationships in—and outside—TA, I also took the opportunity to include a section on this. Although, in many ways, I consider the chapter somewhat dated, I also think it's accurate in its analysis, and makes some points that are still pertinent. Finally, it also marks my early thinking about therapeutic relating, which I develop in the next chapter.

The following chapter, Chapter 5, takes forward and makes more explicit some of the themes that emerged (at least for me) from the 'I'm OK, you're OK...' chapter, notably, the shift in thinking about *the* therapeutic relationship to therapeutic

DOI: 10.4324/9780429398223-6

relating. Chapter 5 also marks my decreasing interest in transference and countertransference and my increasing interest in working therapeutically in and with the present, including with the past in the present. The second part of the chapter focuses the theme of context by means of a meta-analysis of therapeutic relating, based on Stark's (1999) taxonomy of modes of therapeutic action.

Chapter 6 reproduces an article 'The state of the ego: then and now', which was originally published in the *Transactional Analysis Journal* (*TAJ*) *40*(3&4), July and October issue, pp. 261–277, © International Transactional Analysis Association (ITAA), and is also reprinted with permission. This article was inspired by a disagreement I had with Claude Steiner, a TA elder and a friend of mine, about the nature of ego states and, specifically, how Eric Berne, Claude's mentor and friend, had defined ego states. I enjoyed doing the research that forms the basis of this chapter, and consider that the summary of ego state theory and the analysis I made of it is still relevant—and, therefore, hope that it is useful to students/trainees and trainers alike. Claude himself was complimentary and, having read it, said: 'Now I get what you integrationists are on about'.

The title of the next chapter, 'We've had 66 years of ego states and the world's getting worse', is inspired by James Hillman and Michael Ventura's (1992) book *We've had a Hundred Years of Psychotherapy and the World's Getting Worse*. In it, I take the opportunity to take another meta-perspective on ego state theory, this time, looking back at its origins in American ego psychology, and looking out to ideas about self, environment, integration, past and present, and state and process.

Chapter 8 reproduces an early piece of writing about script theory, 'Shame, shaming and "shame": a transactional analysis', which was originally published in 1995 in the *ITA News*, the magazine of the UK's Institute of Transactional Analysis and is reproduced with permission. It is the oldest paper in the book, which at 28, represents a generation. Although, I would explain shame in different terms now, the chapter does offer a TA analysis of shame, using TA proper, script and impasse theory, and, as such, demonstrates a way of addressing using TA theory. Published just one year after I qualified as a certified transactional analyst, it represents the graduation from apprentice to (early) master—and previews my interest in research and language.

This is followed by a new chapter on script. In the first part of Chapter 9, inspired by my work with Graeme Summers in developing co-creative TA (Summers & Tudor, 2000; Tudor & Summers, 2014), and parallel to my work on ego states in Chapter 6, I clarify the two sets of views in TA on script theory. In the second part of the chapter, in a kind of meta case study, I then apply this to the concept of growth; and, in the third part of the chapter, identify some challenges of growth and to the concept of growth, doing so by means of four reflexions, framed in terms of scripts, as well as ego states, transactions, and games.

Game theory is the area of TA about which I have written the least. In part, this is because *Games People Play* (Berne, 1964/1968a) is my least favourite of Berne's books (about which I say more in Chapter 11). Firstly, Chapter 10 reproduces an article 'Recognition, regulation and registration: protection or protectionism? A plea for pluralism', which was originally published in 2010 in *The TAttler*, the magazine of the New Zealand Association of Transactional Analysis.[2] I have long been a proponent of professional regulation, and a critic of the statutory regulation of psychotherapy and the state registration of psychotherapists. This included leading a discussion of this in a group of TA trainers as long ago as 1999 (see Tudor, 2011e, 2011f, 2017/2020f). In Aotearoa New Zealand, the New Zealand Association of Psychotherapists had, for a long time, lobbied the government for such registration (Bayley & Tudor, 2017/2022; Dillon, 2017/2020; Sherrard, 2017/2020), which was approved in 2009 (the year I emigrated/immigrated here). I decided to reproduce the article from *The TAttler* as a chapter in this section of this book as part of my analysis in this article, is that seeking such regulation and registration, against the evidence of research is—or, at least in the New Zealand context, was— an organisational, psychological game. This was not necessarily a popular analysis; nevertheless, and in the interests and the TA principle of open communication, was one which, in my view, needed—and still needs—to be made explicit and debated. In doing so, I was grateful for the support of the late Evan Sherrard, TSTA, a colleague and friend (and an initial supporter of statutory regulation).

This is followed by the final paired chapter in this part of the book. Again, inspired by my work with Graeme Summers on co-creative TA, and my clarification of different meta-views of ego states (Chapter 6) and scripts (Chapter 9), and on the basis of re-reading *Games People Play*, in Chapter 11, I examine game theory. Specifically, I consider its context; the implications of its various and varying definitions; and, in the last third part of the chapter, and, as something of an antidote to games, I turn my attention to play.

Notes

1 Another ITAA conference, also sponsored by the Latin America Transactional Analysis Association (ALAT), and the Asociación Psicológica de Desarrollo Humano, which was held in 2009, chose the theme of 'New Life from Old Roots' which, while acknowledging the title of the earlier San Francisco conference, also referred to the birth of a community of transactional analysts from ALAT.
2 Now the Transactional Analysis Association of Aotearoa New Zealand.

Chapter 4

'I'm OK, you're OK—and they're OK'

Therapeutic relationships in transactional analysis (1999)

Understanding the nature of the therapeutic relationship, from whatever theoretical orientation, is a crucial endeavour for therapists as in most therapeutic contexts it is the experience of the relationship which is considered to be therapeutic or healing—'terapia' meaning healing. In considering the therapeutic relationship from the perspective of transactional analysis (TA), this chapter firstly and principally reviews the concept of relationship, referring to different traditions within TA, i.e., the three 'Schools' of TA, each of which are briefly introduced; secondly, explores the issue of dual relationships and TA's contribution to this controversial area of the therapeutic field; and, thirdly, extends the (largely individual) concept of *the* therapeutic relationship to a number of therapeutic relationships experienced in groups and transacted as members of communities and, ultimately, of society. This chapter does not assume familiarity with TA on the part of the reader and TA-specific terminology is defined in the endnotes.[1] For those wishing to gain further knowledge of TA by reading, Stewart and Joines (1987), Stewart (1989, 1992), Lapworth et al. (1993), and Clarkson et al. (1996) are recommended as useful introductory texts; those who prefer knowledge by experiencing, accredited TA trainers regularly run recognised introductory TA '101' courses.

A note on terms

One of the problems in discussing the concept and practice of the (or a) 'therapeutic relationship' is that the phrase is commonly used to describe two different referents: it describes the contact between therapist and client—in effect a self-defining definition, i.e., 'I have a therapeutic relationship by virtue of being *in* therapy'; at the same time it is used to refer to relationships which are therapeutic, thereby allowing the possibility that some therapeutic relationships (in the first sense) are not therapeutic. In a paper defining the process of definition, Money (1997) identifies three modes of defining: stipulative (prescriptive and authoritative), reportive (reflecting common usage), and mythogenic (expressing radical reconceptualisations of concepts); and three strategies of defining: using words (verbal), pointing (ostensive), and doing (performative): thus yielding nine types of definition. Drawing on this, we may distinguish between the first, self-defining use of the

DOI: 10.4324/9780429398223-7

term 'therapeutic relationship' as a verbal, reportive (VR) definition and the second, based as it is on the experience of the relationship as to whether or not it is therapeutic, as a performative, stipulative (PS) use and application of 'therapeutic relationship'. In this chapter I thus distinguish between the two uses (VR and PS).

Therapy and relationship in transactional analysis

TA has a rich, if somewhat dispersed literature on the therapeutic relationship, though mostly post Berne. In some personal reflections on TA, Stewart (1996) makes the point that the therapeutic relationship is *presupposed* and 'a sine qua non of effective therapy' (p. 198). In this section I draw out the various strands of this tradition by acknowledging the influence of three 'Schools' within TA: the Classical, the Cathexis, and the Redecision Schools—see Barnes (1977) and Stewart and Joines (1987) for further reading on these (and Chapter 12). Whilst all candidates seeking qualification and accreditation as transactional analysts are required to demonstrate that they draw on all traditions within TA, the different Schools represent different emphases in thinking, treatment—and therapeutic relationship. All, however, describe the therapeutic relationship (VR) in relation to transference— and it is the therapist's view of transference which is central to their intention and practice in all therapeutic relationships in TA. Further views about the therapeutic relationship, however, and especially the therapeutic attitude of the therapist, and ones which are agreed by all TA practitioners, may be drawn out from Berne's writing about the philosophy, principles, and practice of TA (see Table 4.1).

TA maintains the contractual basis of all relationships between therapist and client. For a relationship to be therapeutic in TA terms (i.e., VR *and* PS), four elements need to be present:

1. The therapist subscribes to the philosophy, methods, and attitudes described above (Table 4.1).
   This locates and identifies the therapist as a TA therapist.
2. The client has agreed goals which are therapeutic, i.e., which are positive and life-enhancing (and not life-threatening).
   This takes account of the fact that the client's initial goals and contract may not be therapeutic and that contracts both reflect and define an ongoing, organic process (see Lee, 1997), and that within TA, suicide, homicide, and going crazy are generally viewed as forms of escape from life to be confronted rather than supported.
3. The client's achievement of their goal/s requires the involvement of a therapist (as distinct from anyone else such as a friend or partner).
   This recognises the significance, although not necessarily the presence, of the therapist as crucial to the therapeutic process.
4. The above three elements are defined and agreed by the contract and the contractual method.
   See Steiner and Cassidy (1969), Steiner (1979), Stewart (1989), and Chapter 2.

Table 4.1. The implications of TA philosophy and method for the therapist's attitude to the therapeutic relationship

TA—Philosophy, method, and therapeutic attitude	Implications for the therapist's attitude to the therapeutic relationship
Basic philosophy	
• People are OK[2]	Positive and mutual regard/respect (I'm OK, You're OK)[3]
• Everyone has the capacity to think	
• People decide their own destiny and these decisions can be changed	...and a belief in self-responsibility A belief in personal responsibility and autonomy[4]
Therapeutic slogans (Berne, 1966a)	
• *Primum non nocere*: Above all do no harm	The principle from moral philosophy and ethics of non-maleficence
• *Vis medicatrix naturae*: The curative power of nature	Respect for the client's health, potential for health, and for developmental obstructions to health, e.g., defences
• *Je le pensay, & Dieu le guarit*: I treat them and God cures them[5]	A factual (not false) humility[6]
Therapeutic method	
• Contractual method (a mutually agreed statement of change)	Commitment to a clearly defined relationship in which there is joint responsibility for the process of change
• Open communication	Commitment to open communication, e.g., regarding client case notes,[7] case conferences, references, etc.
Therapeutic attitudes (Berne, 1966a) A fresh frame of mind:	
• In good health, physically and psychologically	Respect for self and others Authenticity *as a therapist* (as distinct
• Well-prepared, clear, and open	from as a friend)

The Classical School

Exponents of the Classical School of TA follow most closely the approach to treatment of Eric Berne and his immediate associates. This focuses on the diagnosis of ego states (Parent, Adult, and Child);[8] the use of analytic models to facilitate Adult understanding in the client (the Classical School is closest to the psychodynamic tradition) including their life script[9] and the psychological games they play in order to maintain that script;[10] and the use of contracts to make behavioural changes and to achieve cure (see Berne, 1961/1975a, 1972/1975b).

Berne writes only briefly about the therapeutic relationship as such (see Berne, 1966a). In doing so he suggests that, before and in the first few minutes of each session or meeting with client/s, the therapist should ask themselves 'some fundamental questions about the real meaning of the therapeutic relationship' (pp. 63–64). He views this firstly, with regard to the therapist's own development: 'Why am I sitting in this room? Why am I not at home with my children... What will this hour contribute to my unfolding?' (p. 64). Secondly, Berne suggests reflecting on the client and their motivations: 'Why are they here? Why are they not at home with their children or doing what their fancy dictates. Why did they choose psychotherapy as a solution? Why not religion, alcohol, drugs, crime, gambling... What will this hour contribute to their unfolding?' (p. 64).

On the basis of its philosophy, TA in practice is essentially an actionistic and highly interventive form of therapy.[11] It is based on diagnosis of the client and, arising from the contractual method, having a treatment planning sequence which aims to achieve cure or some specific change in the client. To this end, Berne (1966) identifies eight 'therapeutic operations'—interrogation, specification, confrontation, explanation, illustration, confirmation, interpretation, and crystallisation—which are used by the therapist as interventions (and interpositions). As such, and especially in its classical form, TA is often experienced as a confrontational and challenging form of therapy. Berne (1966) regards 'supportive therapy' as 'intrinsically spurious' and regarded the word 'relationship' as vague or borrowed terminology and asked clients what they meant by the word. From this, 'relating' for its own sake is generally downplayed in TA. Stewart (1992) makes the point that Berne's views on the person of the psychotherapist, the necessary personal and professional training and preparation, as well as their assets, therapeutic attitude, and responsibilities all imply that '*the establishment of a relationship, in and of itself, is not necessarily therapeutic*' (p. 74), a perspective which is consistent with our two definitions of the therapeutic relationship. Berne encourages clients to operationalise the meaning they give to psychological jargon and what Berne referred to as 'institutional concepts' such as 'relationship' and especially the 'therapeutic relationship'.

In his first book on the principles of TA, Berne (1961/1975a) outlines his structural analysis of personality. In doing so Berne lays the foundation not only for the transactional analysis of personality, but also for a transactional model of relationships—and of communication (see Figure 4.1).

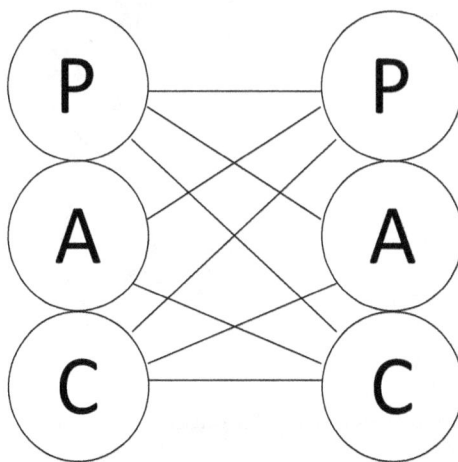

Figure 4.1. A theoretically ideal relationship
(Berne, 1961/1975a).[12]

In defining the Parent and Child ego states, Berne offers a transferential model of relationship: thus, a Child to Parent or Parent to Child transaction is, *by definition* transferential, e.g.:

Therapist (to Client):   'Hello...'
Client (to Therapist):   'You're not interested in how I am; you're just concerned with checking that I won't do anything silly' (A Child reaction to a projected Parent).

Therapist: 'Hello.'
Client: 'You look tired. Are you OK? Are you sure you're well enough to see me today?' (A Parent reaction to a projected Child).

Developing Berne's exploration of the dynamics underlying transference transactions, Moiso (1985) defines the transference relationship in TA terms: '*a relationship in which the patient, in order to reexperience parent-child or primitive object relationships projects onto the therapist his own Parental ego states... These are* projected onto a screen superimposed on the therapist (Child → projected Parent messages)' (pp. 194–195) (Figure 4.2).[13]

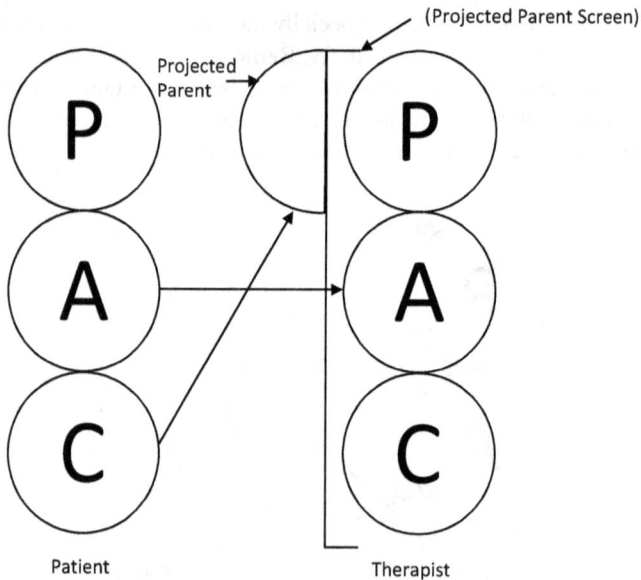

Figure 4.2. Analysis of transference relationship
(Moiso, 1985).

For further reading on the analysis and use of transference and countertransference in TA, see Novellino (1984), Moiso (1985), Barr (1987), Erskine (1991), and Clarkson (1992).

Within TA, especially in its early days, there was a strong tradition of social and radical psychiatry based on the concept of alienation as the essence of all psychiatric conditions which was defined as '*the result of oppression about which the oppressed has been mystified or deceived*' (Steiner, 1971b, p. 5). Steiner and colleagues in the Radical Therapist Collective were at the forefront of critical perspectives and practice in therapy about relationships, particularly those between men and women but also between clients and therapists (see The Radical Therapist Collective, 1971; Roy & Steiner, 1988; Wyckoff, 1976b). This tradition has led to a consistent concern within TA to consider the power issues involved in the therapeutic relationship (see Friedlander, 1987; Jacobs, 1987; Massey, 1987). Boyd (1976), for instance, introduced the concept of 'therapeutic leverage' to describe 'both the here and now attempts of the patient to manipulate the balance of interpersonal power and the second by second maneuvers of the therapist to keep the therapy effective' (p. 402).

The Cathexis School

This School of TA is based on the work of the Cathexis Institute, founded by Jacqui Schiff, as a centre for the treatment of psychotic clients, including those diagnosed as having schizophrenia (see Schiff, 1969; Schiff et al., 1975). Based on their analysis of symbiosis,[14] discounting,[15] and passivity,[16] they developed the theory and practice of reparenting the 'crazy Parent' ego state of disturbed clients who, in regression, 'decathect' (i.e., withdraw energy) from their introjected crazy Parent, replacing it with their introjections of the positive and consistent (re)parenting of the therapist/s.[17] Another way to understand this process, therefore, is that the therapist replaces the Parent and reparents the Child. Due to the regressive nature of the work and the necessary dependency of the client on the therapist, this work usually takes place in residential settings and requires a high level of commitment on the part of both therapist and client (see Robinson, 1998). These requirements and some of the early methods and techniques used by the Schiff family were—and are—also controversial and have led to much debate within the TA community (see Azzi, 1998; Jacobs, 1994). The particular contribution of the Cathexis School to our understanding of the therapeutic relationship is in terms of parenting: radical reparenting, spot reparenting, and self-reparenting.

Therapists working within the Cathexis School of TA positively use the transference by stepping into the Parent role in order to do the reparenting. In the original Schiffian *radical reparenting* model, the client's historical parent figures are excluded from the Parent ego state because they were—and are still experienced as—so damaging. In clients diagnosed as schizophrenic and in the context of a residential therapeutic community, clients regressed and lived in early developmental stages for extended periods; the therapists then parented them, including holding, feeding—and punishing—them so that the client incorporated new, positive experiences of parents into their Parent ego state.[18] In this context regression refers only to 'going back' for extended periods. It is possible to do similar work by 'cathecting young' or 'getting little' for short periods and on an outpatient basis—what Osnes (1974) refers to as *spot reparenting*. Drawing on Berne's (1961/1975a) original work on regression analysis, Osnes suggests that clients go back to an actual and specific experience and relive it up to the point of the original negative parenting (criticism, humiliation, abuse) at which point the therapist intervenes with a new positive, nurturing message, for instance, in response to an early experience of physical abuse:

Therapist (to regressed client):   'Your father is wrong. You deserve to be loved' (Reconstruction of Parent ego state). 'I love you. You don't have to be afraid' (New message for Child ego state).

Both radical reparenting and spot reparenting are based on the contractual method. Both take place in groups and the former almost exclusively in residential settings: all of which provide safety, monitoring, and regulation—for both client and therapist. Nevertheless, this work is problematic in that it places a lot of power, authority, and influence in the hands of the therapist, particularly at the moment of reparenting. It thus requires therapists to 'know thyself' and 'heal thyself': to be absolutely clear about their motivation for doing this kind of work and to be able to leave any of their own issues to one side not least as 'a difficulty may arise ... if unresolved problems in the therapist's ego states are also incorporated' (M. James, 1974, p. 33). Working in this reparenting relationship requires the therapist to work in the transference without identifying themselves with it. Of course, criticisms of this form of therapeutic relationship equally apply to any therapy interventions or transactions which give permission ('It's OK for you to...', 'Well done', or a pleased smile) and affirmation ('You think well') as, at best, they may be experienced as patronising and, at worst, may encourage dependency. Although therapeutic parenting necessarily involves a developmental dependency, even if for only a moment, as with all good parenting, it aims to foster independence and autonomy, that is spontaneity, awareness, and intimacy. A third form of parenting is *self reparenting* (M. James, 1974; James & Goulding, 1998). It differs from radical reparenting in that it takes a more phenomenological and cultural perspective on parenting, parental behaviour, and the Parent ego state; it does not exclude the historical parents, seeing something OK about them, and thus restructures rather than reconstructs the client's Parent ego state. Furthermore, in the process of self reparenting the client's Adult ego state is in charge. Self reparenting involves a specific procedure which may be facilitated by a therapist:

1. Awareness of the need for a new Parent which will compensate, supplement, or diffuse the parent of the old Parent.
2. Historical diagnosis of each childhood figure.

3. Education about parenting.
4. Inner dialogue between the Adult and the inner Child—with a view to discovering what each part of the Child ego state needs.
5. Evaluation of the data by the Adult.
6. Contract on the part of the Adult to be a substitute parent to the inner Child and practice of specific identified parenting behaviour.
7. Recognition of the new Parent (M. James, 1974).

The Redecision School

This School of TA takes its name from the decisional aspect of TA's basic philosophy (see Table 4.1) and the belief and practice that, just as we make decisions about our life, based on our life script, so we may re-decide and change our influences, behaviour, beliefs, experiences, fantasies, and feelings. This school is associated with the work of Bob and Mary Goulding who combined TA with techniques from Gestalt therapy such as 'two chair' work. The Gouldings' main contribution to our understanding about therapeutic relationships is in confronting and redirecting the client's transference to its original source. Whilst recognising and accounting for the existence of 'transferring from the past' in everything we do and thus in every helping relationship, the Gouldings advocated stepping out of the transference role as far as the client is concerned, e.g.,

Client (to Therapist):   'I'd like *you* to be my Dad'.
Therapist: 'Put your Dad there (pointing to a cushion next to the therapist) and tell him what you'd like from him'.

Dialogues between two chairs representing the transferred past and the real present and early scene work replaying scenes from childhood are both techniques used in TA redecision therapy which may be used to work *with* but not *in* the transference. In terms of the therapeutic relationship (PS) *as experienced* the therapist acts more as a facilitator and the client is encouraged to take a meta-perspective on their problems (see M. M. Goulding & R. L. Goulding, 1979).

The different approaches of the different schools of TA to the transference relationship may be viewed as on a continuum, thus:

Working *in* the transference   Working *with* but outside the transference

Cathexis School	Classical School	Redecision School

Integrative TA: an emerging 'School'?

Over the 15 years (1984–1999) in the generic counselling and psychotherapeutic literature, there has been an emerging interest in therapeutic integration; this extends to debates within different 'schools' or 'forces' of therapy and is no less true within TA, although I have argued that TA needs to concern itself more with integration *within* TA, that is, '*intra*gration' (Tudor, 1996), rather than integration (inter-gration) of material into TA.[19] Nevertheless, there is a developing integrative *tradition*—it is not yet a 'School' according to Barnes' (1977) definition—within TA (Erskine & Moursund, 1988; Clarkson, 1992; also see Novey, 1996) and indeed, a significant 18% of Certified Transactional Analysts (CTAs) define themselves in the United Kingdom Council for Psychotherapy's (UKCP) register of psychotherapists as 'integrative psychotherapists' (UKCP, 1996). One feature of this (along with much of the rest of the therapeutic world) is an emerging interest in the concept, attitude, and practice of empathy. In TA, Clark (1991) links this to Berne's concept of transactions in promoting empathic transactions as a means of deconfusing the Child ego state.[20] Drawing on Gelso and Carter's (1985) components of the therapeutic relationship as an organising framework for integration—the working alliance, the 'unreal' (transference) relationship, and the real relationship—these components may be identified as present in TA:

- The working alliance (Adult–Adult)—the first stage in treatment planning (see Clarkson et al., 1996) and operationalised in the contractual method of TA. In her therapeutic relationship model, Barr (1987) views this as the 'core relationship' between client and therapist 'beginning with the client's capacity to recruit and the therapist's recruitability' (p. 135).
- Transference (and countertransference) (Child–Parent, Parent–Child)—central to a TA understanding of the therapeutic relationship (VR and PS) (as elaborated above) and which includes the reparative/developmentally needed relationship (Barr, 1987; Clarkson, 1992) represented by the reparenting work of the Cathexis School.
- The real relationship (Adult–Adult)—reflected in the existential life position 'I'm OK, You're OK' (I+ U+) and the emphasis in TA on the therapist's authenticity as a therapist.

Dual therapeutic relationships

The issue of dual relationships, i.e., one person (the therapist) having more than one relationship with a client (for example as a trainer or supervisor in addition to that of a therapist) to a client, or indeed a client (being, say, also a supplier of goods or services) to their therapist, is a 'hot potato' both within TA and in the wider field of counselling and psychotherapy. As far as therapists in Britain are concerned, at present the dual relationships of therapist and supervisor and therapist and trainer are prohibited (British Association for Counselling, 1997, B.5.2), while the codes of ethics and practice for supervisors and trainers place responsibility on the supervisor and trainer to be explicit about the boundaries between the two roles (British Association for Counselling, 1995, 1996). However, given such prohibitions, there is surprisingly little written, both within TA and more generally, about the logic of the 'no dual relationships' position or its underlying presuppositions. In this section, therefore, I review some of the arguments against and for dual relationships from the perspective of what is or could be therapeutic about such relationships (and thus PS) rather than simply defining dual relationships (in a circular definition) as inherently exploitative and therefore as bad, mad, or dangerous even to contemplate (VR).

The history of therapy is a history of dual relationships

Whilst history is no justification for unethical or unprofessional practice, it is worth noting that the founding fathers and mothers of psychoanalysis (none of whom would nowadays likely be eligible for membership of the training institutes which bear their names or promote their ideas) worked in and with dual and multiple relationships. Freud analysed all his initial trainees; Jung and Reich both had personal relationships with their clients; and Klein analysed her own children. It is easy to condemn such relationships; it is more complex and rigorous to investigate the therapeutic—or exploitative—nature (or otherwise) of these relationships. Schools (and institutes) in both the analytic and humanistic traditions of psychotherapy have in the past positively advocated and even required dual relationships, i.e., trainees being in analysis and supervision with the same training analyst. The argument for this was—and is—based on the applicability of the psychoanalytic method—analysis, suggestion, and insight—to the client whether they are (in roles of) a trainee or a supervisee or not: whatever their issues are, these will be played out in all roles in their lives; whatever their own clients' issues are, these may be understood in terms of the client/trainee/supervisee's countertransference.

'Relationship is confused with role' (M. Cox, 1997, 2000)

Relationship is defined as 'the state of being related; a condition or character based upon this; kinship' (Onions, 1933/1973, p. 1786). On the basis of this definition, the 'relationship' between client and therapist may more accurately be defined as a role: a part or character one undertakes.

An exercise

Take a moment to write down who you are in your life in terms of relationships—daughter/son, sister/brother, mother/father, partner/lover, etc., trainer, tutor, supervisor, therapist, client, etc.

More particularly, you might do this in relation to any of the authors of the chapters in this book (i.e., Feltham, 1999) or, indeed, any writers cited in the book. You might do it in relation to a training or therapy group you are in.

Now think about these as *roles*.... Is there any difference?

In doing this exercise, some people find that thinking and feeling about roles rather than relationships normalises or makes usual what we do: I am a husband,

father, friend, uncle, brother, son, employer, trainer, colleague, supervisor, therapist, consultant, examiner, client, consumer, etc., etc. These are parts, aspects, or
facets of the whole of me: they define a temporal role, some more long-term or
permanent than others. Taking on the role of examiner does not necessary entail
a relationship or kinship; this applies equally to more personal roles, for example,
there are fathers who are in the *role* of a father but who are not actively or meaning-
fully *in relationship* with their children.

Dual and multiple roles are an inevitable part of life and of therapy

This appreciation that we have many roles in life leads us to two conclusions and
decisions: to avoid them or to meet and deal with them. Trying to avoid or *having*
to avoid dual professional relationships (roles) in order to adhere to particular professional codes of ethics and practice may, indeed, be viewed as neurotic:

- As defensive against anxiety or real contact between people—a 'defensive therapy' position.
- As repressive of complexity—

  to simply outlaw the dual relationships of supervisor/therapist does not adequately address the complex issues involved; rather it imposes a rigidity on a
  complex and often ambiguous profession, reduces the choices and autonomy
  of the supervisee, and does not necessarily ensure the optimal welfare of a
  supervisee's clients.

  (Cornell, 1994, p. 25)

- As phobic—in a chapter on the problems of dual relationships in the education
of therapists Lloyd (1992) referred to 'dual relationship phobia' (p. 60).

As members of the same professional body as our therapist, supervisor, client, etc.,
we are in dual relationship; living in a remote area or being part of a 'minority'
community, we are likely to be in dual and multiple professional and therapeutic
relationships. Codes of ethics and practice which place absolute requirements on
us to avoid dual relationships assume a choice which is usually available only in
larger cities and to 'majority' communities. In terms of anti-discriminatory practice and client autonomy, it may well be more therapeutic for a gay man to work
with a local therapist, another gay man, than to travel to another town to see a
second-choice therapist (for a discussion of the boundaries between and negotiation of different professional boundaries, see Embleton Tudor, 1997).

The criticism of dual relationships is not consistent

For the majority of therapists there is a requirement at some stage of their training
or professional development to be in therapy themselves. Given that we subscribe

to the concept of a professional and collegial community (see, for instance, the British Association for Counselling, 1997), this requires therapists to be in a dual relationship/role, that is, one with a colleague. The logic of completely avoiding dual roles is that therapists should be in therapy with non-therapists! Neither does the criticism of dual relationships extend to dual or multiple *therapeutic* relationships, such as identified by Greenson (1967), Gelso and Carter (1985), Barr (1987), and Clarkson (1990, 1995).

Arguments against dual relationships/roles—and responses

Perhaps the strongest argument against dual relationships is that they muddy the transferential waters. Whilst, for some therapists, depending on their theoretical orientation, such muddying might be viewed as a good thing, and others might take on the challenge of working with this complexity, there is a risk to clients (who might also be trainees or supervisees) of a therapist exploiting their client's positive transference. This is a significant phenomenon in the world of therapist training where a significant number of trainees want to train as therapists with their own therapist, whose facilitative qualities and skills they have experienced. Again, I view this as an issue of possible exploitation and is countered by good therapy, training, and supervision, all of which could and should address, in this frame of reference, the counter-transferential issues involved.

In this context of therapist training, one major practical argument against dual relationships is the current situation of 'in-house' certification of counsellors and psychotherapists. Thus, a trainer who may have been a trainee's therapist and/or supervisor may also be in the position of examining that trainee/(client/supervisee). This is a clear conflict of interests and reflects the incestuous and exploitative reality of some training organisations—for an analysis of various characteristics of abusive mini-cultures of training organisations, see Robertson (1993). This is partially addressed by the presence and role of the external examiner, although their role—and relationship—with the training organisation arguably needs to be monitored, externally. It is also answered by external accreditation systems *in addition to qualification*.[21] In TA practitioners are examined and accredited totally 'out-of-house' and one of the organisational strengths of TA is its rigorous and international examination and accreditation of its practitioners, trainers, and supervisors. Also, from a therapeutic consideration, clients who are also trainees/supervisees may not expose or work through the pathological and/or dysfunctional parts of themselves for fear of being judged and assessed as trainees/supervisees.

Most arguments against dual relationships centre on three issues:

1. *The possible exploitation of the client*
    This appears to be founded on the evidence that the majority of ethics complaints from clients investigated by professional bodies, and certainly by the UK's Institute of Transactional Analysis (ITA), concern dual relationships. However, I consider these to be issues of exploitation, not necessarily of

duality. The response to this problem is for the therapist to have good awareness, training, and supervision about issues of power, influence, exploitation,
and anti-oppressive practice—theory and practice which, for instance, the radical psychiatry tradition of TA informs.

2. *The possible conflict of interests*
    In an unsubstantiated assertion, Bond (1993) equates dual relationships with
conflict of interests (see also Herlihy & Corey, 1992). The response is that this
is for both or all parties to consider precisely what interests are in conflict. In my
view, it is the merging of what are conflicts of interests and the possible erosion
of boundaries which is more common and problematic in this area (as with the
above example from training) and is an argument for establishing and maintaining clear rather than blurred roles—personal and professional roles, e.g., not
being both partner and therapist; or incompatible professional roles, e.g., not
being both a trainer and an examiner of those trainees. The concept of symbiosis
is useful in analysing, understanding, and working with issues of merger and
separation. I define incompatibility in relation to:

- TA philosophy: people are OK, everyone has the capacity to think, and people can decide their own destiny (see Table 4.1);
- General values of caring professions such as integrity, impartiality, and respect (see Bond, 1993); and
- Principles from moral philosophy, e.g., beneficence, non-maleficence, justice, and respect for autonomy.

3. *The possible impairment of the therapist's judgement*
    This is not solely a problem of duality but is an issue of professional compe-
tence and is an argument for self-awareness, high quality training, and ongoing
supervision. Obviously, some therapists on some occasions will make a decision
based on some impaired judgement. As regards dual relationships the checklist
(pp. 87–88, below) may aid such judgement and ethical decision-making.

Therapeutic advantages to dual therapeutic relationships

There are two possible advantages of dual therapeutic relationships to be considered:

- As humans we are organised wholes (holons) in multiple roles and relationships,
  trying to make meaning of our complex lives and worlds. Working within a facilitative and 'holding' dual relationship can help us to make sense of this complexity rather than artificially separating (and splitting) ourselves. The therapist/
  trainer/supervisor working with dual or multiple roles also has the opportunity
  to demonstrate dealing with rather than avoiding complexity.
- A person is a client/trainee/supervisee/etc. People go to therapists as whole
  people, who are damaged and disintegrated in some way; as such their

therapeutic issues will have repercussions in all their roles and relationships. Someone who learned to please others will do this as a client, trainee therapist, and supervisee. There is no difference *therapeutically* between the activities of training, supervision, personal therapy, and personal development, that is from what may be *experienced as therapeutic*. Indeed, in the training context, there are strong arguments for a trainer, observing a particular therapeutic issue in a person (at that moment in the role of a trainee), to counsel that person on that issue. Writing from a person-centred perspective but making a point which is equally applicable to other orientations, Mearns (1994) argues that 'personal development for professional working is so crucial to the person-centred approach that it cannot be left to the vagaries of individual therapy' (p. 35). Personal development is an important part of most training in counselling and psychotherapy and takes place in the training group ('check in', group time, reflection time, community meetings, etc.). It may also take the form of a demonstration of individual therapy sessions in the training group. An absolute ban on dual relationships, therefore, would logically exclude such therapy unless it were redefined as 'personal development'.[22] Within TA, the Gouldings promote dual relationships, for instance, between trainer/therapist and trainee/client, arguing that they are protected by the contractual method of TA therapy (R. L. Goulding & M. M. Goulding, 1975/1978). This is an established tradition within TA (for a discussion of which see Bader, 1994; Clarkson, 1994; Cornell, 1994) and, indeed, a number of TA practitioners have left the BAC on this very issue—ironically, in view of the fact that the ITA is in the process of deciding to prohibit combining the roles of therapist and supervisor and to publish a guideline suggesting that the combined therapist/trainer role is best avoided whenever practically possible.[23]

A dual relationship checklist

In an attempt to stem the flood against dual therapeutic relationships, I offer the following ten-point checklist by which clients *and therapists* could both be protected and take permission to explore the therapeutic value of duality, multiplicity, and complexity. I emphasise 'and therapists' as, in the arguments against dual relationships, little attention is given to the exploitation of therapists by clients.

1. Distinguish between relationship and role and between professional role and personal role—which provides a two-by-two framework for congruence and consistency in therapeutic relationships. Of course, therapists are also personal in their professional role: the real(ity) relationship transcends the role relationship.
2. Develop the concept of 'role fluency' (Clarkson, 1994), which involves a fluidity between roles and a fluency in different roles.

3. Reframe the debate from duality to the issue or question of exploitation of *both* clients and therapists in terms of:

   • Sexual exploitation, a response to which is simply that there are—or should be—no sexual relations between a therapist and her/his client (e.g., American Counseling Association [ACA], 1995, A.7).
   • Financial exploitation—the ACA, for instance, discourages bartering, for a discussion of which see Tudor (1998).
   • Political exploitation—Clarkson (1994) discusses the potential for political exploitation whereby, for example, clients who are also trainees and members of the same professional organisation may be involved in voting for their therapist.

4. Subscribe to an accepted professional code of ethics and practice, although the relative permission or prohibition regarding dual relationships will depend on to which code of ethics therapists subscribe.
5. Have a clear, congruent, and communicable personal ethics, which includes being clear about therapists' personal motivation and issues of power.
6. Be well trained and experienced, especially in dealing with issues of power, oppression, exploitation, and abuse.
7. Ensure that all final accreditation procedures are preferably 'out of house' or at least at 'arm's length', so that the trainer (and/or supervisor/therapist) is never the marker or sole or deciding marker of a trainee's work for final accreditation.
8. Develop an ability to evaluate clinical, legal, and ethical considerations in therapy (see, for instance, Bader, 1994).
9. Take 'professional precautions', thus, 'when a dual relationship cannot be avoided, therapists take appropriate professional precautions such as informed consent, consultation, and documentation to ensure that judgement is not impaired and no exploitation occurs' (ACA, 1995, A.6.a).
10. Appreciate that clients, trainees, and supervisees are consenting adults—*and customers*. Some training organisations—and therapists—infantilise their clients in how they regard and treat them (and conceptualise their development in training), which is not only patronising but also fosters exploitation.
11. Acknowledge the humility of what actually helps and heals, e.g., being held, receiving a postcard, a smile, or an acknowledgement at a conference—often outside the boundary of the 'therapeutic hour'; and acknowledge the humanity of being willing to work with complexity, contradiction, and conflict.[24]

From the therapeutic relationship to therapeutic relating

Finally, in this chapter, I am concerned to indicate ways of applying the (largely individual) concept of *the* therapeutic relationship to a number of therapeutic relationships experienced in groups and transacted as members of communities and, ultimately, of society. I identify two aspects of this. The first moves the client from some form of dependency on one (*the*) therapeutic relationship to other relationships which are therapeutic. Within the therapeutic sphere these could be, and often are, other members of a therapy group and, indeed, other therapists; outside therapy, these may be new, often intense friendship relationships which are experienced as therapeutic and which support the client's changes. The second aspect of this wider application is the movement from the nominal (noun) 'relationship' to the activity (verb) of *relating*.

One of the criticisms of therapy is that it individualises—and privatises—relationships: if you have a problem, go to a therapist. When the concept of therapy is explained to the eponymous hero in the film *Crocodile Dundee* (Faiman, 1986), he asks the person concerned, 'Why? Don't you have any friends?' Despite the advances in our understanding of the psyche and the nature of healing in the last one hundred years (since Freud coined the term 'psychotherapy'),[25] the exclusive nature of the therapeutic relationship remains an important criticism and challenge to this particular helping and healing activity. The relationship with your therapist is viewed as *the* therapeutic relationship and, to some extent, the focus on the concept of the therapeutic relationship encourages this. By focusing on the verb/action *relating* rather than the noun *relationship* we shift attention from the relationship between client and therapist (and others) to how the client relates and, further, to how they establish and maintain relating which is therapeutic in the rest of their lives outside the limited contact with their therapist. In the rest of this section, I highlight a number of ways in which the client may unfold the therapeutic relationship into therapeutic relating.

Extending the frame of reference of 'therapeutic relationship'

One of the ways in which the focus on the primary therapeutic relationship (VR) between client and therapist may be extended is in working in groups. Here the contractual method is open to a series of sub-contracts between the group therapist and clients and between clients themselves (Tudor, 1999a). Inevitably a client's goal in group therapy is facilitated by other members of the group: 'I will respond to each person in the group in each meeting', 'I will ask to sit next to someone in the group each meeting', 'I will ask for feedback from group members at least once each meeting': all rely on at least the presence of other group members if not their active participation for the completion of the client's contract. In terms of TA approaches to therapy groups, the Classical School focuses on the analysis of transaction between group members; the Cathexis School draws on others in the group or therapeutic community especially in confrontation and checking reality; while, in the Redecision School, the approach is more individual therapy *in* the group with other group members as witnesses and participants in any therapeutic drama or re-enactment.

This sub-contracting may be extended to the introduction of other therapists, either in the individual setting or to the therapy group. I have made a number of arrangements whereby clients have chosen to work with another therapist, say a woman or a therapist with a different cultural background, while retaining a therapeutic contract—and occasional contact—with me. This fosters the (developmental) reality that clients may be nourished by more than one care-giver and that the initial 'primary' therapist does not have all the answers. It also opens up the primary therapeutic relationship (and, by implication, the therapist's therapy) to other influences and to outside, independent influence and scrutiny. At times the introduction of another therapist to a group is largely pragmatic when due to, for instance, the illness or unavoidable absence of the group therapist. The advantage of such occasions however is, again, the introduction of another frame of reference on clients' issues, including how they accommodate or assimilate a new therapeutic relationship, however temporary. Those group therapists who never introduce a colleague or who never co-lead a group may find it useful to think about the therapeutic advantages of doing so.

The third area of therapeutic relationship outside the primary client–therapist relationship (and one hardly addressed in the literature) is the effect on existing relationships in the client's life and the development of new, influential therapeutic relationships, possibly with other members of a therapy group but also with other, new friends. One common reported experience of longer-term therapy is that clients change their networks of friendships. This is unsurprising in that people often come to therapy with some disturbance (e.g., a life script which supports certain ego state pathology). Their existing friendships and relationships are founded on or at least exist in the context of this disturbance. In the course of therapy and as a result of 'getting better' and/or 'cured' they are likely to review existing relationships/friendships and to view new ones. As a result of an early script decision, one client who had spent most of her life pleasing others changed this and promptly both gave up and lost a lot of her existing friends who had relied on her to please them. Given this, it is important that clients have opportunities to apply and practise relationships which are therapeutic (i.e., PS)—which is one reason to encourage alternate meetings of therapy groups without the therapist (see Tudor, 1999a; Wolf & Schwartz, 1962) and socialising amongst group members.

Therapeutic relating

Finally, I propose a shift in our collective thinking about the importance of therapeutic relationship/s to the concept of therapeutic *relating*. In discussing the logical relation between therapy and relationship Stewart (1996) suggests that the quality which makes relating therapeutic is discovering 'positive intention' (p. 190). If we learn anything from TA therapy it is how to transact with others with positive, active intention in our everyday lives, independently of a (the) therapeutic relationship. The social contact which members of a therapy group may have outside the group provides an important experience, base, and basis for further social contact beyond even these therapeutic relationships. Symor (1977) argues that the 'I'm OK, You're OK' life position is one of liberation and interdependence, 'characterized by autonomous behavior based on choice' (p. 41). Developing Seymour's argument and taking Berne's (1972/1975b) three-handed life positions, I take the 'I'm OK, You're OK, *and They're OK*' position as a profound existential—and operational—challenge to include 'them' (whoever 'they' are) in the field of my relating (see Chapter 1). In practice, in the physical dimension, this means having regard for my environment, both immediate and global, thus: 'think globally, act locally'. In the social dimension, in our relating with others in our public world, this means having respect for and understanding of others and, for instance, not gossiping about 'them'—which is a powerful contract to make, especially in a group and organisational context but, nevertheless, one which I have seen work effectively and which improves the social environment (also see Tudor, 1997b). In the psychological dimension, this means having or developing an understanding of the 'they' in our lives and the part both they and we played in our psychological development; it is easier to blame than to resolve, easier to look back than to look forward. Finally, in the spiritual dimension, this means developing a sense of others as a supportive network or community for our values and aspirations and the meaning we make of our lives.

Summary

This chapter has offered:

- An understanding of the therapeutic relationship in TA, based on the therapist's understanding of transference and on the contractual method.
- The ego state model of personality, by which therapists may distinguish between transference and non-transference transactions.
- A view of TA therapeutic relationships as encompassing the working alliance, the transferential, reparative (reparenting), and real relationships between therapist and client.
- A view that dual relationships are not necessarily exploitative, but that therapists (and clients) need to distinguish between exploitation and duality, and relationship and role.
- An argument that the contractual method of TA defines roles and protects both client and therapist.
- A dual relationship checklist which identifies key issues for the therapist as regards dual roles and relationships.
- A view that change through therapy requires the client to move from a (the) dependent therapeutic relationship to therapeutic relating with others both within the therapy context and, ultimately, beyond.

Notes

1 In the original chapter these appeared in text boxes throughout the chapter, which, on reflection, I find both distracting and messy!
2 A shorthand statement describing the positive essence of people.

3 In his last book, Berne (1972/1975b) developed this into three-handed life positions—
'I'm OK, You're OK, They're OK' etc., thereby giving eight possible life positions (see
Tudor, 2016c [Chapter 1]).

4 Defined within TA as 'the release or recovery of three capacities: awareness, spontaneity and intimacy' (Berne, 1964/1968, p. 158) and enshrined in the BAC *Code of Ethics*
(1997).

5 Although Berne (1966) defines this as 'getting the patient ready for the cure to happen
today' (p. 63), this slogan contradicts much of Berne's other writing on the subject of
cure.

6 He also reminds us that 'the professional therapist's job is to use his [sic] knowledge
therapeutically [emphasis added]; if the patient is going to be cured by love, that should
be left to a lover' (p. 63).

7 See Tudor and Gledhill (2022).

8 An ego state is 'a consistent pattern of feeling and experience directly related to a corresponding consistent pattern of behaviour' (Berne, 1966, p. 364).

9 'A script is an ongoing program, developed in early childhood under parental influence,
which directs the individual's behavior in the most important aspects of his life' (Berne,
1972/1975b, p. 418).

10 'A game is a process of doing something with an ulterior motive that (1) is outside of
Adult awareness; (2) does not become explicit until the participants switch the way they
are behaving; and (3) results in everyone feeling confused, misunderstood, and wanting
to blame the other person.' (Joines cited in Stewart & Joines, 1987, pp. 242–243)

11 The original chapter was published in a volume in a series of books for counsellors and
so, in the original, although I was referring to both counselling and psychotherapy, I
used the terms 'counsellor(s)' and 'counselling'. In republishing this, I have taken the
opportunity to change the language to the more generic 'therapy' and 'therapist'.

12 Based on a three ego state model of health, for a critique of which, see (Tudor, 2003b)
and Tudor and Summers (2014).

13 'A Parental ego state is a set of feelings, attitudes, and behavior patterns which resemble
those of a parental figure ... The Child ego state is a set of feelings, attitudes and behavior patterns which are relics of the individual's own childhood.' (Berne, 1961/1975a,
pp. 75–77; see also Chapters 6 and 7)

14 'A symbiosis occurs when two or more individuals behave as though between them they
form a whole person. The relationship is characterized structurally by neither individual
cathecting a full complement of ego states.' (Schiff et al., 1975, p. 5)

15 'Discounting is an internal mechanism which involves people minimizing or ignoring
some aspect of themselves, others or the reality situation.' (Schiff et al., 1975, p. 14).

16 Passivity is defined as 'how people don't do things (respond to stimuli) or don't do them
effectively.' (Schiff et al., 1975, p. 5)

17 'Reparenting... involves the total decathexis of the originally incorporated Parent ego
state, and the replacement of that structure with a new Parent structure.' (Schiff et al.,
1975, p. 88)

18 There has been considerable debate within TA about some of the original practice of
Cathexis and its theory (see Cornell & Deaconu, 2022; Jacobs, 1994; Mountain, 2022;
Robinson, 1998, 2003).

19 Indeed, one of Zalcman's (1990) concerns about the development of TA theory and
practice since Berne's death (20 years previously) is 'the adoption of concepts and techniques from other methods without sufficient critical evaluation or integration into TA
theory and practice' (p. 5); see also Chapters 12 and 13.

20 Deconfusion is the identification and expression of 'unmet needs and feelings in the
Child ego state which were suppressed at the time of the script decision in the interests
of psychological and/or physical survival.' (Clarkson at al., 1996, p. 241)

21 However, while this can provide some separation, it can also be fertile ground for even more complex dual and multiple relationships and conflicts of interest. In Aotearoa New Zealand, we had a situation where one person was, simultaneously: the programme leader of a training course at a tertiary institution (accountable to that institution and its external regulations); the President of a national professional association (which has specific views about the approach to training psychotherapists), and restricts membership to psychotherapists adhering to that specific theoretical orientation; and the Chair of the regulatory authority which defined scopes of practice for psychotherapists—which restricts registration to those psychotherapists adhering to that specific theoretical orientation.

22 Talking about this in the context of his experience of a marathon with the Gouldings, and in other training he experienced and conducted in the 1970s, '80s, and '90s, Evan Sherrard (personal communication, 2014) said that people used to refer to such demonstrations and experiences as 'work', not therapy. Thus, in setting up a demonstration, the trainer would say: 'OK, who'd like to come and do a piece of work?'

23 This did come in—see the (now) UK Association for Transactional Analysis' (2020) *Dual Relationships Policy*.

24 In the course of writing this original section, at one point I typed 'duel' instead of 'dual' relationships, a Freudian slip which reminds me of the complexity of working with duality and duelling relationships.

25 Since I wrote the original chapter, I have traced this word further back – to 1811, when Johann Heinroth was appointed as a full (and the first) professor of Psychic (Psycho) Therapy at the University of Leipzig (see Steinberg, 2004; Steinberg & Himmerich, 2012).

Chapter 5

From transactional analysis to transactional relating

The gift of the present, and the reality of context

Following on from and reflecting on the previous chapter (which was published 25 years ago), in this chapter I develop the thesis of transactional relating in order to emphasise what I argue is the present-centred purpose of transactional analysis (TA), that is, analysing transactions.[1] As Berne (1966) himself puts it: 'The object of group treatment is to fight the past in the present in order to assure the future' (p. 250).

Re-reading Chapter 4, I was pleasantly surprised to see the last section on therapeutic relating as, although I have been talking about this for some time, I hadn't remembered that I'd articulated it as long ago as 1999. In some ways this isn't surprising as, around the same time, I was also engaged with Graeme Summers in developing the ideas that led to our article on co-creative transactional analysis, which was published in 2000. In that article, we critiqued Clarkson's (1990, 1992) taxonomy of therapeutic relationships;[2] offered an alternative based on present and past relating; and emphasised the co-creative nature of such relating from a transactional perspective. Since then, I have emphasised the present-centred nature of such relating in other work: on person-centred therapy (Embleton Tudor & Tudor, 2009; Tudor & Worrall, 2006), the nature of therapy (Tudor, 2008b), verbal being (Tudor, 2008d), empathy (Tudor, 2011b, 2011g), and the method(s) of psychotherapy (Tudor, 2018b).

Building on that work, and especially my outline of the methodology and method of co-creative relating (Tudor, 2011b),[3] in this chapter, I elaborate a relational TA as a therapy of and with the present moment. Thus, in the first part of the chapter, I revisit and reflect on transactional relating and especially present-centred relating in the context of the work of Daniel Stern, and, specifically, his book *The Present Moment: In Psychotherapy and Everyday Life* (Stern, 2004). In the second part of the chapter, I review different ideas within TA about the therapeutic relationship and therapeutic relating since 1999 (the publication date of the previous article/ chapter), across different approaches within TA, framing them in terms of Martha Stark's (1999) taxonomy of one-person, one-and-a-half-person, and two-person psychology, with my addition of a two-person-plus psychology (Tudor, 2011g).

In both parts of the chapter, I carry forward the same interest that informs my thinking and writing in Part 1, especially Chapter 2, that is, in looking for and at the

DOI: 10.4324/9780429398223-8

philosophy that informs ideas about therapeutic relating (Stern), and the practice and categories described by different modes of therapeutic action (Stark).

The presenting moment

In the preface to his book, *The Present Moment*, Stern (2004) refers to 'the small momentary events that make up our worlds of experience' (p. xi), which is similar to Berne's (1972/1975b) statement that 'Each person is the product of a million different moments' (p. 87). What interests Stern (2004) most is 'when these moments enter one's awareness and are shared between two people' (p. xi). He continues: 'These lived experiences make up the key moments of change in psychotherapy and the nodal points in our everyday intimate relationships' (p. xi).

By way of introducing his discussion of the various aspects of the present, Stern shares the various changes he made to the working title of the book, which, here, I take as headings that frame my elaboration of Stern's ideas.

'A world in a grain of sand'

Stern's reference to William Blake's (1863/1958) poem captures the sense of seeing the large and general in the small and particular. Stern himself acknowledges 'the size of the small world revealed by microanalysis and... the fact that one can often see the larger panorama of someone's past and current life in the small behaviours and mental acts making up this micro-world' (p. xiv). The importance and significance of this is being able to extrapolate from the analysis of a specific transaction in therapy to a broader analysis (for instance, in terms of transactions, ego states, scripts, and games) of how a client thinks and feels about and operates in their world(s). Again, this echoes Berne's (1961/1975a) idea about TA as a social psychiatry, that is, 'the study of the psychiatric aspects of specific transactions or sets of transactions which take place between two or more particular individuals at a given time and place' (p. 12) (for further discussion of which see Tudor, 2020g, and Chapter 12). The correlation between a grain of sand (as a microcosm) and the world (as the microcosm) is also represented in Rogers' (1961/1967) thinking when he writes that '*What is most personal is most general*' (p. 26). Here Rogers is writing about expressing himself in ways that are personal, in a sense, particular and private, and perhaps even incomprehensible (at least initially), and then discovering that it is precisely that (the personal) which resonates and speaks most deeply to others (and, in that sense, is most general). The importance and significance of this is in the reaction of others: it is precisely the acknowledgement of the generality of the personal experience that helps the person being personal feel less alone and alienated (Rogers, 1975/1980). Taking this further in terms of viewing 'The world in an individual' (Tudor, 2016d), I advance a perspective that acknowledges and welcomes the world, that is, the client's present world, into therapy, however that is manifested in the particular grain of sand.

In practice, I am particularly interested in the microcosm that is the first moment: how people come into the room; how they great me; whether they shake my hand, and, if so, how; how they sit; their first breath; the first thing they say, and don't say—and also what my first moments were in response to them. For a number of years (in the UK), I worked in a room with a very light carpet and soft furnishings, on entering which most clients (and supervisees and trainees) took off their shoes. I remember the response of one particular new client as follows:

Client: [Pauses at the door] Oh, I didn't realise I had to take my shoes off.
Keith: You don't have to take shoes off.
Client: [Bending down and taking off her first shoe.] Oh, I've got a hole in my tights.
Keith: [Pause] ... It's an imperfect world.

This exchange, which lasted less than a minute, turned out to be a symbolic microcosm of my client's experience of the general, that is the wider world, both present and past; and my last comment, which was entirely intuitive, turned out to reflect my client's experience of an unpredictable, uncertain—and imperfect— human world.[4] Clearly, different therapists will respond differently to any initial stimulus; the most important thing is to notice. Discussing the requirements of the group therapist, Berne (1966) states that visual observation 'is the basis of all good clinical work, and takes precedence even over technique' (pp. 65–66).

The obscure side of the moon

This second of Stern's proposed titles refers to the awareness of 'the experienced microworld' (Stern, 2004, p. xiv) being more to do with implicit than explicit knowing. Stern himself defines this as 'non-symbolic, non-verbal, procedural, and unconscious', contrasting it with explicit, verbalised knowledge which is 'symbolic, verbalizable, declarative, capable of being narrated, and reflectively conscious' (p. 113). He elaborates this with reference to literature from communication studies, psychology, and, specifically, developmental psychology, including infant observation, the latter of which is particularly significant because, as Stern (2004) points out:

> Babies do not communicate in the verbal explicit register until after 18 months or so, when they begin to talk. Accordingly, all the rich, analogically nuanced, social and affective interactions that take place in the first 18 months of life occur, by default, in the implicit nonverbal domain.
>
> (p. 113)

Stern refers to implicit knowing as comprising non-verbal communication, body movement, sensation, affects, expectations, shifts in activation and motivation, and styles of thought, and acknowledges its representation in words or, at least, what lies between lines—and, interestingly, for transactional analysts, uses the example of someone repeatedly saying 'Yes, but...' (see Berne, 1964/168a). Stern's (2004) own analysis of this is 'that the "yes" is a Trojan horse to get inside your walls. The "but" releases the soldiers' (p. 114), an image which describes the kick that one can feel from the 'but'—and, indeed, the anxiety that builds up when one is anticipating the 'but' in someone's statement, especially the longer it continues.[5]

In TA, implicit knowing is found in the concept of intuition, the subject of Berne's (1949/1977f) early interest and research and which he defined as 'knowledge based on experience and acquired through sensory contact with the subject, without the "intuiter" being able to formulate to himself or others how he came to his conclusions' (p. 4). In their article on intuition, and drawing on both Berne and Stern, Bove and Rizzi (2009) underscore the affective dimension of the intuitive process, concluding that:

> our way of being with another person can allow emotional communication and a sense of connection with others... [and that] it is through such intimate and genuine contact that the interpersonal relatedness is cocreated in which it is possible to share experience.
>
> (p. 42)

For Moustakas (1990), intuition is 'a kind of bridge... between the implicit knowledge inherent in the tacit and the explicit knowledge which is observable and describable. [It] is the realm of the between, or the intuitive' (p. 23). I quote Moustakas as he founded heuristic research (which was closely aligned with the early development of humanistic psychology), and which, according to McLeod (2003), is 'a powerful discovery-oriented approach to research' (p. 97). Alongside indwelling and personal knowledge (from Polanyi, 1962), and the tacit dimension of knowing (also from Polanyi, 1964, 1966, 1969) and the felt sense (from Gendlin, 1981, 1991, whom Stern cites but whose work he does not elaborate on), intuition is a key concept in Moustakas' heuristic research methodology. Importantly for our present purpose and focus, Moustakas (1990) suggests that: 'Such knowledge is possible through a tacit capacity that allows one to sense the unity or wholeness of something from an understanding of the individual qualities or parts' (pp. 20–21), and that 'Intuition makes possible the perceiving of things as wholes' (p. 23). Thus, if we can see only a part of someone—or, more accurately, *as* we can only see only a part—such as a crescent moon, we can know that it is a part of whole, and intuit that which is obscured.

I am interested in Stern's use of the image of the moon and of the word 'obscure', which suggests being unseen rather than lacking light. Nevertheless, I think that the dark side—whether of the moon or the Force—is also a useful metaphor for implicit knowing; indeed, in some mythologies, religions, and wisdom traditions, the light (and known) comes from the dark (and unknown). For instance, in

Māori mythology, the second major myth cycle concerns te Pō—form, the dark, the night—the whakapapa (or genealogy) of which is:

> Na Te Kore Te Pō (from the void the night)
> Te Pō-nui (the great night)
> Te Pō-roa (the long night)
> Te Pō-uriuri (the deep night)
> Te Pō-kerekere (the intense night)
> Te Pō-tiwhatiwha (the dark night)
> Te Pō-te-kitea (the night in which nothing is seen)
> Te Pō-tangotango (the intensely dark night)
> Te Pō-whawha (the night of feeling)
> Te Pō-namunamu-ki-taiao (the night of seeking the passage to the world)
> Te Pō-tahuri-atu (the night of restless turning)
> Te Pō-tahuri-mai-ki-taiao (the night of turning towards the revealed world).
>
> (see Walker, 1990)

I suggest that these nuanced descriptions of the night offer a rich sense of implicit knowing—whether in the consulting room or the whare nui (meeting house); in therapy or everyday life; in awakening or dreamtime; in the morning, afternoon, evening, or night. Moreover, the heuristic discovery of this implicit knowing relies not on the truth being 'out there' and discoverable through the use of a telescope or microscope, but, rather, 'in here' and discoverable through a self-reflective lens.

A phenomenological view of psychotherapeutic experience

The third title Stern considered for his book refers to the philosophical basis of his work. In the Introduction to *The Present Moment*, Stern (2004) states that:

> change is based on lived experience. In and of itself, verbally understanding, explaining, or narrating something is not sufficient to bring about change. There must also be an actual experience, a subjectively lived happening. An event must be lived, with feelings and actions taking place in real time, in the real world, with real people.
>
> (p. xiii)

He refers to this as the 'basic assumption' (of his work), a phrase that points to the methodology of his method, that is, that it is experiential and phenomenological—which, as denominators in common with TA, form another theoretical connection between Stern and Berne. From phenomenological philosophy, Stern acknowledges the importance of now, of taking directly lived experience in the present as a starting point, and of 'consciousness, rather than the unconscious, [being] the key mystery' (p. xv).

Stern puts forward the idea of the present moment 'to deal with the problem of "now"' (p. 3), and emphasises the importance of now for three reasons:

1. Because, Stern argues, 'we are subjectively alive and conscious only *now. Now* is when we directly live our lives' (p. 3). Berne (1964/1968a) expresses something similar when he asserts that 'Awareness requires living in the here and now, and not in the elsewhere, the past or the future' (p. 179). Here I offer a brief example of what Stern (2004) refers to as a 'phenomenologic perspective' on how things appear to consciousness, 'as they seem when they are in mind':

As I write this, right now, at 11:41 on 13th October 2018, looking out from the window of my practice room in Titirangi (West Auckland), my eyes move from the screen of my laptop, down to the keyboard, back to the screen, and then out to the beautiful view out over the Manukau Harbour, and back down again. My stomach rumbles. I take another sip of the rich black coffee I am drinking. My stomach rumbles again. I think about lunch, another hour away. Maybe I shouldn't drink more coffee. I do like it, however; I take another sip. My stomach stops rumbling. Good. I'll have another drop of coffee before midday (which is my cut off point for drinking anything with caffeine in it). I do my usual thing of taking a mini break while I'm on a roll (in terms of writing) so that I know that I will be able to continue on my roll after the break. I take my shoes off. I love walking in bare feet, especially outside in public areas. I feel grounded.

As I settle back, I re-read and review the previous paragraph. I type in a comma after 'rich' and then take it out again.[6] At Junior School (in the UK in the early 1960s), I was taught to put in a comma after the first or two or more adjectives; these days it appears that you only insert commas in longer lists of adjectives. I wonder when it changed. I text my daughter to check if she's OK. She hasn't got my previous messages. I resend them. I go back (seven sentences) and insert the parenthesis '(in the UK in the early 1960s)'. I notice the movement between myself (my thoughts, bodily sensations, my feelings), the external world (the view, my daughter), and thinking about writing for the reader and explaining the context of place (Titirangi) and time (the early 1960s), a thought which represents a present concern about a future moment in time. I come back to my stomach which is enjoying the coffee and telling me that I'm on my limit. I look at the time. It's 12:02. Wow, that's uncanny. I wonder if I can include a picture in this text, but then think that maybe I already have. My iPhone buzzes: my latest message to my daughter has been sent but my previous messages still haven't been. This particular past is still waiting to be sent, in the future... I change the order of the parts of this chapter. It's time for lunch. I put my shoes on. I feel sad. It's 12:28—or at least it was!

In addressing the problem—or, perhaps better, meeting the challenge—of living what is now in our lives, we might think about this as helping us to focus as much on the 'is' as the 'now'. This radical focus on the present addresses one of Hilman's criticisms of therapy: 'Why can't therapy be interested in each hour as it appears and not try to thread those hours together into what's called a process, a journey, [or] developmental growth?' (in Hilman & Ventura, 1992, p. 241).

2. Because 'therapeutic work in the "here and now" has the greatest power in bringing about change' (Stern, 2004, p. 3).

   This is what Eckhart Tolle (1997) refers to as *The Power of Now*. Stern (2004) describes this as 'where and when mutually aware contact between the minds of the therapist and patient takes place' (p. 3), though I also notice this in an educational/training context in which the most powerful learning/teaching takes place when and as a result of reflecting on exchanges or transactions that take place in the here-and-now in the classroom/group, exchanges which, of course are often concerned with and or influenced by the there-and-then— and the over-there. Stern himself draws on the work of Edmund Husserl in phenomenology especially with regard to his use of the concept of epoché (cessation), a process of suspending judgement or setting aside assumptions, in this case, about the present, precisely in order to *be* in the present, which is why co-creative TA emphasises the importance of present-centred relating, therapeutic or otherwise (Summers & Tudor, 2000). This perspective has influenced my own work with clients in which, as I am interested in the present, I pay attention to when a client is experiencing something, that is, that they are *in* their experience, as distinct to talking *about* their experience in a way that explains it away. In practice, I seek to help clients focus on their experience, often doing this by asking them to pause (before rushing into an explanation), and, I realise, often indicating this by an accompanying gesture of my hands that indicates an enclosing bracket and some containment. As Stern (2004) puts it:

> *The present moment is not the verbal account of an experience.* It is the experience as originally lived. It provides the raw material for a possible later verbal reasoning....
>   *The felt experience of the present moment is whatever is in awareness now, during the moment of being lived.* On this point we must return to the phenomenological perspective. The content of a present moment is simple— it is what is on the mental stage now.
>
> (p. 32)

This focus on the present doesn't mean that, as a therapist, I ignore the impact of the past or the client's history, or that I don't work with the past (Parent and Child ego states). I do; however, my interest in the past is as the—or a—history of the present. Foucault explained this concept to an interviewer in 1984: 'I set out from a problem expressed in the terms current today and I try to work out its genealogy. Genealogy means that I begin my analysis from a question posed in the present' (quoted in Kritzman, 1988, p. 262).

3. Because, while psychodynamic theories of therapeutic change have emphasised the role of the past in determining present, as Stern (2004) puts it: 'we have not paid the same attention to the nature of present experience as it is being influenced and is happening' (p. 4).

Later in his book, Stern writes about forms of the past that encounter unfolding events in and of the present, stating that:

> The present comes under much control of the past, and the past may be realized or altered or even surprized by the present. Equally, the present determines which pieces of the past will be chosen to be reanimated and assembled.
>
> (p. 31)

Stern cites as examples of forms of the past schemas, representations, models, and so on, to which, from a TA perspective, I would add: unhelpful and unhealthy transactions; Introjected Parent and Archaic Child ego states; self-limiting scripts; and negative games. This particular aspect of Stern's work has also influenced co-creative TA, I would say, especially its emphasis on present-centred development (Tudor & Summers, 2000). Žvelc (2009, 2010) uses the concept of 'relational schemas' in two articles in which he integrates Stern's ideas with TA.

Kairos

The nature of time has preoccupied human beings for as long as we have existed, and has been explored by theologians and philosophers, determined by scientists and politicians, and analysed by psychologists and psychotherapists. From Greek, we derive two words for time: kairos, which is usually translated as appropriate time, and chronos, from which we get chronological time, or clock time (see Tudor, 2001, 2002a, 2008e). Reflecting on the present moment, Stern (2004) acknowledges that 'Another feature... that intrigued me was that it has psychological work to do. It has to chunk and make some sense of the moment as it is passing, not afterwards. It has to lean toward a next action' (p. xv). Hence he draws on the concept of kairos, which he describes as follows:

> *Kairos* is the passing moment in which something happens as the time unfolds. It is the coming into being of new state of things, and it happens in a moment of awareness. It has its own boundaries and escapes and transcends the passage of linear time. Yet it also contains a past. It is a subjective parenthesis set off from chronos. *Kairos* is a moment of opportunity, when events demand action or are propitious for action.
>
> (p. 7)

More specifically, Stern draws on Edmund Husserl's proposal that the present moment has a duration and consists of three parts:

• A present-of-the-present-moment—a present instant of chronos, the passing point of moving time.

- A past-of-the-present-moment—an immediate past that is still echoing (and which, therefore, doesn't need to be recalled), which Husserl referred to as retention.[7]
- A future-of-the-present-moment—which Stern (2004) describes as 'the immediate future, which is anticipated or is implied in what has already occurred during the past- and present-of-the-present-moments' (p. 27).

Reflecting on this, Stern suggests that: 'the most essential point about this three-part present moment is that all of its parts stand together, subjectively, as a single, unified, coherent, global experience occurring in a subjective now.' (p. 27). This equally describes the integrating Adult—or, at least, how I think of the integrating Adult or neopsyche (Tudor, 2003b): a powerful metaphor for a constantly evolving co-creative personality that is processing the present, past, and future in the here-and-now. Neville (2018) articulates this from a person-centred perspective, arguing that the 'self', 'with which we are inclined to identity, is simply our recollection of our past moments of experience, a recollection which, of course, is part of our current moment of experience' (see Neville & Tudor, 2024, and Chapter 7).

The moment of meeting

Stern's (2004) penultimate working title acknowledges the importance of intersubjectivity and, as he puts it, 'the nature of cocreativity and the enlargement of the intersubjective field that served as the main context of the changes in treatment' (p. xvi). He is interested in 'the small momentary events that make up our worlds of experience' (p. xi) and 'when these moments enter one's awareness and are shared between two people'. He continues: 'These lived experiences make up the key moments of change in psychotherapy and the nodal points in our everyday intimate relationships' (p. xi). He also suggests that 'The moment is a whole happening, a gestalt. The psychological subject matter is the whole, not small units to make it up' (p. 14).

Some years before Stern, Rogers (1959) wrote a paper on 'The essence of psychotherapy' in which he refers to 'moments of movement' and such a moment as a 'molecule' of therapy and personality change (p. 53). For Rogers, such moments are existential, experiential, integrated, physiological, complete, real, and acceptable (see also Tudor, 2008e). Developing Rogers' ideas, O'Hara (1999) (who was influenced by both person-centred and gestalt psychology) applies what she refers to as 'moments of eternity' (p. 63) to brief therapy, a perspective which offers a challenge to the notion that effective psychotherapy has to be long-term. For Guglielmotti (2008), such moments require a real relationship (for further discussion of which, see the next part of the chapter); as she puts it: 'A real relationship cures and leads to intense experiential "meeting moments"' (p. 104).

Stern (2004) himself argues that intersubjectivity in itself constitutes 'a major motivational system essential for human survival—akin to attachment or sex' (p. xvi), and that it reflects a new form of consciousness, 'a form of reflectivity arising when we become conscious of our contents of mind by virtue of their be-ing simultaneously reflected back to us from the mind of another' (p. xvi). I think this is a beautiful description of the methodology of therapy and, specifically, its epistemology, that is, how we (come to) know what we know. Indeed, Stern (2004) discusses this with reference to awareness, 'a mental focusing on an object of expe-rience' and consciousness, 'the process of being aware that you are aware' (p. 123), both of which he views as a necessary condition for the present moment. This view of intersubjectivity, awareness, and consciousness also points to an ontology of therapy: that we are relational beings (Macmurray, 1957/1969, 1961/1991), dialog-ical beings (Buber, 1937; Frankl, 1963; Friedman, 1992; Levinas, 1982/1985), and beings who meet and encounter each other (Levinas, 1982/1985; Schmid, 2006).

In terms of therapeutic practice, such moments require the therapist to be open to all stimuli and fully present. Different theoretical approaches have various ways of conceptualising and practicing this, including Freud's (1912/1924) idea that the therapist needs to maintain 'the same "evenly-suspended attention"... in the face of all that one hears' (p. 111). Being fully present is implied and enhanced by the concept of contact in both gestalt and person-centred psychology, and is well-articulated in a recent volume on integrative psychotherapy by Žvelc and Žvelc (2021), who take a mindfulness- and compassion-oriented approach to their inte-gration of this form of therapy.

Having examined therapeutic relating from a present-centred perspective, I now broaden this enquiry to encompass the focus of therapy as described by Martha Stark in her book *Modes of Therapeutic Action* (Stark, 1999).

Modes of therapeutic action

In the introduction to her book, Stark (1999) acknowledges the influence of Steven Mitchell's (1988) work on *Relational Concepts in Psychoanalysis*, in which he synthesises three perspectives on the psychotherapeutic process: the drive–conflict model, the deficiency–compensation model, and the relational–conflict model. Drawing on Mitchell's taxonomy as well is the work of others, Stark identifies three models—or what she refers to as modes—of therapeutic action which she names as:

- Model 1—in which the therapeutic action or activity focuses on the enhance-ment of knowledge, and which Stark names as 'one-person psychology'.
- Model 2—in which the focus is on the provision of experience, which Stark names as 'one-and-a-half-person psychology.
- Model 3—in which the focus is on engagement in relationship, which Stark names as 'two-person psychology'.

In effect, each model describes a range of approaches to psychotherapy, mainly informed by psychoanalytic and psychodynamic thinking, 'though Stark also in-cludes some humanistic theorists such as Carl Rogers. However, in my view, the real strength of the model is the fact that it is a meta-model that offers a coherent (and still contemporary) categorisation of different therapeutic models, based on different conceptualisations of the perceived and/or experienced problem, the person of the patient or client, the goal of treatment and focus of therapeutic action, the person and role of the therapist, and the therapeutic relationship itself, all of which are summarised in Table 5.1. Stark herself views this as an integrative model, a position with which I disagree (see pp. 113–135 below). I think its importance is precisely in the delineation of differences and distinctions between the different models or modes. As Stark (1999) herself puts it, when discussing the difference between Models 1 and 2:

> I would like first to highlight the distinction between a drive–conflict model of therapeutic action that conceives of insight as the treatment of choice for the patient's structural conflicts and a deficiency–compensation model of therapeutic action that conceives of experience/relationships as the treatment of choice for the patient's structural deficits.
>
> (p. 8)

I have used Stark's meta-model to discuss different modes of empathy (Tudor, 2011g); other transactional analysts have drawn on her work to frame different 'Schools' of TA (Widdowson, 2010), and relationships relevant to ethics in clinical practice (Eusden, 2011). Indeed, according to Berlin (2019), Stark's approach 'has been widely accepted and integrated into the contemporary relational TA literature' (p. 169).

Table 5.1 summarises Stark's three modes,[8] as well as my own addition of a fourth mode (Tudor, 2011g), and includes different traditions or approaches to TA (updated from the previous chapter [see also Chapter 12]), following which I discuss in some more detail each of the modes with reference to different approaches within TA, especially with regard therapeutic relating, and conclude this part of the chapter with some comments and critiques of Stark's model.

One-person psychology

Influenced by Mitchell's (1988) work, Stark's (1999) first model is based on structural conflict, with the main goal of treatment being strengthening of the ego by way of insight. As Stark puts it:

> Whether expressed as (1) the rendering conscious of what had once been unconscious (in topographic terms); (2) where id was, there shall ego be (in structural terms); or (3) uncovering and reconstructing the past (in genetic terms), in Model 1 it is 'the truth' that is thought to set the patient free.
>
> (p. xv)

In this model and mode, the therapist is 'an objective observer of the patient' (p. xvi), which is why the principal example of therapeutic 'action' in this model is the interpretive model of classical psychoanalysis, though any therapeutic approach that focuses on the one-person of the patient or client and, as Stark puts it,

Table 5.1. Modes of therapeutic action

Model	Description Association (with approaches in TA)	Problem focus	The person of the patient/client	Goal of treatment/ Focus of therapeutic action	The person and role of the therapist	The therapeutic relationship
One-person psychology	The enhancement of knowledge, 'the interpretive model of classical psychoanalysis' (Stark, 1999, p. xv) Associated with Classical TA (psychodynamic), relational TA (psychodynamic)	On human nature; structural conflict; impaired capacity; relationships within the person	Patient (usually)	Strengthening of the ego through insight: the 'truth' sets the patient free, whether topographically, structurally, or genetically	As a neutral object, outside the therapeutic fields; an objective observer of the patient's internal dynamics	Patient/ client-centred; 'you' relationship; unidirectional, i.e., within[9]
One-and-a-half-person psychology	The provision of experience, for instance, based on self psychology (Morrison, 1994) Associated with Classical TA (cognitive behavioural), Cathexis reparenting (and rechilding), Redecision, and integrative TA	On nurture in the formative years, either the presence of bad (Fairbairn, 1954) or the absence of good (Balint, 1968); structural deficit	Patient or client as subject	Providing a corrective experience by way of the relationship between the patient and therapist	As an empathic self object, joining the patient 'in order to immerse herself in the patient's subjective reality' (p. 4); a good object or parent	An 'I–It' relationship; unidirectional, i.e., for
Two-person psychology	Engagement in relationship Associated with radical psychiatry, integrative TA, constructivist (narrative) TA, and relational TA (both psychodynamic and co-creative)	On enactments in the therapeutic relationship, both failures and ruptures	Client (more usually) or patient as intersubjective subject and agent, i.e., as proactive, and able to have an impact on the other	Focusing on the here-and-now interactive engagement, e.g., by changing the stroke economy in the relationship (Steiner, 1971c), or in terms of relational needs (Erskine, 1998)	As an authentic subject, centring on their own experience in order to deepen their understanding of the client	An 'I–Thou' relationship; or a 'Thou–I' relationship (Schmid, 2006); bidirectional, i.e., with, and between
Two-person-plus psychology	Engagement and action in relationship-in-context, and with the world Associated with radical psychiatry and EcoTA	On enactments in relationships in and with the world, and in the world itself	Client, person- and agent-in-context/ activist, i.e., as proactive, able to have an impact, and mindful of their environment	Acknowledging the social/ political dimension of therapy and its impact on the client, e.g., by changing the stroke economy in the client's world	As an authentic subject-in-context, centring on their own experience as well as that of others in order to deepen and widen their appreciation of the client-in-context— and of the context	'I-You-It', 'we-in-context' relationships; bidirectional; multidirectional, i.e., with, between and beyond

Based on Stark (1999), and developed from Tudor (2011g).

'the internal workings of her mind' (p. 3), would fall within this model. This is represented within TA by Berne's own interpretative understanding and style—after all, he himself undertook psychoanalytic training, which included training analyses with Paul Federn (1941–1943) and Erik Erikson (1947–1949). The influence and development of psychoanalytic and psychodynamic thinking in TA may be seen in Berne's own contribution to theory, i.e., ego states (from ego psychology) and games (repetition compulsion), and in the writing of Bob Drye (1980), Carlo Moiso (1990, 2000), Michele Novellino (1987, 1990, 2000, 2003, 2005, 2008, 2010, 2011), Bruce Loria (1990), Ken Woods (1995, 1996, 2003), Ulrike Müller (2000, 2002), Bill Cornell (2000, 2005, 2008, 2013, 2016), Helena Hargaden (2002, 2005), Charlotte Sills (2002), Ray Little (2005), Servaas van Beekum (2005, 2006, 2009, 2016), Maria Teresa Tosi (2008), Anna Emanuela Tangolo (2015), Jo Stuthridge (2015), and others.

In terms of practice, there are a number of methods and techniques in TA that are or can be delivered by the 'objective' transactional analyst/therapist to the patient or client, including:

- The bull's-eye operation (Berne, 1961/1975a), and the bull's-eye transaction (Karpman, 1971).
- All eight therapeutic operations (Berne, 1966a), i.e., interrogation, specification, confrontation, explanation, illustration, confirmation, interpretation, and crystallisation.
- Group rules (Berne, 1966a), which, by definition, are unilateral (see Chapter 2, n7).
- Allowers (Kahler with Capers, 1974).
- The carom transaction (Woollams & Brown, 1978).
- Mindfulness-based TA (Žvelc et al., 2011).[10]

In the context of the present discussion, I think it is particularly interesting and certainly significant that the therapeutic operations which, according to Berne (1966a) 'form the technique of transactional analysis' (p. 233) reflect the image of an analyst 'operating' with regard to the client, and specifically with regard to their ego states. Moreover, Berne's description of the operations, which he divides into two categories—interventions, which are those operations that intervene 'in the conflict between two ego states' (p. 364), and interpositions, which interpose something 'at the boundary between two ego states' (p. 365)—is highly technical, including 'do's, 'don't's, and caveats for the therapist, and there is no sense of a therapeutic relationship. In the light of research that acknowledges the importance of the therapeutic relationship, it is perhaps not surprising that, with some exceptions,[11] Berne's therapeutic operations are not discussed much in contemporary TA literature, although Hargaden and Sills (2002) transpose and reclaim them as empathic transactions, arguing that:

> It is not too difficult to recognize how Berne's style and use of language, steeped as it is in the 'masculine', with an emphasis upon 'manoeuvres', 'decoys' and

'smartness' and the supposed virtue of incisiveness (almost as though therapist and patient are engaged in a game of chess), could be shame inducing. This is another major reason for the emphasis upon the concept of transactions rather than operations.

(p. 117)

One might say, and given his psychoanalytic training, it is perhaps unsurprising, that, in TA, Berne focuses more on the analysis than the transactional.

Finally, on one-person psychology, and although their work would generally be more associated with one-and-a-half-person psychology (see Table 5.1 and the next section, below), in advocating the view that the power is in the patient, Robert (Bob) and Mary Goulding (1975/1978) were, in effect, representing a one-person psychology. Bob Goulding puts (t)his philosophy succinctly: 'I see the power being in the patient, not in the therapist, and that the therapist's real job is to *allow* the patient to find his own power, and to put that power to use in a service, not a dis-service' (in R. L. Goulding & M. M. Goulding, 1975/1978, p. 10). He contrasts this approach to what he saw as Eric Berne's overemphasis on the scripting of patients by their parents and reports challenging him about this regarding the autonomy of the individual. I agree with Goulding's critique of Berne but would equally apply this to his own overemphasis on a kind of reified view of individualised power in the patient, and, more seriously, the unexamined assumption that the therapist still has the power to 'allow' the patient's discovery, and, therefore, prefer to view the power as *in the relationship* (see below).

One-and-a-half-person psychology

In contrast to Model 1 which is based on structural conflict, Stark's Model 2 is based on structural deficit, that is, 'an impaired capacity to be a good parent unto herself' (Stark, 1999, p. xviii); and, whereas the focus of therapy in Model 1 thera-pies is on the enhancement of knowledge, in Model 2 therapies it is on the provi-sion of experience, and, specifically, a corrective or different experience. As Stark (2004) puts it:

When the etiology shifted from nature to nurture, so, too, the locus of the thera-peutic action shifted from insight by way of interpretation to a corrective experi-ence by way of the real relationship (that is, from within the patient to within the relationship between patient and therapist).

(p. xvii)

Stark herself cites self psychology and object relations as informing the theory and practice of 'the therapist's restitutive provision' (p. xvii) although, I and others would argue that humanistic psychology and its various therapies have also contributed to our understanding of the importance of this aspect of the therapeutic relationship, notably Carl Rogers and his theory of the necessary and sufficient conditions of therapy (Rogers, 1957, 1959), and, not least, ideas and practice developed within TA. These include:

- Permission (Crossman, 1966) and the permission transaction.
- Reparenting (Schiff & Schiff, 1971; J. Schiff et al., 1975).
- Spot reparenting (Osnes, 1974).
- Stroke city/Trashing the stroke economy (Schwebel, 1974).
- The Parent interview (McNeel, 1976).
- Parent resolution (Dashiell, 1978).
- The developmentally needed relationship (Barr, 1987).
- Rechilding (Clarkson & Fish, 1988).
- The reparative relationship (Clarkson, 1993).
- Relational needs (Erskine, 1998).
- Empathic transactions, including holding as an empathic operation (Hargaden & Sills, 2002).

From this list, it is clear that the provision of experience—corrective, developmentally needed, reparative, and, in any case, different (in a positive way)—can take many forms; indeed, this list represents concepts and practice across a number of approaches to TA, i.e., Classical, Cathexis, radical psychiatry, Redecision, and integrative (see also Chapter 12).

One of the key techniques in such provision is empathy, which, in recent times and in a Western intellectual context, derives both from person-centred psychology (Rogers and others) and self psychology (Kohut and others), and, as such, takes different forms (for a description and analysis of which see Tudor & Worrall, 2006; Tudor, 2011g). In TA, empathy as a provision of experience is most associated with the work and empathic transactions of Clark (1991), Erskine and his associates (Erskine, 1993; Erskine et al., 1999), and Hargaden and Sills (2002).

Another way of thinking about this provision is to focus on the environment in which transactions take place. Bob Goulding concludes the short chapter in which he critiques Berne (as noted above) by suggesting that:

> the therapist's job is to create an environment in which that person can make new decisions in his life and get out of a script—to live autonomously, responding to the new environment in a way appropriate for this time and place, not hanging onto old feelings from the past, and looking for reasons to justify them.
> (R. L. Goulding & M. M. Goulding, 1975/1978, p. 11)

The view of the therapist's role as creating—or, I prefer, co-creating—an environment that supports new decisions and, ultimately, new ways of relating is close to Rogers' (1957, 1959) theory of the necessary and sufficient conditions of personality change, and, thereby, reflects more of a one-and-a-half-person psychology (Tudor, 2011d).

Commenting on recent developments in TA ego state theory that have emphasised intersubjective and relational models (e.g., Fowlie & Sills, 2011; Hargaden & Sills,

2002; Tudor & Summers, 2014), Anthony (2018) suggests that 'One consequence of this reconceptualisation has been to obscure some of the therapist's parental functions and the potential value of parental transactions in the therapeutic process' (p. 365). He continues: 'These major contributions have undoubtedly facilitated a significant new approach with benefits for the TA psychotherapy practitioner', viewing them correctly as 'arguments against emphasizing techniques' (p. 365). 'However', he argues,

> at the same time, this emphasis on reconsidering transactional analysis concepts in a two-person self-in-relationship context leaves unaddressed various questions regarding the practical operation of Parent functions in the therapy room: Are parental interventions useful? If so, when? How might clients understand and respond to such transactions? Are such transactions always in the domain of one- or one-and-[a-]half-person therapeutic processes?
>
> (pp. 365–366)

In terms of my own practice, to these questions I would say, respectively, 'No, and, therefore no', 'As parental ones', and 'Yes'. More importantly, however, I suggest that the answers depend on your model of ego states, and how you view and work with the parental/Parental metaphor (Lomas, 1987/2001). Thus, while Anthony attributes a number of contributions to the therapeutic process to the therapist's Parent ego state—namely, boundary setting, permission giving, and modelling—I would see these as equally, though differently, attributable to the integrating Adult ego state (see Tudor, 2003b, 2016b). Anthony attributes two other contributions—the object of attachment, and focus for transference—to the therapist's Parent ego state but, here, again, it depends on how you think about objects, attachment, transference, and the nature of psychotherapy. Simply put, if you hold a three ego state model of health (for both client and therapist), then it follows that you may well conceptualise the client's desire for attachment and the understanding of transference, along with boundary setting, permission giving, and modelling as Child–Parent and Parent–Child transactions. If, however, you have a one (integrating Adult) model of health, then you would not foster Child–Parent attachment or transference. I'm not saying I'm right or that I'm right for all therapists; I'm more interested in being theoretically and philosophically consistent—and in fostering consistency (to which I hope this book contributes). This is why I don't agree with Anthony's accusation that, in developing intersubjective and relational theory, I and others have obscured some of the therapist's parental functions, but would assert that, rather, I/we have shed light on different ideas about Parental—and, for that matter, Child—transactions, and, thereby, have unobscured them.

Two-person psychology

In terms of the history of Western psychology, Stark's Model 3 represents what is commonly referred to as 'the relational turn': in other words, a shift from a view that the patient is healed by insight and/or a corrective experience to one which asserts that what heals is 'interactive engagement with an authentic other' (Stark, 1999, p. xix). Psychoanalytic thinkers and practitioners date the relational turn to the work of Greenberg and Mitchell on *Object Relations in Psychoanalytic Theory*, published in 1983. I have argued that this dates back to the work of Jessie Taft (1933/1973), who coined the phrase 'relationship therapy'; Carl Rogers and others, who were researching and writing about the therapeutic relationship in the 1940s and 1950s (Tudor, 2022b)—and that the humanistic psychology movement of the 1950s and 1960s, which was founded in order to offer something different to psychoanalysis and behaviourism, was, in fact, the original relational turn in psychotherapy.

According to Stark (1999), 'in a relational model of therapeutic action, all experience is thought to be co-created, with contributions from both participants' (p. 209). She goes on to apply this to transference and countertransference:

> So, too, countertransference (which is the therapist's experience of the patient) is never just a story about the therapist; nor is the transference (which is the patient's experience of the therapist) ever just a story about the patient. Rather, both experiences involve the here-and-now of the therapeutic interaction.
>
> (p. 209)

So, whether the therapist is more informed by psychoanalytic/psychodynamic or humanistic thinking, we may be able to agree that therapeutic relating is co-created by client and therapist, takes place in and involves the present, and is processed in the present. Examples of this in TA include:

- Ego state diagnosis, specifically as it involves the client, in terms of determining the historical and phenomenological criteria, as originally identified and required by Berne (1961/1975a).
- Co-operative contracts (Steiner, 1974), and contracts and contracting in which the bilateral nature of contracts is emphasised (Rotondo, 2020; see also Chapter 2).
- Game theory that emphasises the bilateral nature of games (Hine, 1990; see also Chapter 11).
- Empathic transactional relating (Tudor, 2011b, 2011g).
- Taking permission (Tudor, 2016b) (as distinct from being given permission).

Stark summarises the difference between one-and-a-half and two-person psychology as follows: although, as she acknowledges, in the corrective provision/model, relationship is involved, 'it was more of an I–It than an I–Thou relationship—more a one-way relationship between someone who gave and someone who took than a two-way relationship involving give-and-take, mutuality, and reciprocity' (p. xviii). This relies on the genuineness or authenticity of the therapist and the client, as well as that of the relationship—and I suggest that, just as every client deserves a new theory, which Kramer (1995) wrote about Otto Rank's work, so every client deserves a new relationship. As Guglielmotti (2008) puts it, referring to Stern's work also with others: 'A real relationship cures and heals through intense experiential "meeting moments"' (pp. 103–104). This kind of relationship also relies on the attitude and intention of the therapist; in other words, that the therapist is focused on and in the relationship, not what they can correct or repair through the relationship. Thus, the therapeutic relationship may be one in which, Guglielmotti (2008) continues:

> the client's procedural unconscious experience can be reorganized through new experiences... [and] new forms of attachment enable the client to experience himself or herself in a new emotional climate with a new feeling of belonging and being together with the other... [which] allows him or her to overcome his or her emotional pain
>
> (p. 104)

—but, crucially, this is undertaken by the client, not the therapist. In terms of empathy, this is the difference between the empathic transaction as described by Hargaden and Sills (2002), with the *intentional* ulterior transaction from the Adult ego state of the therapist to the Child ego state of the client, and the empathic transactional relating of co-creative TA as I describe elsewhere (Tudor, 2011b), with no intentional ulterior transaction. I emphasise the word intentional as, commenting on this passage and the difference between Hargaden and Sills' (2002) model of the empathic transaction and my view of co-creative empathic transacting or relating (Tudor, 2011b), Gregor Žvelc (personal communication, 7 July 2023) asked how they differ—and for an example. Reflecting on Gregor's question, and reflecting on examples, I consider that the social level of therapist to client transactions could be exactly the same ('You look sad', 'That must have been difficult for you', etc.); the difference lies in the intentionality (the ulterior transaction)—and in the underlying model of ego states.

Writing about his different viewpoint on diagnosis, Rogers (1951) summarises this two-person psychology well:

> Therapy is basically the experiencing of the inadequacies in old ways of perceiving, the experiencing of new and more accurate and adequate perceptions, and the recognition of significant relationships between perceptions.
>
> In a very meaningful and accurate sense, therapy *is* diagnosis, and this diagnosis is a process which goes on in the experience of the client, rather than in the intellect of the clinician.
>
> (p. 223)

Two-person-plus psychology

In the original article in which I proposed this additional mode to Stark's taxonomy (Tudor, 2011g), I offered the following justification:

> Two-person psychology, psychotherapy, and other activities [that] help healing and change take place in a social context, and that social context has an evident

effect on what happens in the consulting room—and, indeed, even on whether the client gets to and continues to attend therapy. Furthermore, for some therapists... the context that clients bring into the consulting room is an important focus for therapy. Given the significance of client factors and extratherapeutic factors, and in acknowledgement of an interest in the social context of therapy... I propose a fourth mode of therapeutic action: a *two-person-plus psychology*. This phrase and mode acknowledges the significance and impact of these factors and of the social context of the client, the therapist, and the therapy—and of the therapist's and client's empathic relationship with such factors.

(p. 52)

Theory and practice that contribute to what I conceptualise as two-person-plus psychology, include: indigenous therapies; Marxist psychoanalysis; anti-psychiatry; radical therapy; red therapy; pink and queer therapy; social action psychotherapy; social therapy; ecotherapy; and wild therapy, for further details of and references to which, see Tudor & Begg (2016) and Tudor (2018b). Within TA, this form of psychology may be seen in the praxis of and writing about:

- Radical psychiatry (The Radical Therapy Collective, 1971; Steiner, 1975b; Wyckoff, 1976b).
- Social action (Schiff, 1975).
- Cultural scripting (White & White, 1975), cultural scripts (J. James, 1983a, 1983b), and their various applications since (for references to which, see Tudo, 2020g).
- Socially responsible therapy (Steiner, 1976), and social responsibility (Cornell & Monin, 2018).
- Racism (Batts, 1982, 1983).
- Nuclear disarmament (Trautmann, 1984).
- The Master–Slave relationship (English, 1987; Jacobs, 1991).
- Social applications (Novey, 1996).
- Gay and lesbian issues (Cornell & Simerly, 2004).
- Oppression (Rowland, 2016), and systemic oppression (Minikin & Rowland, 2022).
- Sexuality (Cornell & Shadbolt, 2009), gender, sexuality, and identity (McLean and Cornell, 2017).
- Normativity, marginality, and deviance (Deaconu & Rowland, 2021).
- EcoTA (Barrow & Marshall, 2023a; Marshall, 2021a, 2021b).[12]
- Intersectionality (Baskerville, 2022).

In this fourth mode of therapeutic action, the aetiology of a person's condition is primarily viewed as alienation—in its various forms (see Steiner, 1974; Tudor, 1997a), and, therefore, that focus of the therapeutic action, both in and outside the consulting room, is on disalienation (see Bulhan, 1979), and any and all therapeutic engagement that addresses this. For example, Rogers (1975/1980) argues that 'empathy dissolves alienation' (p. 151). This mode also acknowledges the importance of extra therapeutic factors that impact on the effectiveness of therapy (Lambert, 1992), such as the qualities of the client themselves, as well as their environment. Lambert himself notes that therapists need to 'draw upon the natural helping systems that are abundant in the environment to assist them in their efforts to improve psychological therapies' (p. 99), a comment that echoes Karen Horney's (1945/1999) statement that 'Life itself still remains a very effective therapist' (p. 240). Another aspect of this mode is the therapist's willingness and interest to work explicitly with material in and from the world outside the consulting room, including the client's own external world, as well as the external world of social and political events.

Echoing Starks' summary of her modes and models—enhancement of knowledge (Model 1), provision of experience (Model 2), and engagement in relationship (Model 3)—I would say that two-person-plus psychology (Model 4) is characterised by engagement and action in relationships-in-context and in the world (see Table 5.1). Using the word 'engagement' links this mode with two-person psychology, on which it builds, and, by including the word 'action', extends the sense and work of engagement to making an active difference in the world, whether in the immediate world of the client or the wider social/political world and environment. As the radical psychiatrists put it: 'therapy is about change not adjustment' (The Radical Therapy Collective, 1971, book cover). As I summarised this in the initial article, in this mode:

> The therapist pays attention to the client sense of connection with and/or disconnection from her or his world and belonging to and/or alienation from the world, including relationships with her or his faith, ancestors, and natural environment. Some therapists explore these relationships with the client by physically moving out of the frame of the consulting room into the environment [itself].
>
> (Tudor, 2011g, p. 53)

The model itself

Finally, I briefly consider the nature of Stark's model or meta-model.

Stark herself refers to her model as 'an integrative model of therapeutic action' (p. xv), and does so, I think, as she goes on to suggest that, in order to be 'optimally effective', the therapist 'must be able to work comfortably within all three models of therapeutic action—sometimes using first one approach, than another, sometimes using two or three approaches simultaneously' (p. xxiii). However—and whilst I respect Stark's ambition for therapists' skill(s) and effectiveness—there is a major problem with this perspective.

The problem or issue is that these different approaches or modes are significantly different—practically, theoretically, and philosophically—and, therefore, I would say, should be viewed as distinct (see also Berlin, 2019). Indeed, there are times when Stark herself presents them as distinct and not simultaneous, thus: 'the therapist can optimize her effectiveness if she has the capacity to hold in her mind an intuitive sense of whether the therapeutic action in the moment involves *knowledge, experience,* or *relationship*' (p. 5). Whilst I agree with Stark's intent 'to demonstrate the clinical usefulness for the therapist of *thinking* [emphasis added] in terms of enhancement of knowledge, provision of experience, and engagement in relationship as three primary agents for therapeutic growth and change' (p. xxiii), I think she underestimates the significance of the meta-theoretical assumptions underlying the different *practice* in these different modes.

These differences—and the disagreement about the extent to which these differences matter—are important not only with regard to Stark's integrative vision for her model but because, as Berlin (2019) points out:

> This [Stark's] approach has been widely accepted and integrated into the contemporary relational TA literature... [and has formed] the basis from which to TA practitioner believes that she or he may choose to move back and forth between a relational stance and a classical, redecision, or Cathexis one.

> (p. 169)

This question of being able to move back and forth between different approaches is of relevance within TA, as the descriptors of various criteria in three of the four (Level I) certifying examinations make specific references to the candidate's ability to conceptualise different TA theoretical concepts/models and to select and apply them to practice (see ITAA IBoC, 2022). This suggests that candidates understand both the differences between various concepts and models in TA, and, in terms of metaperspective and coherence (consistency) (terms that appear in descriptors of the rating scale(s) for the written exam in all four fields—see ITAA IBoC, 2022), also the underlying assumptions of concepts and between models.

As I acknowledge at the beginning of this part of the chapter, I consider one of the strengths of Stark's model is precisely its categorisation of distinct modes of therapeutic action and the distinctions it draws with regard to different aspects of therapeutic theory and practice. Elsewhere, I have suggested that the therapist's adoption of an 'all modes' approach can be confusing 'because there is a significant difference in the therapist's role, attitude and method between the modes... that may compromise the repertoire or at least make the transition between these modes more difficult for both therapist and client' (Tudor, 2011b, p. 326). For example, I would suggest that it is confusing to the patient that, at one moment, they would be seen as the source of their psychopathology, expressed as internal conflict (Model 1), while, at another moment or point in their therapy, the therapist would hold the patient's parents as responsible for their pathology, in terms of their failure of the child/patient (Model 2). In terms of the therapeutic relationship, it is confusing for the client for the therapist to position themselves outside the therapeutic field, as an objective, neutral therapist (Model 1) and, at the same or a later time, in the relational field, as a subjective or intersubjective engaged therapist (Model 3). Berlin (2019) also takes issue with Stark on her all modes approach, observing that 'changing from one model or mode to another would involve the therapist fundamentally changing her or his beliefs about the reality of the therapeutic relationship in order to make it fit with the therapeutic intervention choice' (p. 170) in addition to asking—and answering—the question 'Can a therapist ever choose to step outside therapeutic field?' In his excellent article, Berlin (2019) goes on to pose other questions that challenge other aspects of Stark's all modes, integrative approach: 'Can a therapist remain aware of and respond to countertransference in real time?', 'Can a therapist intention define which ego state she or he is in?', and 'Are differing TA conceptualisations of how change occurs compatible?'

Now, I would go further and, drawing on Steiner's (1981) point that 'every transaction has political consequences, every message has a meta-communication, a message about the message' (p. 171), suggest that it is anti-therapeutic to move across modes. For example, in the scenario where a client is working on (or through) their grief of the absence of a good parent in their childhood, Stark's modes provide us with different understandings of therapeutic actions—and the meta-communication of those actions, thus:

- A therapist working on the internal conflict that this loss evokes (Model 1) might focus on the distinction between mourning and melancholia (Freud, 1915/1984b). The meta-communication here would be something along the lines that this conflict (or confusion) lies within the patient and their past relationships, predominantly and most importantly with their parents, which, ultimately, is for them to resolve.
- A therapist working to provide a corrective or reparative experience for the client (perhaps on the basis that 'It's never too late to have a happy childhood') (Model 2) might invite the client to see them (the therapist) as a benevolent parent(al) figure who can provide and fulfil the client's attachment needs. The meta-communication here is that the patient or client is (more or less) dependent on the therapist's provision of this experience.
- A therapist working in an intersubjective and relational way (Model 3) might focus on how the client's grief, loss, and anger is also expressed in the present therapeutic relationship, and might share some of her own experience of this. The meta-communication here is that the client can rely on the therapist's present engagement in the relationship.
- A therapist working in an intersubjective, relational, and contextual way (two-person-plus psychology [Model 4]) might acknowledge the client's experience of grief and loss in the world, perhaps linking this to some social/political world events to which the client has referred. The meta-communication here is that the client can connect with and rely on people, places, and objects in the world to resolve their grief and/or to accept that grieving is part of a continuing bond with the loved object/subject; and that grief doesn't preclude their engagement with(in) the present (and) in the world.

From even these brief summaries, it is clear that these different modes represent different and differing paradigms, in terms of ontology (the essence of things, including human beings and, therefore, human nature), and epistemology (theories of knowledge), methodology (theories and philosophy of practice), as well as the method (practice itself).

Summary

In this chapter, I have explored the importance of the present moment as a way of working therapeutically and transactionally, and suggested that, as transactional analysts, we bring our analytic skills to bear on analysing *with* our clients our ways of being-with each other and, therefore, not our (therapeutic) relationship but, rather, our ways of relating therapeutically. In this sense, to paraphrase but contra Berne, I would say that: transactions were first systematically studied by transactional analysis, and they are its foundation stones and its mark. Whatever deals with the analysis of transactions is transactional analysis, and whatever overlooks them is not.

Notes

1 In her work in eco-TA, Marshall (2001b) puts this more fundamentally when she writes: 'The ecological self is also relevant in our more present-centred *being* [emphasis added] in the world—those ways in which we are constantly incorporating the life around us' (p. 34).

2 In fact, Clarkson's taxonomy of relationships is based on Gelso and Carter (1985) who identified the three elements of the therapeutic relationship as the working alliance, the real relationship, and the unreal relationship, and on Barr's (1987) identification of the reparative or developmentally needed relationship, to which Clarkson added the transpersonal relationship; thus, the citation to this model should rightly read 'Gelso & Carter, Barr, & Clarkson'.

3 In that article I identified the methodology of co-creative transactional analysis as 'certainly phenomenological and arguably hermeneutic' (p. 326), and the principal method as transacting empathically. Specifically, I identified as methodology, that the therapist works in partnership with the client; that the therapist works with what is present in what is past in the present; and that the therapist works with the client's present-centred neopsychic functioning/integrating Adult. Also, I proposed in terms of method, that the therapist facilitates the client in expanding their neopsychic functioning; that the client abstracts empathic knowledge from the experience of their emotional resonance at both social (conscious) and ulterior (unconscious) levels; that, when this present-centred process is interrupted in whatever way, the therapist and/or client re-experiences some past relational patterns; and that, when the client expands their Adult, in effect, they decontaminate and/or deconfuse their Introjected Parent and Archaic Child ego states.

4 For some further details about my work with this client, see Tudor and Worrall (2006).

5 My daughter, who is very direct, introduced me to a variation on this ('No, but...'), when, as a teenager, she used to say: 'No offence, but...', a statement which, of course, signalled that what she was about to say was likely to give offence!

6 No doubt inspired by Oscar Wilde, who is reported to have said that: 'I was working on the proof of one of my poems all the morning, and took out a comma.... In the afternoon—well, I put it back again' (see Cooper, 2022).

7 Carroll (1872/2021) expresses this well when he says, through the character of Alice: 'I could tell you my adventures—beginning from this morning,' said Alice a little timidly: 'but it's no use going back to yesterday, because I was a different person then.'

8 I am aware that, since the publication of her book on *Modes of Therapeutic Action*, Stark has formulated another two other models (Stark, 2016, 2017, 2021): model 4, which she describes as 'the existential-humanistic perspective' (Stark, 2021, p. 34), and model 5, 'a quantum-neuroscientific approach to symptomatic relief and behavioral change' (p. 42). However, these additions (to which she refers as both models and modes), are part of her 'Psychodynamic Synergy Paradigm' (p. 12) and, therefore, do not constitute part of a meta-model, which is why I do not include them in this present work and analysis.

9 In designating this and the other prepositions to the different therapeutic relationships, I follow (for the most part) Stark (2021) when she writes: 'the preposition *within* (Model 1), *for* (Model 2), *with* (Model 3), *between* (Model 4) and *beyond* (Model 5) are specifically designed to speak, roughly, to the directionality of the therapeutic action' (p. 29).

10 I place this here as, according to G. Žvelc (personal communication, 7 July 2023), 'mindfulness-based TA involves mindfulness meditation practice, which is more one-person concept', while mindfulness- and compassion-oriented integrative psychotherapy (Žvelc & Žvelc, 2021), with its emphasis on co-creation and the importance of present relating, would clearly be a two-person psychology.

11 As supervisory operations (Tudor, 2002c), as educational operations (Joseph, 2012), and as therapeutic transactions in clinical work with children (Morena, 2019).

12 Although never formally part of the TA community, Beth Roy, an early radical psychiatrist, did add to Steiner and Wyckoff's (1975) formulation of alienation (from our body, our mind, and our love), that of our alienation from the Earth (Roy, 1988).

Chapter 6

The state of the ego

Then and now (2010)

This chapter considers the state of ego state theory in transactional analysis (TA). Based on the hypothesis that there is a confusion in practice and the TA literature based on different and differing structural models of ego states, I clarify Berne's concept of the ego and of ego states by drawing on the earlier work of Federn (1952d), Weiss (1950), and Glover (1955). Following the work of Trautmann and Erskine (1981), Erskine (1988, 1991), Gobes (1990), Oller-Vallejo (1997, 2003), and Wadsworth and DiVincenti (2003), and a close reading of Berne's (1961/1975a) *In Psychotherapy*, I clarify the distinction between two sets of structural ego state models with regard to definitions of ego states, theories of human development, the concept of integration, and views about the goal or end of therapy. While the chapter is informed by my work as a clinician, the clarification of the two sets of models, and especially the differing views of the Adult, has implications for all applications of TA.

Transactional Analysis in Psychotherapy was Berne's (1961/1975a) first statement about TA in which he outlines 'a unified system of individual and social psychiatry' (p. 11). While the book fulfils its promise to outline 'a unified system', it also reflects some divergence—and some confusion—in Berne's thinking (at least as represented in the book) about the nature of ego states, in particular and most significantly the Adult ego state, and about the nature of integration. Stewart (1992) comments on Berne's inconsistency with regard to definitions of ego states and, with reference to Berne's contribution of ego states, Oller-Vallejo (1997) acknowledges that there are 'conceptual inconsistencies and confusion in Berne's writing' (p. 290). Most differences and disagreements among transactional analysts about ego states and their implications for practice can be traced back to *Transactional Analysis in Psychotherapy* and, therefore, Berne's text warrants further study and heuristic analysis. This chapter represents an attempt to outline, clarify, and acknowledge these inconsistencies and confusion as they influence and impact how, as transactional analysts, we think about ego states and human development, what integration is and, therefore, how we conceptualise and practice TA not only as psychotherapists but as practitioners in all fields of application. I suggest that the identification of the two sets of models helps to resolve, or at least clarify, certain debates and controversies.

DOI: 10.4324/9780429398223-9

The first part of the chapter places Berne's contribution in the context of the work of Federn (1952d), Weiss (1950), and Glover (1955). While transactional analysts may be relatively familiar with Federn and Weiss through Berne's reference to their work, Glover's work on the ego is perhaps less well known. Based on a close reading of *Transactional Analysis in Psychotherapy*, the second part of the chapter outlines what I refer to as two 'sets' of ego state models and, with reference to Berne's (1961/1975a) text, elucidates the differences between these different conceptualisations with regard to ontology (the 'essence' of being, in this case, of ego states), development (i.e., human development), and 'cure' or the ideal(ised) end of therapy, as well as integration and functioning. The third part of the chapter considers some of the differences and confusions in the literature on these aspects of theory, addresses some points made by Oller-Vallejo (1997, 2003) on these two sets of models, and takes issue with the primacy that Oller-Vallejo (2003) has given to one ego state model. The then and now of the title refers not only to the sense of historical review in the context of the special issue (of the *Transactional Analysis Journal* in which this chapter was first published), but also and specifically, to the view that in the integrating Adult model—James and Jongeward (1971), Erskine (1988), Erskine and Moursund (1988), Trautmann and Erskine (1999), Lapworth et al. (1993), and Tudor (2003b)—the Parent and Child ego states represent the 'then' or 'there and then', while the integrating Adult represents the 'now' or 'here and now'.

The ego and its states

From the Latin word for 'I', the ego is conceptualised, at least from psycho-analytic and psychodynamic perspectives, as the central core around which all psychic activities revolve and resolve. In classical psychodynamic theory, the ego represents both a cluster of conscious cognitive and perceptual processes, such as memory and problem solving, as well as specific defence mechanisms that serve to mediate between the id and the superego. Berne's conceptual-isation of ego states and ego state analysis stands in this tradition and the subsequent development of ego psychology (see Chapter 7). In his book on conceptual domains of psychoanalysis (that is, drive, ego, object, and self), Pine (1990) acknowledges both Hartmann (1939/1958) (whose earlier work in the early 1920s was published in German) and Freud (1937/1964) as hav-ing offered theories of ego development that were the early seeds of an ego psychology.

Drawing originally on a biological metaphor, Berne (1961/1975a) describes as-pects of human mental activity as 'organs' or, more precisely, 'psychic organs' whose function is to organise external and internal material. Berne drew on and ac-knowledged both Federn's (1952d) work identifying states of the ego and Weiss's (1950) clarification of ego psychology: 'Every ego state is the actually experienced reality of one's mental and bodily ego with the contents of the lived-through pe-riod' (Berne, 1961/1975a, p. 141).

The discrepancy in chronology between Federn's (earlier) work and Weiss's is due to the fact that the majority of Federn's early work was published in German; indeed, only 17 out of 80 of his publications between 1901 and 1938 were published in English, compared with all but two of 16 works published between 1940 and 1952. His pupil and later colleague, Eduard Weiss, organised the editing and posthumous publication of a collection of Federn's work, including unpublished papers, and thus the reference to Federn (1952d). Although Federn had published papers in English on various aspects of the ego in 1926, 1928, 1932, 1934, and 1949, Berne's (1961/1975a) references to Federn were based on the volume of collected papers, and his knowledge of Weiss's (1950) work, as well as his own contact with Federn, with whom he was in analysis in New York between 1941 and 1943. However, it is also clear that Berne was familiar with Federn's earlier work on the nervous system (Federn, 1938) as Berne cites this in an early paper published in 1949 (Berne, 1949/1977f) (for further discussions of which see Tudor, 2003b; and Chapter 7).

Insofar as the concept of ego states is a part analysis of the personality—that is, one based on the conceptualisation of parts—its lineage can be traced back to the work of Glover (1932/1956b, 1943/1956a). Berne was clearly aware of Glover's (1955) work as he cited him in *Transactional Analysis in Psychotherapy*, although Berne's citation and note links Glover's statements on transference neurosis with the idea of script; Berne does not mention Glover's work on the ego. Elsewhere, Berne (1972/ 1975b) acknowledges Federn as 'the first psychoanalyst... to make a specific study of internal dialogues' (p. 273); he also acknowledges what Federn (1934/1952a) refers to as 'a mental duologue between two parts of the ego' (p. 93), in this case, 'the adult and the infantile, with its different stages and results being visually represented' (p. 93). Both Federn (1929/1952b) (in a chapter based on a paper read before the Vienna Psychoanalytic Society in 1928) and Weiss (1950) also cite Glover, although each only with one passing reference. Nevertheless, the antecedents are there. Glover identifies the 'ego system' or 'ego-nucleus' (1932/1956b) and, later, the 'ego-nuclei' (1943/1956a) and defines them with regard to their dynamic function in terms that prefigure Berne's later descriptions:

> Theoretically an ego-nucleus can be defined as a psychic organization which (a) represents a positive relation to the objects of any important instinct, (b) secures the discharge of reactive tension consequent on frustration by objects of that instinct, (c) promotes the relation to reality through gratifying impulses of self-preservation, and (d) in one or other of these ways reduces anxiety within the psyche.
>
> (pp. 316–317)

Glover (1943/1956a) goes on to state that 'although these nuclei have a good deal in common, *they have in their earliest phases a partial autonomy*' (p. 317) that derives from the fact that not all self-preservative drives have the same object, a point that is consistent with and anticipates Berne's distinction between the Child and the

Parent ego states. Glover also writes about a nucleus being able '*to seize the psychic apparatus and occupy the approaches to perceptual consciousness*' (p. 318), a statement that finds echoes in Berne's (1961/1975a) view that an ego state has 'executive power', by which it has psychic energy or cathexis, and that each ego state 'gives rise to its own idiosyncratic patterns of organized behavior' (p. 75).

Berne takes Weiss's (1950) definition of an ego state as 'the actually experienced reality of one's mental and bodily ego with the contents of the lived-through period' (p. 141) and his tripartite division of the ego (see below) and adopts Federn's (1929/1952b) observation that the person could experience either a current ego state or a past one. Berne, however, makes one main amendment to Federn's model: as well as being experienced internally or intrapsychically, each category of ego states is shown in a distinctive set of behaviours (see Stewart, 1992).

For his own part, Berne (1961/1975a) defines ego states 'phenomenologically as a coherent system of feelings related to a given subject, and operationally as a set of coherent behavior patterns, or pragmatically, as a system of feelings which motivates a related set of behavior patterns' (p. 17). So far, so good—or, at least, so far, so consistent. The confusion arises when Berne goes on to describe ego states in more detail.

In the early part of *Transactional Analysis in Psychotherapy*, Berne (1961/1975a) quotes Weiss (as noted above) and links this to the work and findings of Penfield, the surgeon and neuropathologist on whose work Berne drew. Berne argues that Weiss pointed out exactly what Penfield had proved, that is, in Berne's words, 'that ego states of former age levels are maintained in potential existence within the personality' (p. 19). What Weiss refers to as a sort of 'child ego', Berne names 'the Child ego state'; what Weiss refers to as a 'psychic presence' or 'the mental image of another ego', Berne names 'the Parent ego state'; and what Weiss refers to as the current ego state, Berne names 'the Adult ego state'. In this sense, Berne is simply dividing the personality into three denoted states of mind and their related patterns of behaviour and suggesting that all three exist as psychic organs (the archeaopsyche, the exteropsyche, and the neopsyche, respectively), phenomena, and substantives. Here Berne is implying what Novey (in Novey et al., 1993) refers to as the 'three-ego-state model' (p. 125) or, at least, a definition of ego states that supports the idea of the three ego states (Parent, Adult, and Child) as the total or complete personality and structure of personality (see Berne, 1961/1975a; Figure 6.1b; and Table 6.1).

Elsewhere in the same book, however, Berne (1961/1975a) refers to these different states more pejoratively, especially when he writes about ego states and their associated postures, manner, facial expressions, and other physical characteristics. At times he characterises—even caricatures—them as, in a particular instance, 'tittering coyness' (p. 30) (Child), 'primly righteous' (p. 30) (Parent), and as having an 'ability to think logically' (p. 30) (Adult). In a reference to the concept of a 'constant ego state', Berne caricatures clergymen as the Parent, diagnosticians as the Adult, and clowns as the Child. He refers to Child and Parent ego states as having an archaic quality 'inappropriate to the immediate reality' (p. 30) and compares these with the Adult ego state, in which a particular patient 'showed considerable skill in marshalling and processing data and perceptions concerning her immediate situation: what can easily be understood as "adult" functioning' and, in another passage, as 'rational reckoning' (p. 31).

Later, when discussing symptomatology, Berne (1961/1975a) refers to the Child as 'a purgatory, and sometimes a hell, for archaic tendencies' (p. 60), to hallucinations as exhibitions of the Parent, and to character disorders and psychopathies as manifestations of the Child. In this sense, Berne appears to imply that it is more desirable to be Adult. Indeed, he describes the Adult as 'characterized by an autonomous set of feelings, attitudes, and behavior patterns which are adapted to the current reality' (p. 76). Later, he refers to 'this "integrated" person [who] *is* charming, etc., and courageous, etc., in his Adult state, whatever qualities he has or does not have in his Child and Parent ego states' (p. 185). He clarifies what he means by this by way of a contrast in the next sentence: 'The "unintegrated" person may *revert to* being charming, and may feel that he *should* be courageous' (p. 195). Elsewhere, Berne refers to a patient who 'is able to feel and express the autonomous Adult anger and disappointment at her husband's behavior' (pp. 157–158), thus clearly acknowledging that the Adult ego state encompasses appropriate emotions. He also distinguishes Adult sexuality, in which:

> the sexual fantasies seemed to be free of pregenital elements. They were intrusive, considerate, and well adapted to the current reality possibilities of each situation; in principle they met the criteria for realistic genital sexual 'object interest', if not love, and they were based on healthy biological instinctual pressures. Since they were neither inhibitions nor archaic elements, they could not be regarded as anything but Adult, free from exterospsychic and archaeopsychic influences, and controlled by reality-testing.
>
> (p. 238)

This Bernean view of personality represents an approach to ego state theory that emphasises the Integrated Adult (Erskine, 1988, 1991) or integrating Adult (James & Jongeward, 1971; Trautmann & Erskine, 1999; Tudor, 2003b).

From this summary (see also Table 6.1), it is clear that Berne defines ego states in different ways and in ways that had—and have—different implications. An appreciation of this, as well as the controversies about ego state theory—see Trautmann and Erskine (1981), Erskine et al. (1988), Novey et al. (1993), English (1998), and Novey (1998)—and a number of conversations with Claude Steiner over the past five years, led me to undertake a close re-reading of *Transactional Analysis in Psychotherapy* in order to identify precisely what it was that Berne had written. (In undertaking the background research for this chapter, I discovered that this close reading paralleled a similar process undertaken by Steiner at the request of Trautmann and Erskine, as reported by Wadsworth and DiVincenti, 2003.) Tables 6.1, 6.2, 6.3, and 6.4 summarise this textual reading with regard to the differences as well as some similarities between the two sets of models in Berne's (1961/1975a) work. I refer to 'sets of models' because there are a number of models of ego states that fall under each 'set'.

Two sets of ego state models

In this heuristic research I have identified a number of areas of difference regarding ontology or the 'essence' or nature of things, in this case, the nature of ego states, summarised by means of different definitions of ego states (Table 6.1); human development (Table 6.2); integration (Table 6.3); and cure or the end result of therapy (Table 6.4).

Ontology

The ontology of things is often implicit in definitions. Table 6.1 summarises and draws out the ontological differences in the views of ego states in the two sets of models, that is, differences about the 'essence' or nature of ego states, illustrated by means of the different—and differing—definitions of ego states in general, and specifically of Adult, Parent, and Child ego states. In all the tables, all the quotes, unless otherwise stated, are taken from Berne (1961/1975a).

Central to these ontological distinctions is the question of whether Child and Parent ego states 'contain' archaic experiences and introjects that are script free (set 1 models) or whether the Child ego state is defined as comprising fixated material only and the Parent ego state introjected material only. Indeed, in the interests of clarifying such distinctions between the models (or sets of models), Oller-Vallejo (2003) makes a plea for proponents of the Integrated/integrating Adult model to use terms such as 'integrating ego', 'introjected ego', and 'fixated ego' as substitutes for Adult, Parent, and Child ego states—which some of us do (see Figure 6.1b). As far as the Adult is concerned, the issue is whether it is viewed as a residual state left over after all the elements of Child and Parent have been detected and, according to Berne (1961/1975a), is concerned only 'with the earthly realities of objective living' (p. 60) (Table 6.1, set 1), or whether it is an expansive ego state that 'characterises a pulsating personality, processing and integrating feelings, attitudes, thoughts and behaviours appropriate to the here-and-now—at all ages from conception to death' (Tudor, 2003b, p. 201): in other words, the now (Adult) and the then (Child and Parent) (Table 1, set 2).

Figure 6.1b refers to Parent and Child ego states (plural). This follows Berne's view that there are three categories of ego states: Parent, Child, and, arguably, Adult, each of which refers to a plurality of feelings, attitudes, and behaviour patterns. As Stewart (1992) points out, 'The word "Child" on Berne's full definition does not refer to "one ego-state". It denotes a whole category of ego-states. All the ego-states in that category share one defining feature: they are archaic relics of the person's own childhood' (p. 26).

Table 6.1. Two sets of ego state models in TA: definitions

	Set 1 *Models representing the three ego states as the total or 'complete' personality*	Set 2 *Models representing the Integrated Adult/ integrating Adult*
Definition of ego states	**Similarities** 'The uniformity of a character rests on the existence of some firmly established, invariable ego states, in which the main boundaries are unchangeable as to their content and extent' (Federn, 1936/1952e, p. 332) 'The permanence of previous ego states extends Freud's concept of ego fixation to the field of normal psychology' (Federn, 1952c, p. 218) 'Every ego state is the actually experienced reality of one's mental and bodily ego with the contents of the lived-through period' (Weiss, 1950, p. 141) 'Phenomenologically as a coherent system of feelings related to a given subject, and operationally as a set of coherent behavior patterns, or pragmatically, as a system of feelings which motivates a related set of behavior patterns' (p. 17) **Differences** 'In structural terms, a "happy" person is one in whom important aspects of the Parent, the Adult, and the Child are all syntonic with each other' (p. 57)—although Berne acknowledges the limitations of this analysis by suggesting that this could describe a 'happy' concentration camp commandant. 'The characteristics of the archaeopsyche is what Freud calls primary process; that of the neopsyche, secondary process; and that of the exteropsyche, something akin to identification' (p. 240)	
Adult ego state/ neopsyche	**Similarities** 'Reliability or commitment is regarded as an inherent social quality of the Adult' (p. 111) Berne describes the Adult mediating between Parent and Child to prevent depressions (p. 155) **Differences** Is concerned with 'data-processing as a way of life' (p. 46) 'Is concerned with the earthly realities of objective living' (p. 60)	An integrating organ 'which is felt as the unified ego' (Weiss, 1950, p. 17) 'Is principally concerned with transforming stimuli into pieces of information, and processing and filing that information on the basis of previous experience' [emphasis added] (p. 37)

	Neopsychic judgment can be impaired—Berne gives the example of hypomania (p. 66) The neopsyche can become disorganised (p. 185) Berne described the 'Professor' (later, 'Little Professor') as 'the shrewd (second-order) Adult component of [a patient's] Child' (p. 185) 'The ethical Adult, "Ethos", may be regarded functionally as the Parent-programmed Adult.... The feeling Adult, "Pathos", may be understood as a Child-programmed Adult' (p. 242) 'Is a data-processing computer, which grinds out decisions after computing the information from three sources: the Parent, the Child, and the data which the Adult has gathered and is gathering' (Harris, 1967, p. 53)	'In her healthy state... the Adult is charged with free cathexis and is therefore experienced as her "real Self"' (p. 41) 'Is characterized by an autonomous set of feelings, attitudes, and behavior patterns which are adapted to the current reality' (p. 76) Has 'the "instinct of mastery" and [strives] towards such qualities as responsibility, reliability, sincerity, and courage' (p. 77) 'Is noted to be organized, adaptable, and intelligent, and is experienced as an objective relationship with the external environment based on autonomous reality-testing' (p. 77) 'There are moral qualities which are universally expected of people who undertake grown-up responsibilities, such attributes as courage, sincerity, loyalty, and reliability' (p. 195) 'This "integrated" person is charming, etc., and courageous, etc., in his Adult state, whatever qualities he has or does not have in his Child and Parent ego states. The "unintegrated" person may revert to being charming, and may feel that he *should* be courageous' (p. 195) 'The neopsychic ego—at every age—is a continually contacting, integrating, and emerging process' (Erskine, 1993, p. 185)
Parent ego state/ exteropsyche	**Similarity**	
	'Is a set of feelings, attitudes, and behaviour patterns which resemble those of a parental figure' (p. 75) and is exhibited in the form of the prejudicial or prohibitive Parent.	
	Differences	
	'Is the guide for ethical aspirations and empyrean esuriences' (p. 60)	'Is judgmental in an imitative way, and seeks to enforce sets of borrowed standards' (p. 37)

(Continued)

Table 6.1. (Continued)

	Set 1 *Models representing the three ego states as the total or 'complete' personality*	Set 2 *Models representing the Integrated Adult/ Integrating Adult*
	'Is a set of feelings, attitudes, and behavior patterns which resemble those of a parental figure' (p. 75) and is typically exhibited in two forms: the prejudicial or prohibitive Parent and the nurturing Parent. Berne describes the therapist making 'Parental demands' (p. 146) and adopting a 'Parental... attitude' (p. 150) 'If [the therapist] decides that a certain patient needs Parental reassurance, he does not play the role of a parent; rather he liberates his Parental ego state' (p. 233) The basis of certain therapeutic interventions, i.e., support, reassurance, persuasion, and exhortation (Berne, 1966a)	
Child ego state/ archeopsyche	**Similarities** 'Is a set of feelings, attitudes, and behavior patterns which are relics of the individual's own childhood' (p. 77)	
	Differences Has both 'natural' and adapted states (p. 32) Comprises (all) 'the relics of childhood' (p. 36) 'Charm, spontaneity, and fun which are characteristics of the healthy child' (p. 46) 'Means an organized state of mind which exists or once actually existed' (p. 61) Provides meaning by means of its 'archaic data-processing' (p. 64) 'The therapist's Child [was] working intuitively and subconsciously' (p. 69) Is exhibited in one of two forms: the adapted Child and the natural Child (pp. 77–78) Berne described the Child cooperating with the Adult (p. 146) 'The therapist... must be half Child and half Adult observer of both his own and the patient's behavior' (p. 227) Berne refers to the Adult in the Child (throughout)	Is 'distinguished by autistic thinking and archaic fears and expectations' (p. 31) 'Tends to react... abruptly, on the basis of pre-logical thinking and poorly differentiated or distorted perceptions' (p. 37) 'Is a warped ego state which has become fixated' (p. 54) 'Is a purgatory, and sometimes a hell, for archaic tendencies' (p. 60) Is 'confused and loaded with unconstructive feelings' (p. 235)
Parent and Child ego states	**Difference**	Have 'an archaic quality in that were appropriate to some former stage of... experience, but were inappropriate to the immediate reality' (p. 30)

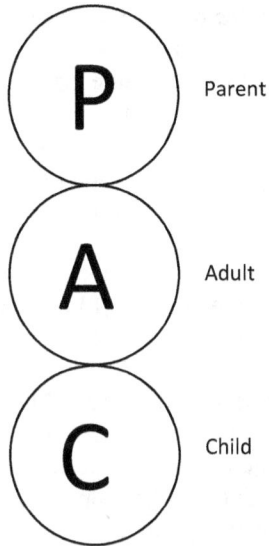

Figure 6.1a. Traditional model of ego states

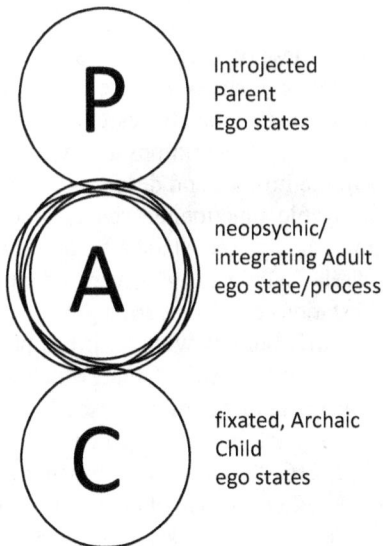

Figure 6.1b. Integrating Adult model of personality
Based on Tudor (2003b).

There is, however, a difference between, on the one hand, Parent ego states and Child ego states or the introjected and archaic (fixated) aspects of the personality and, on the other, the Adult ego state. While clearly we experience a plurality of here-and-now feelings, attitudes, and behaviours, one difference between Parent and Child in contrast to the Adult is in the difference in their respective time dimensions. As Stewart (1992) puts it, 'Child and Parent ego-states are both "stored" from the person's own past. By contrast, Adult is experienced in the ever-moving present' (p. 27).

The second difference is one of function and process. In making this distinction, I draw on Federn's (1949) argument that, 'To recognize the central ego-function as separate from the single ego-performances, theoretically and practically, is of great value for the clinical, therapeutic, and hygienic approaches' (pp. 290–291). Thus, Parent and Child represent plural—that is, multiple 'ego performances' or experiences—while the central function of the Adult is that of integrating both our experience/s of the present and those of the past. In the interests of clarity, then, I suggest that it is helpful to distinguish the neopsyche as the integrating (Adult) ego state (singular) or, better, integrating process, a clarification that offers a different conceptual apparatus for understanding the personality and its development (see Tudor, 2003b; and Figure 6.1b).

From these ontological differences, other differences follow. As R. Cox (1992/1996) puts it, 'ontology lies at the beginning of any enquiry' (p. 145). At the same time, ontology no longer refers to an essentialist notion of a fixed essence of things. According to Cox, 'the ontologies people work with derive from their historical experience and in turn become embedded in the world they construct' (p. 145). In this sense, we can see that these two sets of views about ego states represent not only different ontologies about ego states but also different views about ontology: definitions in set 1 reflect a certainty about the essence or nature of the ego; in set 2, while some of Berne's (1961/1975a) definitions also appear quite certain, Erskine's (1993) and Tudor's (2003b) definitions and descriptions of the Integrated/integrating Adult or, better, neopsychic functioning, reflect a constructivist and deconstructivist view of relational being (see Marshall, 2000; Stewart-Harawira, 2005; Figures 6.1a and 6.1b), while Temple's (1999) view of functional fluency focuses on the behavioural manifestations of the integrating Adult ego state.

One implication of this difference is with regard to physis (or phusis). Berne (1968/1971) describes this as 'the force of Nature, which eternally strives to make things grow and to make growing things more perfect' (p. 98). In the TA literature from Berne onward, physis is diagrammed as a force, urge—Berne refers to physis as a 'growth force' (pp. 142, 216, 228) and as a 'growth urge' (p. 114)—or motivation originating in the Child ego state. This makes sense from a set 1 perspective on ego states (see also Table 6.3). From a set 2 perspective, however, it makes no sense that this growth force is diagrammed as emanating from the Child, which represents archaic, fixated ego states. Since physis represents neopsychic motivation, from a set 2 perspective, it should properly be diagrammed as an aspect of the integrating Adult (see Tudor, 2003b; and Chapter 7).

Human development

As far as human development is concerned, some TA theorists and practitioners take the view that, developmentally, the Child and Parent develop first and that this is followed by the Adult at ten months (Harris, 1967), 12 months (Levin, 1974; Schiff et al., 1975), or 18 months (Klein, 1980). These perspectives represent different models within the three ego states model (set 1) (see Table 6.2). Other transactional analysts, who follow Berne's definition of the Adult as adapted to the current reality, argue that this applies to a baby (e.g., Gobes as cited in Novey et al., 1993; James & Jongeward, 1971; Sprietsma, 1982) and, indeed, to a foetus adapting to its current reality in utero (Tudor, 2003b). These perspectives represent models based on different views of the Integrated/integrating Adult (see Table 6.2, set 2). As models and metaphors, they are significant in that they influence the way we think about human development, and, of course, how we think about development influences, and perhaps even determines, the way we construct models, which, in turn influences or determines practice.

Techniques such as reparenting and rechilding,[1] and the permission transaction are based on helping to develop or 'grow' Parent and/or Child ego states and thus represent set 1 models of human development and growth, whereas set 2 models aim to enhance or expand the integrating Adult principally through empathic transactions or transacting (see Tudor, 2003b, 2011b).

Integration

These differences about human development (foetus, infant, child, and adult) are also based on differences about the nature of integration. In the first set of models (set 1), integration takes place as human beings develop and distinguish between natural and adapted states (in all three ego states) through a process of decontamination (although, arguably, this concept derives from a set 2 model of ego states) and as they move through various identified stages of development in an epigenetic sequence reminiscent of Erikson's (1968) 'eight ages of man'. Erikson's influence on Berne, who was in analysis with Erikson between 1947 and 1949, is documented and discussed by Cheney (1971), Jorgensen and Jorgensen (1984), Stewart (1992), and Barnes (2007). The idea that development takes place through the resolution of a series of psychosocial crises means that, in effect, set 1 models are based on a conflict model of development and integration.

The second view of integration (represented by set 2 models) also derives from Berne (1961/1975a), who suggests that 'it appears that in many cases certain child-like qualities become integrated into the Adult ego state in a manner different from the contamination process' (p. 194). He goes on to acknowledge that 'the mechanism of this "integration" remains to be elucidated' (p. 194). This is a significant passage because it hints at an integrative process or mechanism whereby qualities, attitudes, feelings, behaviours, and thoughts are integrated from the environment into the Adult in an uncontaminated and unproblematic way and not

Table 6.2. **Two sets of ego state models in TA: human development**

Set 1	Set 2
Differences	
Stage models	Process models

	Set 1	Set 2
Human development	Stage models 0–5 years—Parent and Child 10 months onward—Adult (Harris, 1967) 0–6 months—Natural Child (C_1) 6–8 months—Little Professor (A_1) 18 months–3 years—Adult (A_2) 3–6 years—Supernatural Child (P_1) 6–12 years—Parent (P_2) 12 years onward—Recycling (Levin, 1974) 0–6 months—me, not me (C_1) 6 months–1 year—Little Professor (A_1) 1–2 years—what do others do? (A_2) 2–3 years—terrible twos (A_1/ A_2) 3–4 years—trusting threes (P_1) 4–5 years—fearful fours (P_1) 5 onwards—A_2 and P_2 (Schiff et al., 1975) 0–6 months—Natural Child (C_1) 6 months–1 year—C_1 and Little Professor (A_1) 1–3 years—development of Adapted Child (P_1) and formation of A_2 3–6 years—and P_2 6–7 years—equal energy in all three ego states 7–13 years—increase in A_2 skills 13–18 years—surge of sexual/ aggressive energy in C_1 18 years onward—equal energy in all three ego states (Klein, 1980)	Process models Healthy development is viewed as a process that may be described in terms of an Integrated/ integrating Adult: 'The Adult ego state is ageless' (James & Jongeward, 1971, p. 277) 'A person is actually "Born Adult"' (Sprietsma, 1982, p. 228) The neonate has an Adult ego state (Gobes, as cited in Novey et al., 1993) People are conceived Adult (Tudor, 2003b) When this development is interrupted in some way, we may think about this in terms of undigested Parental introjects and fixated, archaic Child experiences: Conception In utero Birth At any age (Based on Gobes, as cited in Novey et al. 1993; Tudor 2003b)[2]

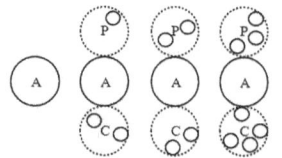

via Archaic Child or Introjected Parent states. In his work *Ego Psychology and the Problem of Adaptation,* Hartmann (1939/1958) argues that:

> not all adaptation to the environment, or every learning and maturation process, is a conflict. I refer to the development outside of conflict of perception, intention, object comprehension, thinking, language, recall-phenomena, productivity, to the

well-known phases of motor development, grasping, crawling, walking, and to the maturation and learning processes implicit in all these and many others.

(p. 8)

According to Hartmann (1939/1958), psychoanalytic ego psychology up to 1939 had been predominantly a conflict psychology, with the conflict-free aspects of what he referred to as 'reality-adapted development' (p. 13) peripheral or underdeveloped. In this sense, set 2 models may be viewed as a development from Hartmann's views on adaptation and to represent a growth model of development and integration. In terms of the provenance of ideas and influence, it may be significant that, in his work, Berne does not refer to Hartmann. However, as Federn (1928, 1932) refers to Hartmann, and to Glover (Federn, 1929/1952b), and Weiss (1952)

Table 6.3. Two sets of ego state models in TA: integration

	Set 1	Set 2
View of integration	**Similarity**	
	'Anyone functioning as an Adult should ideally exhibit three kinds of tendencies: personal attractiveness and responsiveness, objective data processing, and ethical responsibility; representing respectively archaeopsychic, neopsychic, and exteropsychic elements "integrated" into the neopsychic ego state' (p. 195)	
	Differences	
		'Integrated personality... means maintenance of control not only of the partial ego reactions but also of different ego states. This maintenance requires the reliable and strong cathexis of the lasting, mature ego state' (Federn, 1952c, p. 218)
		The integrating organ synthesises and integrates all the dynamic factors that arise as a result of inner tension, controls the perceptive-motor system, and takes into account external contingencies or reality. (Weiss, 1952)
		'It appears that in many cases certain child-like qualities become integrated into the Adult ego state in a manner different from the contamination process' (p. 194)
		'This "integrated" person *is* charming, etc., and courageous, etc., in his Adult state, whatever qualities he has or does not have in his Child and Parent ego states. The "unintegrated" person may *revert to* being charming, and may feel that he *should* be courageous' (p. 195)

refers to Hartmann in his introduction to Federn's papers, we may surmise that it is likely that Berne was aware of Hartmann's work.

The concept of the neopsyche as an elaborative system connected to the mental-emotional analysis of the here and now is a perspective that acknowledges the importance of the plasticity of the ego and the fluidity of the Adult ego state (represented in Figure 6.1b). This plasticity is consistent with recent developments in neuroscience and development psychology. As Hartmann (1942) argues, 'The mobility or plasticity of the ego is certainly one of the pre-requisites of mental health, whereas a rigid ego may interfere with the process of adaptation' (p. 314). There is a link between this developmental integration and the nature of psycho-therapy, which Rogers (1942) defines thus:

> It aims directly towards the greatest independence and integration of the indi-vidual.... The aim is not to solve one particular problem, but to assist the indi-vidual to grow, so that he can cope with the present problem and later problems in a better-integrated fashion.
>
> (p. 28)

Cure

Finally, these different sets of ego state models differ in their view of the ideal (or idealised) goal of therapy or cure in terms of ego state analysis. As Stewart (2001) points out succinctly, one's view of cure depends on which of the two definitions— or two sets of definitions —is adopted, that is, whether the totally cured person

Table 6.4. Two sets of ego state models in TA: cure/goal of therapy

	Differences	
'Cure'/ ideal end of therapy	A 'complete' set of functioning ego states, that is, the presence of functioning Parent, Adult, and Child ego states	The Integrated Adult/ integrating Adult only

may be characterised as having all three ego states or only an Integrated/integrating Adult. Stewart concludes, 'It's purely from this difference in definition that the difference between the two models arises' (p. 144).

Difference, confusion, schism, and reconciliation

In one of his articles on this topic, Oller-Vallejo (2003) suggests that the controversy over these two (sets of) models 'is generating an epistemological schism that could have serious consequences for the future of transactional analysis' (p. 162). He argues—and I agree—that these differences are serious 'not only because many people are confused, which could cause the method to suffer a loss of credibility, but also because of the theoretical lack of rigor that the two models and the controversy reveal' (p. 162). Indeed, I would extend Oller-Vallejo's concern and analysis to include differences (if not a schism) based on different views about the ontology of ego states, of human nature, and about therapeutic method. In my work as a trainer and supervisor, I observe that many TA trainees, as well as a good number of TA practitioners, use models from both sets without distinction and often without awareness. Significantly, this theoretical confusion—and conflation—leads to confusion in practice. For example, in response to a client who is anxious, one TA practitioner might say, 'It's OK to be anxious' or 'You don't have to feel anxious here'; another TA practitioner might say, 'You look anxious'. These represent different responses based on the different understandings and models outlined in this chapter (see Table 6.5).

Given that TA values consistency (see EATA PTSC, 2022; ITAA IBoC, 2022), it is important that practitioners know what they are doing—and why. Moreover, as Warner (2000) observes with regard to different levels of 'interventiveness' in

Table 6.5. Analysis of different responses to a client feeling anxious

Response	'It's OK to be anxious' or 'You don't have to feel anxious here'	'You look anxious'
Transaction	Permission transaction	Empathic transaction
Purpose	To give permission and temporary reassurance, to reChild (and reParent)	To make contact, engage, and invite reflection and dialogue
Implication for human development	To repair and grow the Child	To expand the Adult
Epistemological implication	Knowledge (and certainty) lies with the therapist	Knowledge rests with the client, accessed and enhanced by means of encounter and dialogue
Ontological implication	That anxiety is or was difficult and problematic	That anxiety is an existential reality of life
Set of ego state models	Set 1	Set 2

person-centred therapy, 'there are very real dangers in trying to mix interventions and theories at different levels of intervention, since these therapies are grounded in quite different types of therapeutic relationship' (p. 252). The same is true with regard to the use of different sets of models of ego states in TA: to mix models is dangerous in that it is confusing for the client and, ultimately, can undermine the process and progress of therapy or change. Difference is not a problem. Indeed, differences such as those outlined in Table 6.5 are understandable given the different and differing theories within TA and their implications, and, in any case, TA encompasses a number of different schools or traditions and considerable divergence in theory and practice. Difficulties arise, however, when differences are not acknowledged or articulated or when one 'side' or sect claims priority on intellectual territory and/or a monopoly on truth.

One cause of these differences and confusion is Berne's own writing, as can be seen from this present analysis. It is evident that Berne defines ego states in various ways at different times and that some of his later definitions of ego states were not as complete as those in his earlier writing (for a brief summary of which, see Wadsworth & DiVincenti, 2003). As Stewart (1992) points out,

> when Berne wrote about ego-s[t]ates, he did not always describe them in ways that were consistent with his own definitions. Not surprisingly, this has sometimes been a source of confusion, both for transactional analysts and for commentators from other disciplines.
>
> (pp. 25–26)

In attempting to account for this confusion, Stewart (1992) suggests that subsequent to his 1961 work, Berne often used partial definitions—for example, in *Games People Play* (Berne 1964/1968a)—but that he did this in the context of referring to his original and more elaborated definitions. In this sense, Berne himself may have contributed to the oversimplification of certain aspects of his own theory.

In his 2003 article on the three basic ego states, Oller-Vallejo refers to a schism. This word refers to a breach of unity, divided allegiance, or sects formed by divisions, originally within the context of the Christian Church. However, his own argument and language, especially in his 2003 article, is that of division, sectarianism, and schism. Here I address three of his arguments.

The primacy of the three ego state model

In both of his articles, Oller-Vallejo (1997, 2003) asserts the primacy of the three ego states model and dismisses the Integrated/integrating Adult model, concluding (in 2003) that 'my proposal is to continue developing and disseminating the three ego state model as the single appropriate TA model of personality, thus ending, for the benefit of TA, a controversy that I find futile' (p. 166). From this, it is clear that Oller-Vallejo simply wants to erase the Integrated/integrating Adult (set 2) model of ego states rather than to accommodate both models and, not least, some of Berne's own definitions and specifically those about the Adult being adapted to the current reality. This dismissal reflects a more general move on the part of some in the TA community to discount (at T_2) (Schiff et al., 1975) the significance of the stimulus, that is, the definitions of ego states that are the basis of the Integrated/ integrating Adult model and the integrative approach in TA (for a history and summary see Wadsworth & DiVincenti, 2003). Simply to assert the primacy of one model over another and to use that as the basis for dismissing a particular model is an ad hominem argument. Moreover, to claim that one is doing so for the benefit of the TA community may be considered somewhat arrogant.

The positive Parent and Child

In both of his articles on the subject, Oller-Vallejo (1997, 2003) makes much of Berne's positive use of Parent and Child, referring to them (1997) as 'positive operations in the here and now' (p. 291), including Berne's (1966a) Parent interventions of support, reassurance, persuasion, and exhortation. However, Oller-Vallejo does not acknowledge that Berne himself mixed his models and here was clearly using these interventions in the context of a three ego state and functional model (set 1). Furthermore, Oller-Vallejo also omits quoting Berne's (1966a) own cautions about these particular 'other types of interventions' (p. 248):

- Firstly, that 'the transactional analyst may have to fall back on other approaches, but that he should not do so unless he can state his reasons clearly' (p. 248)—hardly an unequivocal endorsement of these other interventions.
- Secondly, that they are to be used (only) in 'special situations' (p. 248), such as the treatment of active schizophrenics—in this context, about which there has been considerable controversy both within and beyond TA.
- Thirdly, that while the Parent—Child relationship between therapist and patient may be effective and gratifying, 'it may in the long run make it more difficult to accomplish the ultimate aim of therapy' (p. 249)—by implication, an Adult–Adult relationship.

To argue in this way is partial.

The invalidation of certain techniques

Echoing a point similar to one made by English (1998), Oller-Vallejo (2003) suggests that the consequence of accepting the view of the Integrated/integrating Adult is the 'invalidation of reparenting, redecision, and rechilding approaches' (p. 163). This is not the case. The logic of the Integrated/integrating Adult (set 2) approach is simply to pursue a different method. Techniques such as reparenting and rechilding are perfectly valid if they are based on consistent ontology, epistemology, theory, and model/s (i.e., Set 1 models). To argue in this way is to rely on a straw argument.

Possibilities

When I have presented these different sets of models,[3] colleagues have generally appreciated and agreed with the differences outlined and have often wanted to find some way of combining or reconciling the two models or sets of models. A number of authors have put forward theories that have points in common with both sets of models. Oller-Vallejo (1997) cites Clarkson with Gilbert (1988) and Clarkson (1992) as contributions that combine the Integrated Adult with positive and changeable aspects of Parent and Child ego states. However, I think this is a further confusion. As Oller-Vallejo (1997) himself points out, 'They [the two models] offer different models of personality... [and] use distinct conceptual perspectives' (p. 291). Oller-Vallejo (1997) himself suggests that the 'positive operations' (Parent and Child) can be considered to be part of the Adult in the Integrated Adult model and, thus, that 'the integrated Adult is a more extensive concept than the Adult of the three ego states model' (p. 291).

Another possibility is that practitioners might draw on set 1 models such as reparenting and rechilding before using set 2 models in promoting the integrating Adult. While this may appear satisfactory, it has the disadvantage of having to make an ontological and epistemological switch in mid treatment, and because this switch would be made by the practitioner, one problem is that it leaves the power with the practitioner and not the patient or client. While I am open to the idea of some reconciliation between the two sets of models, I do not see it myself and, instead, prefer to be clear about the differences between models and sets of models.

Conclusion

Over the past 60 years there has been extensive debate about the nature of the ego and of ego states, including, on this present debate (English, 1998; Erskine, 1988, 1991; Novey, 1998; Oller-Vallejo, 1997, 2003; Trautmann & Erskine, 1981; Wadsworth & DiVincenti, 2003). Given the centrality of ego states to TA, it seems not only inevitable but crucial that this continue. As Gregory (2000) puts it: 'Berne's definitions and operationalization of ego psychology is continuously open to scrutiny, particularly as knowledge of neuropsychology and neurophysiology expands. Definitions of phenomenological realities, the concept of experience, and the psyche will continue to be explored' (p. 152)—and such exploration should not be a problem, or be problematised, pathologised, or cancelled. Neither TA nor its practitioners should be stuck with or in the 'then' past or with previous interpretations of the past. Indeed, one of the problems with this debate is that some of it is based on what Berne said or is said to have said (see Wadsworth & DiVincenti, 2003),[4] which is partly why I chose to return to Berne's (1961/1975a) seminal text.

As for the difference between the two models outlined here, far from the futile controversy Oller-Vallejo (2003) describes, I regard the differences as ground for fertile debate and greater clarity. In this sense, it seems to me that, like the integrating Adult, this debate reflects a critical, reflexive, changing, and expansive present 'now'. While I have a preference, I do not wish to argue for the primacy of one model or set of models over another. My principal concern here is for clarity, consistency, and coherence and that TA practitioners embody and are encouraged to embody a philosophical congruence between personal philosophy, espoused (TA) theory, method, and practice. It is my hope that the distinctions offered in this chapter foster this concern and contribute to that practice.

Notes

1 Or, more accurately, re-Parenting and re-Childing.
2 The representations of the Adult ego state in this Figure should, for consistency, be drawn with multiple circles. They are only represented by a single circle for ease of reading, given their size.
3 Now, over some 15 years.
4 Claude Steiner and I disagreed about this. As I note elsewhere: 'Claude and I had a number of differences and disagreements... [including about] his... insistence that the oral tradition (including his personal knowledge of Berne) took precedence over the written tradition (as in what Berne actually wrote)' (Tudor, 2020d, p. 2).

Chapter 7

We've had 66 years of ego states and the world's getting worse

In 2000, 'Co-creative transactional analysis' was published in the *Transactional Analysis Journal*. The article was the culmination of some two years' work by Graeme Summers and myself, but drew on a critique of various aspects of transactional analysis (TA) which each and both of us had developed over the previous 15 years of experience of and involvement with TA (see Summers, 2014; Tudor, 2014b). The article took a constructivist approach to TA by which we deconstructed aspects of the theories of transactions, ego states, scripts, and games—including deconstructing the usual order in which these four fundamental pillars of TA theory are presented (usually beginning with ego states).[1] We identified our own theoretical influences of this work, i.e., field theory and social constructivism (to which we later added health psychology and critical theory); proposed three principles of co-creative TA (of 'we'ness, shared responsibility, and present-centred development); and, generally, advanced a perspective that acknowledged the psychology of health alongside the psychology of pathology, and emphasised present-centred relating (on which I expand in Chapter 5).

The logic of what Graeme and I had written led me, with Graeme's encouragement, to examine the dominant ego state model in TA, a research project which led, three years after our original article was published, to the publication of a chapter on the neopsyche in which I advanced the argument for and a description of the integrating Adult (Tudor, 2003b). I considered that there was a specific need for an elaboration of the Adult ego state not only as this was significantly underdeveloped within TA theory and practice, but also as it is the aspect of personality which represents the integrating process.

That work and my re-reading of *Transactional Analysis in Psychotherapy* (Berne 1961/1975a) led me to identify two sets of models of ego states (Tudor, 2010c, reproduced in this book as the previous chapter), one of which (set 1, and the dominant model in TA) is based on a three a state model of personality (i.e., Parent, Adult, and Child) and a three ego state model of health: in other words, that the project and outcome of TA interventions in therapy (and, arguably, in all fields of application) is a full and healthy complement of Parent, Adult, and Child ego states. The other set of models (what I referred to as set 2) is also based on the three ego state of personality, but proposes a one ego state model of health, i.e., that of

DOI: 10.4324/9780429398223-10

the integrating Adult. I elaborated the implications of this in terms of methodology and method in two subsequent articles on empathy (Tudor, 2011b; 2011g).

However, as I have been presenting this material, the logic of the neopsyche and of the process of integrating, and the influence of organismic psychology on my thinking (see Tudor, 2003b; Tudor & Worrall, 2006) has led me to question the relevance of framing personality in terms of ego; and, in a number of workshops in the past 20 years, both I and participants have speculated that the neopsyche/integrating Adult is, in many ways, beyond ego. While this journey has been—and is—intellectually stimulating, exciting, and even liberating, it poses a dilemma, for, as Berne (1970/1973) puts it: 'Parent, Adult, and Child ego states were first systematically studied by transactional analysis, and they're its foundation stones and its mark. Whatever deals with ego states is transactional analysis, and whatever overlooks them is not' (p. 223). On this basis, questioning the existence, validity, and/or usefulness of ego states in TA appears as anathema and, therefore, risks ex-communication. At the same time, Berne (1972/1975b) himself also discusses the problem of adapting the clinical situation to theory, what he refers to as 'a danger of Procrustes'—in Greek mythology, a rogue smith and bandit who attacked people by stretching them or cutting off their legs so that they fitted the size of an iron bed. In discussing how to avoid this, Berne also refers to 'the map–ground problem' whereby an aviator flies according to a map but doesn't check this against the ground, as a result of which he gets lost. Berne concludes: 'The moral is, look at the ground first, and then at the map, and not vice versa' (p. 409). Applying this moral or principle to ego states, I consider the ground, including the intellectual and cultural ground which, I argue, has moved away from ego psychology, and then question whether the map of ego states still best describes the territory of the psyche. In this sense, I am not overlooking ego states but, rather, looking them over.

The title of this chapter is inspired by the book, *We've had a Hundred Years of Psychotherapy and the World's Getting Worse* by James Hillman and Michael Ventura (published in 1992), a book which Thomas Pynchon, the American novelist, describes as 'provocative, dangerous, and high-spirited', adjectives which strike me as consistent with the impropriety of this present work. Some question the correlation between the advent, establishment, and contribution of psychotherapy and a deterioration in the world, and, in any case, it is always useful to define terms. Hillman himself addresses this: 'my approach is the world is getting worse [and] that's correlated with therapy's concerns, and if we were less concerned with ourselves and paid more attention to the world, the world wouldn't be getting worse' (p. 229). The point here is to accept the reality of 'worse' and what Hillman and Ventura refer to as 'decline', precisely in order to do something about it. As they put it:

Hillman: The role of therapy, then, is to awaken the patient to the fact that, not only is the society dysfunctional but—

Ventura: —it's going through an absolutely fundamental change.... What is clearly not possible is to find your own little psychologically safe and stable place.

(p. 230)

From this perspective (at least) two questions arise:

1. Are ego states—that is, the concept of ego states—the most useful way for understanding human beings and, specifically, human personality, in the 21st century, in all our complexity and infinite variety, and, not least, accounting for differences and intersectionalities of class, culture, disability, ethnicity, location, race, sexuality, sexual orientation, and so on?
2. Are ego states and the ego state model(s) in TA (still) helpful in helping us to pay more attention to the world?

This chapter attempts at least to address if not answer these questions. In doing so, and in order to contextualise the development of both ego and ego state psychology, I first offer a brief history of ego psychology.

A brief history of ego psychology

As noted in the previous chapter, from the Latin word for 'I', the ego is conceptualised, at least from a psychoanalytic and psychodynamic perspective, as the central core around which all psychic activities revolve. In the classical psychoanalytic theory, the ego represents both a cluster of conscious cognitive and perceptual processes such as memory, and problem-solving, as well as specific defence mechanisms that serve to mediate between the id and the superego.

Most histories of ego psychology acknowledge its origins in Freud's two papers: 'The ego and the id' (1923/1984a), which established the tripartite structural model of the psychic apparatus, and 'Inhibitions, symptoms and anxiety' (1926), in which Freud argues that anxiety is the impetus to the synthesising and executive functions of the ego, ideas that are echoed in Berne's (1961/1975) analysis of the significant properties of psychic organs, namely: executive power, adaptability, biological fluidity, and mentality. However, it should be noted that the translation of Freud's word 'Ich' (meaning 'I') as 'ego' was the work of Strachey, Freud's primary translator. As Holt (1975) points out, it is a British tradition, and not one that Freud particularly liked; and, in fact, he himself seldom used the word. As a result, there is a conflation of the use of the word ego to stand for 'I' as the speaking subject, 'I' as a whole person, and the ego as a structure. For further discussion of the implications of this Latinisation of the original German, see Kernberg (1982), Kirshner (1991), Solms (1999), and Kobrin (2013).

Freud's papers were followed by Anna Freud's *The Ego and the Mechanisms of Defense* (published in German in 1936 and in English the following year), which emphasised the defensive functions of the ego; and Heinz Hartmann's *Ego Psychology and the Problem of Adaptation* (published in German in 1939, though not in English in its entirety until 1958), which focuses on the adaptive functions of the ego. In her tribute to Hartmann (on the occasion of his seventieth birthday) and his contribution to the development of the field of ego psychology, Anna Freud (1966) acknowledges his 'more revolutionary manner, [that is] from the new angle of ego autonomy, which until then had lain outside analytic study' (p. 18). Wallerstein (2000) summarises Hartmann's central conception of a conflict-free sphere of the ego as 'a sphere in which functions of primary autonomy (e.g., perception, motility, language, thinking) grew not out of conflict between the id and the outer world, but rather apart from conflict, on an innate maturational timetable' (p. 137).

Berne (1961/1975a), too, advances a view of the epigenetic origins of the Adult:

> it appears that in many cases certain child-like qualities become integrated into the Adult ego state in a manner different from the contamination process.... it can be observed that certain people when functioning *qua* Adult have a charm and openness of nature which is reminiscent of that exhibited by children.
>
> (pp. 194–195)

Elsewhere (Tudor, 2003b), I refer to this as 'a significant passage, which hints at the integrative process (or "mechanism") whereby qualities, attitudes, feelings, behaviours and thoughts that are integrated into the Adult are uncontaminated and unproblematic' (p. 211), though Berne (1961/1975a) himself acknowledges that 'the mechanism of this "integration" remains to be elucidated' (p. 194). Interestingly, in his next book, *The Structure and Dynamics of Organizations and Groups*, Berne (1963) repeats his definition of the Adult ego state being 'an independent set of feelings, attitudes and behavior patterns that are adapted to the current reality', adding 'and [which] are not affected by Parent prejudices or archaic attitudes left over from childhood.... The Adult is the ego state which makes survival possible' (Berne, 1963, p. 186). Moreover, for many people in the world, the 'current reality' is not something to which it is particularly desirable to adapt. As Victoria Baskerville (personal communication, 8 July 2023) puts it: 'Current reality is changed by the systemic, [and] by the individuals positioning themselves within systemic oppression.' This is another reason why we need a critical Adult (Tudor, 2015).

Wallerstein (2000) goes on to note that 'These conflict-free functions could of course be invaded secondarily by conflict' (p. 137)—which sounds like a description of the Bernean concept of contamination, and is consistent with the one ego state model of health (Tudor & Summers, 2014) in which the Integrated Parent and Archaic Child ego states are metaphors for those aspects of our personality that are secondary and in conflict with neopsychic integrating Adult functioning.[2] Although there is very little discussion in TA about ego psychology, Paul (1970) notes an early contribution that TA had made to this form of psychology: 'The analysis of games has succeeded character analysis in the development of ego psychology' (p. 122).

In his contribution to the symposium 'The ego and the id after fifty years', Holt (1975) identifies two strands to the development of ego psychology: the first, a revised and extended conceptualisation of defences (driven primarily by the work of Anna Freud), and the second, 'the increased role of reality as determined by behaviour' (p. 570) (as expounded primarily in the work of Heinrich Hartman), the latter of which also paved the way for Erikson's (1950, 1958) psychosocial and psychohistorical outlook. Hart (1975), Marcus (1999), and Wallerstein (2000) acknowledge a number of developments in ego psychology:

- Regarding the mental function of thinking—represented by the work of Rapaport (1967) and his colleagues.
- Regarding normal growth and development—by Vaillant (1993).
- Through child observation—by Mahler (1968) and other colleagues, work that Stern (1985) built on, albeit looking at the development of the whole person or self.
- Its integration with object relations—by Jacobson (1954, 1964), Schafer (1968), and Loewald (1980) and other colleagues.
- Its integration with Kleinian mechanism—by Kernberg (1975).

Notwithstanding such developments and interconnections and its influence, as a branch of psychology, ego psychology has declined, and is much less present in the literature in the past 45 years than it was in its heyday in the 1940s, 1950s, and 1960s (see Figure 7.1).

A number of reasons have been advanced for this, including:

- Some theoretical obstacles to the integration of ego psychology in psychoanalysis, especially regarding autonomous ego function (for further analysis of which, see Marcus, 1999).
- Some philosophical problems—in his interesting and challenging paper, Holt (1975) argues that ego psychology, as well as its historical antecedent, soul theory, have a number of philosophical fallacies, including dualism,

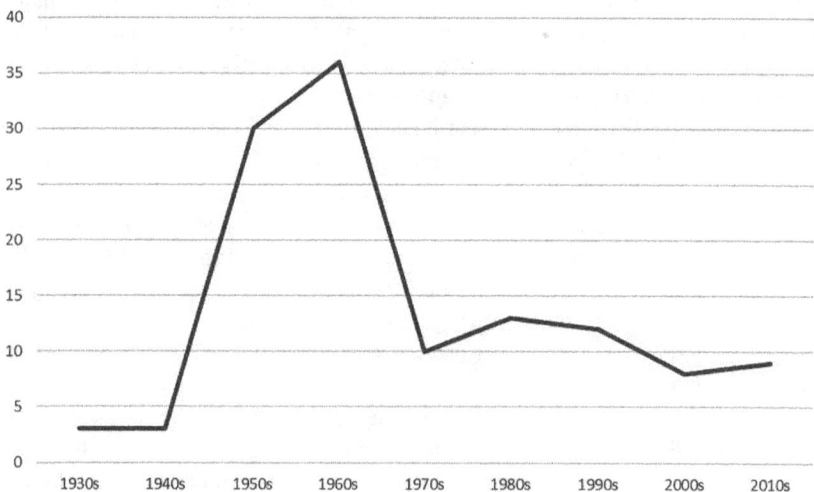

Figure 7.1. Numbers of articles on ego psychology by decade

Source: From the Psychoanalytic Electronic Publishing (PEP) library (PEP, 2024).

anthropomorphism, reification, and essentialism, a critique which I think, is helpful in our present deconstruction of ego states (see pp. 151–160, below).

• The criticism that ego psychology was too focused on structure at the expense of articulating the empathic connection between therapist and client—which led to the development of self psychology (Kohut, 1971). This focus may be found in TA when ego state analysis (as in 'Which ego state are you/your client "in"?') is privileged over the analysis of transactions (TA proper) and especially enquiry into the empathic quality—and experience—of transactional relating.

• The broader movement in psychoanalysis and psychotherapy from drive, ego, and object to self, and from the intrapsychic to the intersubjective, the interpersonal, and relational.

• The relatively local influence of some of its thinkers—as Bergmann (2000) observes: 'The fact is that the Hartmann school remained confined to the United States.... No thinker in Europe or South America drew inspiration from Hartmann' (p. 7). Commenting in 2018 on the ego psychologists of the 1950s, Greenberg said 'I cannot think of any who are still around today' (in Greenberg & Aron, 2018, p. 58).

Hart (1975) himself is pessimistic about the future of ego psychology, as well as that of psychoanalysis, mainly as he doesn't see that either had a metapsychology—a point Marcus (1999) also makes about ego psychology—in the context of the collapse of which, Hart asserts: 'I find it hard to imagine that the concept of the ego will survive the general collapse' (p. 573). Nonetheless, some 25 years later, Marcus (1999) was referring to 'Ego psychology today' (p. 853) and Wallerstein (2000) to 'the current status of American ego psychology' (p. 161). Finally, with regard to this brief history, and notwithstanding the excellence of Holt's (1975), Marcus' (1999), and Wallerstein's (2000) papers on the history and development of American ego psychology, it is surprising, at least to this transactional analyst, that none of them mention Glover, Federn, Weiss, or Berne, or, for that matter, John and Helen Watkins (Watkins, 1978; Watkins & Watkins, 1997; see pp. 147–148, below), though this may be part of the continuing battle over ideas and, not least, history.

Of course, referring to ego psychology as American (as most commentators do) raises the importance of acknowledging the cultural context of the development of ego psychology; as Rogers (1959) puts it: 'No theory can be adequately understood without some knowledge of the cultural and personal soil from which it springs' (p. 185). Thus, ego psychology, including ego state psychology, cannot be understood outside its cultural environment, that is, of the development of psychology in the United States of America, especially in the years after the Second World War. In his study of Rogers' psychology, Van Belle (1980) acknowledges the influence of Protestantism and especially Calvinism, which, Van Belle suggests, from the Puritans, who emphasised the objectively revealed Will of God, stressed submission to law and order, and, from the Wesleyan Evangelicals, who emphasised the personal religious conversion experience, stressed free will. Van Belle suggests that 'it was part of the democratic spirit that was shaping the nation in the eighteen hundreds to place the emphasis on the "individual" and his freedom in choosing a course of action, or forming a society' (p. 17). Van Belle goes on to suggest that, by the early 20th century, this had so much 'become part of the American mind' (p.17), that Dewey (1920/1963) could assert that 'society is composed of individuals; [and that] this obvious and basic fact no philosophy, whatever its pretensions to novelty, can question or alter' (p. 187).

In his paper on 'The growth and transformation of American ego psychology', Wallerstein (2000) refers to this as a 'metapsychological paradigm [which was] developed in the immediate post-World War II period, primarily in America, by a brilliant cluster of European refugee analysts in their adaptation to the scientific and intellectual climate of the New World' (pp. 135–136). If we consider all theory as autobiographical (Valéry, 1958), we can perhaps understand why both adaptation and integration were important to these particular analysts. Commenting on the influence of the social environment on the development of TA, Campos (2003) comments: 'I doubt that transactional analysis could have taken root prior to the late 1950s in the United States, before which U.S. society had been mostly governed by normative standards of conventionality and conformity' (p. 117).

Having reviewed some elements of the theoretical background and some aspects of the cultural background of American ego psychology paradigm, I now focus on its two key concepts—as identified by Rangell (1965), Marcus (1999), and Wallerstein (2000) amongst others—of autonomy and adaptation.[3]

Autonomy and adaptation

Autonomy, or self-determination, is linked to free will and, as we know, is central to Berne's conception of TA, both as something to attain (Berne, 1964/1968a), and as a personal quality (Berne, 1966a). As Holt (1975) puts it: 'a patient with no remaining vestige of free will is not analyzable for he cannot decide to cooperate, to keep his appointments, and to keep working at his problems despite the pull of resistance' (p. 562). As noted above, Anna Freud acknowledges Hartmann's contribution to the concept of ego autonomy. For Holt, the contribution of ego psychology to the development of autonomy is an important one as, for him, Freud's 'commitment to strict determinism limited the degree of ego autonomy he could postulate' (p. 563). He continues: 'I believe that he [Freud] was delayed and generally hampered in accepting the conception of autonomy because of its implication that a person can attain some freedom from the pushes and pulls of his inner necessities and external pressures' (p. 562). In his assessment of Hartmann's contribution to ego psychology, Marcus (1999) acknowledges Hartmann's identification of 'conscious and unconscious neurocognitive capacities... [and of] how they operated *in relative autonomy from dynamic conflict* [emphasis added]' (p. 845). With regard to Berne's view of autonomy, and in a critique that parallels that of Holt's of Freud, Cornell (2010) argues that Berne's underdevelopment of physis and aspiration 'is related to his pessimistic assessment of peoples' willingness to be truly autonomous, that is, that the pressures of script outweigh the desire to pursue one's own nature' (p. 243).

For Hartmann (1939/1958), up to 1939, psychoanalytic ego psychology had been predominantly a conflict psychology, with the conflict-free aspects of what he refers to as 'reality-adapted development' (p. 13), peripheral or underdeveloped. In this sense, what I refer to as set 2 models of ego states may be viewed as a development from Hartmann's views of adaptation,[4] representing a growth model of development and integration (for further details of which see Summers & Tudor, 2014; Tudor, 2003b). Moreover, in his book *Ego Psychology and the Problem of Adaptation*, as noted in the previous chapter, Hartmann (1939/1958) argues that:

> Not all adaptation to the environment, or every learning and maturation process, is a conflict. I refer to the development *outside of conflict* of perception, intention, object comprehension, thinking, language, recall-phenomena, productivity, to the well-known phases of motor development, grasping, crawling, walking, and to the maturation and learning processes implicit in all these and many others.
>
> (p. 8)

This is echoed in TA by Berne's emphasis on transactions or, as he puts it (in the subtitle of his book on *Transactional Analysis in Psychotherapy*, 'social psychiatry' (Berne 1961/1975a), a perspective on which Shmukler (2001) picks up: 'Berne's criticisms of classic psychoanalysis, which he answered by originating transactional analysis, are still answered in part by an ego psychology that stresses social and interactional factors, as does current transactional analysis theory' (p. 95). Hartmann's point about adaptation is also found in Berne's view of uncontaminated integration—and, by implication, adaptation. I refer to these points about development and adaptation not least as they point to and remind us of a more phenomenological, contextual, and fluid approach to ego states (as developed below).

In his article on modern ego psychology, Marcus (1999) summarises its contribution and strengths as follows:

> The adaptational processes of the ego are now also generally accepted. Adaptation to reality experience and to emotional experience is one of the mediating tasks of the ego. The concept of ego integration processes is likewise accepted universally, implicitly or explicitly, as a crucial aspect of the clinical description of patients. Ego integrative processes function at different levels of consciousness and with different levels of organization. Object relations, compromise formations, and self are all synthetic organizations. It is the ego especially that organizes and mediates compromises, integrating each individual's unique psychic reality. Hence the name ego psychology.
>
> (p. 855)

While the contribution of ego psychology was and is a view of autonomy and adaptation based on a growth model of human development (Rogers in Rogers & Russell, 2002) as distinct from one based on conflict—and/or deficit and confusion

(Clarkson & Gilbert, 1990)—there are also tensions between autonomy and adaptation. In his article discussing the unresolved tension in Berne's basic beliefs, Cornell (2010) identifies this unresolved conflict as that 'between the psychological power of aspiration versus adaptation' (p. 243).

Ego psychology and ego states

Although ego psychology had its origins in psychopathology and a conception of defence (see A. Freud, 1936/1937; Pine, 1990), Hartmann (1939/1958) argues that, as a development of psychoanalysis, ego psychology offers 'a *general* [emphasis added] theory of mental life' (p. 4). He also frames his discussion of the concept of health in terms of the ego (Hartmann, 1942). Drawing originally on a biological metaphor, Berne (1961/1975a) describes aspects of human mental activity as 'organs' or, more precisely, 'psychic organs', whose function it is to organise external and internal material.[5] Drawing on Federn's (1929/1952b) work identifying states of the ego, and Weiss's (1950)[6] clarification of ego psychology, Berne (1961/1975a) defines ego states 'phenomenologically as a coherent system of feelings related to a given subject, and operationally as a set of coherent behavior patterns, or pragmatically, as a system of feelings which motivates a related set of behavior patterns' (p. 17). Thus, as Rath (1993) acknowledges: 'ego psychology represents the basis of the theory of personality structure and dynamics in transactional analysis' (p. 208). While acknowledging Berne's debt to Federn, Oller-Vallejo (1997) argues that:

> Berne's specific contribution was distinguishing and defining three types of ego states—Parent, Adult, and Child—as well as his emphasis that "ego states are experiential and social realities" (Berne, 1966a, p. 220), different from the superego, the ego, and the id [and that] this concept represented a milestone in the development of personality theories.
>
> (p. 290)

In his discussion of the contributions of TA to integrative psychotherapy, and arguing that TA began as a process of integration, Christoph-Lemke (1999) notes that 'Berne broadened psychoanalytic structure theory and expanded Federn's (1956) concepts of "past ego states" (archeopsyche) and "acquired ego attitudes" (exteropsyche)' (p. 203). Also commenting on Federn's influence on Berne, Wadsworth and DiVincenti (2003) make an important point about Berne's view of the nature of ego states:

> What is consistent in Berne's definition of an ego state is that it is a system of feelings or a pattern of feelings. This is because the major source of Berne's ideas on ego came from his mentor Paul Federn. In *Ego Psychology and the Psychoses,* Federn (1952[d]) described the ego as a real experienced state of feeling and not simply a theoretical construct.
>
> (p. 154)

Insofar as the concept of ego states is a part analysis of the personality, that is, one based on the conceptualisation of parts (as noted in Chapter 6), its lineage can be traced back to the work of Glover (1932/1956b, 1943/1956a). Berne was clearly aware of Glover's (1955) work as he cites him in *Transactional Analysis in Psychotherapy*, although Berne's citation and note links Glover's statements on transference neurosis with the ideas of script, and does not mention his work on the ego. Elsewhere, Berne (1972/1975b) acknowledges Federn as 'the first psycho-analyst... to make a specific study of internal dialogues' (p. 275) and the develop-ment of what Federn (1934/1952) refers to as 'a mental duologue between two parts of the ego' (p. 93), in this case 'the adult and the infantile, with its different stages and results being visually represented' (p. 93). Federn (1952c)[7] and Weiss (1950) also cite Glover (although each only with one passing reference). Neverthe-less, the antecedents are there. Glover identifies the 'ego system' or 'ego-nucleus' (1932/1956b) and, later, 'ego-nuclei' (1943/1956a), and defines them with regard to their dynamic function in terms that prefigure Berne's later descriptions (Glover, 1943/1956a):

> Theoretically an ego-nucleus can be defined as a psychic organization which (*a*) represents a positive relation to the objects of any important instinct, (*b*) secures the discharge of reactive tension consequent on frustration by objects of that instinct, (*c*) promotes the relation to reality through gratifying impulses of self-preservation, and (*d*) in one or other of these ways reduces anxiety within the psyche.
>
> (pp. 316–317)

Glover goes on to state that 'although these nuclei have a good deal in common, *they have in their earliest phases a partial autonomy*' (1943/1956a, p. 317), which derives from the fact that not all self-preservative drives have the same object, a point which is consistent with, and which anticipates, Berne's distinction between the Child and the Parent ego states. Glover also writes about a nucleus being able '*to seize the psychic apparatus and occupy the approaches to perceptual conscious-ness*' (p. 318), a point which finds echoes in Berne's (1961/1975a) perspective that an ego state has 'executive power' by which it has psychic energy or cathexis, and that each ego state 'gives rise to its own idiosyncratic patterns of organized behav-ior' (p. 75; and see Table 7.1 below).

For another review of Berne's development of ego state theory, which also ac-knowledges the influence of Eugene Kahn (Kahn & Cohen, 1936) and Wilder Pen-field (1952) on Berne's thinking, see Heathcote (2010).

Although my primary focus is on TA, in reviewing ego psychology and ego states, it would be remiss not to mention a strand of thinking and practice about ego states that was developed entirely separately from TA.

In the 1970s, 1980s, and 1990s, John Goodrich Watkins and Helen Watkins de-veloped what they referred to as ego states theory and therapy, which, like TA, drew on both Federn's work, and on psychoanalysis, but also and unlike TA, on hypnosis, and the concept of dissociation as first proposed by Janet (1907). John Watkins' primarily clinical orientation was that of a hypnotherapist (Watkins, 1947), but, together with Helen Watkins, developed ego states theory and therapy (Watkins & Watkins, 1988, 1997). Watkins and Watkins (1997) define an ego state 'as an organized system of behavior and experience whose elements are bound together by some common principle, and which is separated from other such states by a boundary that is more or less permeable' (p. 25). The similarity with Berne's definition should, perhaps, not be surprising, given the common ancestry with Federn (Berne was analysed by Federn and John Watkins by Weiss). What is more surprising is that neither the Watkinses or their followers (e.g., Leutner & Piedfort-Marin, 2021) reference Berne or TA. Leutner and Piedfort-Marin (2021) even claim that 'ego states theory and therapy were developed by John and Helen Watkins in the 1970s, 1980s and 1990s' (p. 2), without any acknowledgement of the fact that Berne's original paper on ego states was published in 1957 (Berne, 1957b/1977d), and despite that fact that John Watkins said that he knew of TA (as reported in Clark, 1998).

The key features of the Watkinses' ego states theory are:

- An emphasis (from Federn) on the cathexis of the ego with energy, and the flexibility and strength and inflexibility and weakness or impermeability of the boundary of the ego.
- An emphasis (from Weiss) on the stratification of the repressed ego states, for access to which they emphasised the use of hypnosis.
- The concept of the dissociated ego state which, in its extreme form, may become the alter of a multiple personality.
- A system of ego states which partly overlap, are partly hidden, and which exist around a centre which is referred to as the core ego or core self.
- A focus (from Hilgard, 1973) on dissociation, and on hypnosis as the principal way to work with it.

It is clear that the Watkinses and their followers developed their ego states theory separately from Berne and other transactional analysts. However, when these ego states theorists refer to three possible ego states that might exist in a husband and wife and that this area of couple work might be studied one day (Watkins & Watkins, 1997); the adult ego state (Reddemann, 2011); and categories of ego states that include the inner critic, the (inner) aggressor, and the child part (Fritzche, 2013), their separation seems almost wilful and somewhat dissociative. In any case, and especially as John Watkins knew of Berne's work, it does seem strange that the Watkinses didn't acknowledge Berne's original development of ego states, even if only to draw some distinctions and differences between the two developments. Nonetheless, in his review of the Watkinses (1997) book, Clark considers that the parallel development of their ego-state theory 'validates transactional analysis theory especially in terms of Berne's structural model of ego states' (p. 176).

So, having acknowledged the tradition of American ego psychology and its manifestation in models of ego states, I now turn to consider four dilemmas posed by the ego state model of the ego, which I introduce with some thoughts on the problem of the self.

From ego to self and beyond

The problem of the self

As philosophers have been debating the concept of self, or the self, for centuries, when psychoanalysis proposed the concept of the ego, it raised the question of the self. Berne (1961/1975a) himself discusses what he refers to as 'The problem of the self', with reference to one of his clients, Mrs Tettar. Analysing her compulsive hand-washing, he suggests that:

> When it was said that Mrs. Tettar's hand-washing was ego dystonic, this meant specifically Adult-ego dystonic. In her overt psychotic state, however, when her 'real Self' was the Child, the hand-washing became *ego syntonic*.... In other words, her hand-washing was Adult-ego dystonic and Child-ego syntonic, so whether at a given moment she perceived it as dystonic or syntonic depended upon which was her 'real Self' at that moment.
>
> (p. 40)

Thus, he resolves the problem of the 'real Self' by postulating three states of cathexis (or energy): bound, unbound, and free (which I summarise in Table 7.1).

While this may resolve the question of the *real* Self, i.e., that it can be described in terms of any ego state, in relation to free cathexis, muscular energy, and, arguably, free choice, it doesn't resolve the nature of the self. Indeed, as he himself acknowledges, ten years later, 'the feeling of the Self is independent of all other properties of ego states and of what an ego state is doing or experiencing' (Berne, 1972/1975b, p. 249)—which raises the question of where the self/Self is if independent from and, therefore, outside the ego state structure. As Ghan (1977) puts

Table 7.1. Berne's analysis of Mrs Tettar in terms of ego states, cathexis, executive power, and Real Self

Mrs Tettar's state	Child ego state	Adult ego state	Real Self
In her healthy, 'old self'	Bound cathexis	Active (unbound + free)	Adult
In her neurotic hand-washing state	Unbound cathexis, Executive power	Free	Adult
In her psychotic state	Unbound and free cathexis, Executive power	Relatively depleted of cathexis	Child

From Berne (1961/1975a).

it, Berne's three psychic organs, and their attendant ego states raise a number of problems:

Theoretical—Where and what is the Self[?]
Conceptual—How is the Self to be reconciled with the current Transactional Analysis tradition of three stacked circles[?]
Clinical—How to confront with patients the vital issue raised in the articulation, 'I cannot control myself.'[?]
Phenomenological—If I discovered my Parent, my Adult and my Child, then who is me and who is the knower[?]
Existential—What is it that moves within, yet is not visible to the external world except in manifestations of voice, gesture and behavior, etc., known as Parent, Adult and Child[?]

(p. 228)

Writing from a Buddhist perspective, Porter-Steele (1990) also raises issue about the self, putting it (in her own word) 'baldly':

That there's a huge flaw in the assumptions upon which almost all psychotherapy theory is based.... [which is] the notion that there is or has ever been such a thing as a self, or ego, whatever we may choose to call it. Can't be found, can't be found.

(p. 56)

She goes on to suggest that ego states are—or represent—'habitual patterns' (p. 56), and that Berne's description of ego states 'provide a particularly useful handle for working with those of our patterns which are the most painful' (p. 57).[8]

In their review of the psychology of the self in TA, Clarkson and Lapworth (1992) identify six, interrelated concepts of the self in TA, each of which they relate to models of ego states:

- Wholeness—in terms of Berne's (1972/1975b) diagram (see Figure 7.1), with regard to which they acknowledge the body-awareness 'skin' of the whole self.
- A multiplicity of selves—in terms of the various structural and functional models of ego states in TA.
- The moving self—in terms of the sense of self in different ego states (after Berne 1961/1975a [as noted above], 1972/1975b).
- The interpersonally-developed self—in terms of the incorporation of object relations into the internal structure of ego states, especially the Child ego state (for the further development of which, see Hargaden & Sills, 2002).
- True self and false self—in terms of splits in the self and impasses (see Clarkson, 1989; M. M. Goulding & R. L. Goulding, 1979; Mellor, 1980).
- The self as organising principle of physis—in terms of the implications of a healthy 'inner core' and a 'universal Self' (James & Savary, 1977).

Clarkson and Lapworth's review is comprehensive and, although written 30 years ago, stands the test of time. Nevertheless, I think it's difficult if not impossible to map the self on to the ego—and vice versa—as such terms describe different ideas, experiences, and conceptualisations of ourselves, which also includes: I, me, and we; organism, self, and person (for discussions of which see Tudor & Worrall, 2006); mind, body, and brain; and character, characteristic, disposition, habit, humour, personality, temperament, and trait—and much more! Notwithstanding the fine work that various colleagues have undertaken to expand the conceptualisation of self in terms of ego states, especially with regard to culture—notably Hargaden and Sills (2002), who provide a cultural reading and model of the development of the self (in C_2); Shivanath and Hiremath (2003), who offer an extension of Steiner's (1974) script matrix as a cultural script matrix which encompasses script messages from culture, religion, and the wider society; and Baskerville (2022), who builds on Hargaden and Sills' work, in her transcultural and intersectional ego state model of the self—fundamentally, the concepts of ego and of self are too associated with the individual, and with the reification of the individual, at least in Western psychology, which has created the dilemmas to which I now turn.

Outside—in

> **James Hillman:** We've had a hundred years of analysis, and people are getting more and more sensitive, and the world is getting worse and worse. Maybe it's time to look at that. We still locate the psyche inside the skin. You go *inside* to locate the psyche, you examine *your* feelings and *your* dreams, they belong to you... but look what's left out of that.
>
> (Hillman & Ventura, 1992, p. 3)

For all its simplicity and accessibility, in proposing ego states as *the* way of describing personality, Berne created a number of problems, the first of which is that, as a theory, it encourages us to think of ourselves as somewhat separate from our environment. In both *Games People Play* (Berne, 1964/1968a) and in *What Do You Say...?* (Berne, 1972/1975b), Berne emphasises this visually, when he draws a 'skin' around the three ego states (Figure 7.2), describing the result as 'the complete personality diagram of any human being whatsoever, encompassing everything he may feel, think, say, or do' (Berne, 1972/1975b, p. 12). Apart from this being a somewhat grandiose statement based on the assumption—and fallacy—of universalism, it also raises a number of questions about the nature of the ego (and the self and the person), and its (and their) relation with their environment.

One problem raised by this diagram is that, by creating a visual representation of the whole personality, Berne actually creates some gaps between the ego states and the skin, promoting the obvious—though, perhaps, unasked—questions: 'What's in the gaps?' and/or 'What do the gaps represent?'[9] (see Figure 7.3).

As neither Berne nor others have addressed this, the gaps remain untheorised.

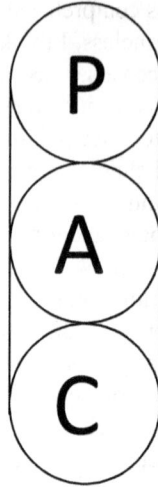

Figure 7.2. Structural diagram of a personality
Source: (Berne, 1972/1975b).

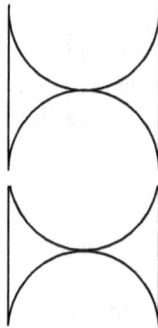

Figure 7.3. The gaps between ego states and the complete personality
Source: Based on Berne (1972/1975b).

A second problem is this 'skin' diagram emphasises the separation of the person(ality) from their environment and that the psyche (Hillman) or the ego or personality (Berne) is inside the skin. This concept of the 'skin-bound ego' (Anzieu, 1989) is the dominant model of the self in Western psychology. The traditional, open ego state diagram at least suggests that the ego states are in the environment. Taking inspiration from the gestalt conceptualisation of self, environment, and the contact boundary, I offer a modified version of the traditional ego state diagram which acknowledges the relationship with the environment (Figure 7.4).

One of Hillman's criticisms of therapy is that it internalises emotions. He reports an incident in which a truck nearly ran him off the road (as he was on his way to

Environment

Parent ego
states and
sense of self

Environment

Adult ego
states and
sense of self

Environment

Child ego
states and
sense of self

Environment

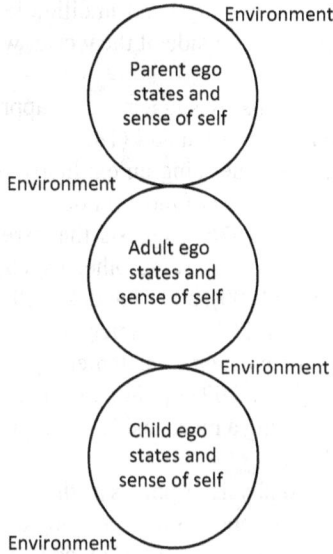

Figure 7.4. Structural ego state model, acknowledging its relationship with the environment

therapy), and he was feeling terrified. His therapist's response was to help Hillman make links to his father; his fragility and vulnerability in relation to men; his power drive; and so on, about which Hillman comments:

> We convert my fear into anxiety—an inner state. We convert the present into the past, into a discussion of my father and my childhood. And we convert my outrage—at the pollution or chaos or whatever my outrage is about—into rage and hostility. Again, an internal condition, whereas it starts in *outrage*, an emotion. Emotions are mainly social.
>
> (Hillman & Ventura, 1992, p. 11)

This example represents the dilemma about the ego and state states to which I refer as 'outside—in'. As Hillman argues: 'By going inside we're maintaining the Cartesian view that the world out there is dead matter and the world inside is living' (p. 12). In TA, the radical psychiatry tradition and others who represent and apply TA as a social psychology draw on the view that the world 'out there' is living and relevant to people, not least in its impact (see, more recently, Chinnock & Minikin, 2015; Minikin, 2018; 2023; Minikin & Tudor, 2016; Sedgwick, 2021).[10]

Socrates' advice 'To know thyself' (as the beginning of wisdom) has been widely adopted by the human potential movement as an invitation, an imperative even, to look inward and inside (for instance, through Inner Child work), and to become more self-actualised. Barad (2003) offers a counterpoint to this: 'Knowing is a matter of part of the world making itself intelligible to another part.... We do not obtain knowledge by standing outside of the world; we know because "we" are *of* the world' (p. 409).

Some have tried to resolve this by suggesting an approach based more on 'we psychology', a term coined by Fritz Künkel (1889–1956), who drew on the work of Freud, Adler, and Jung in synthesising an explicitly religious psychology (see Künkel, 1984), but which is the basis of most if not indigenous psychology (which predates Künkel). G. S. Klein (1976) suggests that 'wego' comes before ego, a suggestion that has been taken up by some other psychoanalysts, namely, Emde (1988a, 1988b), Blatt & Blass (1990), and Thandeka (1999), and the group analyst Dalal (1998). Elsewhere (Tudor, 2016e [Chapter 1]), I suggest that 'We are' is the fundamental life position—or existential statement; and, as Victoria Baskerville (personal communication, 8 July 2023) points out, it is also a statement used in activism. One way of representing a more inside out approach to ego or wego is the integrating Adult (Figure 7.5).

Berne (1947/1971) refers to physis or phusis as the 'force of Nature, which eternally strives to make things grow and to make growing things more perfect' (p. 89), and, in *A Layman's Guide...* (Berne, 1969/1971), as 'a fourth force of personality besides the Ego, the Superego and the Id.' (p. 98). In *What Do You Say ...?*, he diagrams it as a vertical arrow of aspiration originating in the Child ego state. The advantage of the integrating Adult model is that it not only represents a different model of health, it also recognises that the force of Nature lies not only in the individual (and, more specifically, their ego or ego state), but in life itself—hence the arrows in Figure 7.4 directed into the integrating Adult. Another way of representing this more outward looking, integrating perspective is the more recent use of the term 'eco states' coined by Marshall (2021a, 2021b; see also 2023).

Taking this a step further, just as, following Klein, 'wego' comes before ego, I would also suggest that the environment comes before the individual. Totton (2011) puts this well: 'That aspect of individuality which is an organismic and energetic

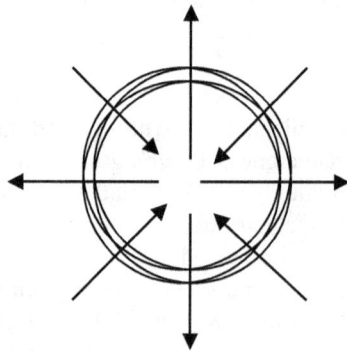

Figure 7.5. The integrating Adult, including physis

signature—the *impersonal* aspect of self—is part of nature, which precedes and grounds culture' (p. 44). Ultimately, prioritising the environment focuses us on the outside rather than the inside. In other words, it's not all about you—or me. A Māori whakataukī (proverb) summarises this well: whatungarongaro te tangata, toitū te whenua | people disappear, but the land remains.

Top—down

In presenting his three ego state model of personality, Berne (1961/1975a) writes that 'The Parent was put at the top and the Child at the bottom intuitively' (p. 80) He goes to state that 'This intuition had good moral origins' (p. 80).[11] In doing so (and as the English language is not only read from left to right but also from top to bottom), Berne, in effect, prioritises and privileges the Parent and the Parent(al) metaphor, which, for some of us, represents a second dilemma: that of a top–down approach to the psychology of people and relationships. For instance, in his work on the limits of interpretation, Lomas (1987/2001) expresses his misgivings about 'the paternalistic leanings of psychoanalysis' (p. 9), and the overuse of the metaphor of parenting to describe psychotherapy. Commenting on the legacy of this conventional ego state model in TA, Barrow (2007) argues that 'it supports the notion of the Parent as suppressing the capacities of the Adult and Child ego states' (p. 207). Clearly, psychotherapy that offers a 'corrective emotional experience' (Alexander & French, 1946), or a reparative experience such as a permission, and which operates on the basis of a deficiency-compensation model (and, therefore, represents a one-and-a-half-person psychology), does place the psychotherapist in a parental or quasi-parental role (see Chapter 5). The problem with this is that is places the client (or patient)—and, for some, the student/trainee—in the position of a child, and Child. In response, Barrow (2007) suggests an inversion of the conventional model, placing the Child on top and the Parent on the bottom, arguing that 'By inverting the metaphor, its growth-promoting potential is more fully revealed' (p. 208). Elsewhere (Tudor, 2013a, 2014/2017c), I discuss what Foulkes (1975) refers to as 'symmetrical and horizontal relationships' (p. 3), and the advantages of thinking horizontally rather than vertically, for instance, about transference, and relationships beyond therapy. In this spirit, I offer a horizontal version of the co-creative ego state model (Figure 7.6).

Two further problems arise from this top-down perspective on ego states.

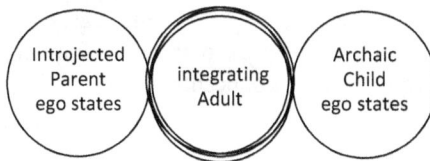

Figure 7.6. A horizontal model of ego states

The first is nominalisation. Berne and others, specifically when referring to the functional model of ego states, named certain functions such as the Adapted Child, the Controlling Parent, the Critical Parent, the Free Child, the Natural Child, the Nurturing Parent, and the Rebellious Child. The problem with this is that it associates adaptation, control, criticality, and so on, with certain ego states in a fixed and rigid way—and, moreover, one which does not meet the requirements for ego state analysis identified by Berne (1961/1975a, 1963) himself. This is particularly problematic as adaptation (as discussed above) is an important aspect of ego psychology and one which Berne (1961/1975a) associates with the Adult ego state. Similarly, control, criticality, freedom, naturalness, nurturing, and rebellion are all qualities which, on the basis of a thorough ego state analysis, may turn out to be Parental, Child, and/or Adult. This certainty about naming ego states and encouragement of understanding ego states as things in themselves also extends to ego state theory itself. For instance, Claude Steiner, with whom I had a number of vigorous debates about ego state theory, insisted that there were three ego states and only three ego states, and, thus, he didn't like models or theories that proposed anything else, including the integrating Adult ego state model, which proposes a one ego state model of health.[12] In 1517 a German pastor nailed 95 theses to the castle church door in Wittenberg, an act that began and symbolised a religious revolution that swept Europe. In 1905 an Englishwoman chained herself to the railings outside the British Prime Minister's residence in support of women's suffrage. In 1937 a French painter exhibited a work of art painted in response to the bombing of Guernica in the Basque country, a painting which epitomises the tragedy of war and the resistance against fascism. Not many would argue that Martin Luther, Emmeline Pankhurst, or Pablo Picasso were, in terms of ego states, acting anything other than from a conscientiously objecting, critical, integrating Adult. As Hartmann (1939/1958) observes, 'Luther's, "Here I stand—I cannot do other…" is not pathological behaviour' (p. 94). For further discussion of the Critical Adult, see Tudor (2015). Moreover, viewing ego states as mutable metaphors (Barnes, 1999; Gobes, 1990; Jacobs, 2000; Tudor, 2003b) avoids the danger of such nominalisations.

The second is anthropomorphism. Holt (1975) argues that 'anthropomorphism points to the redundant and confusing custom of postulating an additional entity beyond the observable organism and then giving this abstraction many of the properties of an entire person' (p. 553). This appears in TA when people talk about their Child, Parent, or Adult in a way that distances them from themselves, e.g., 'my Child's scared', 'my Parent's being critical', 'my Adult's making good decisions', etc. Along with tautology, concretism, and infinite regression, Holt (1975) argues that 'the very concept of ego exposes us to all these temptations' (p. 554). A close cousin to anthropomorphism is anthropocentrism (see p. 160 below).

Past—present

In his comments on his therapist's focus following his near accident (referred to above, pp. 152–153), Hillman says: 'We convert the present into the past' (in

Hillman & Ventura, 1992, p. 11). Referring to the inner child, he comments: 'That's the therapy thing—you go back to your childhood. But if you're looking backward, you're not looking around' (p. 6).

The majority of psychotherapies focus on the past as the source of the conflict, deficit, or confusion, though, interestingly, when discussing the object of group treatment, Berne (1966) wrote that it is 'to fight the past in the present in order to assure the future' (p. 250), a statement that clearly centres therapy in the present. In Chapter 5, I make the case for a present-centred view of therapy and of TA. Hillman argues that:

> this way of thinking suggests a completely different method for psychotherapy. Instead of starting with the small (childhood) and going toward the large (maturity), consider starting with causal traumas and external claims that determine what is to come, we start with the fullness of maturity, who and where what you are in communal world now, and read from the tree's leaves and branches and dead wood backwards to younger phases as foreshadowings, as smaller mirrors of the larger person.
>
> (Hillman & Ventura, 1992, p. 67)

The privileging of childhood as primary and determining represents for Hillman a psychology based on an 'upside-down premise' (p. 68) and he continues:

> The early scars become suppurating wounds or healed-over strengths, but not necessarily prunings for the shape of the tree, a shape ordained by the seed itself. Not only is childhood thus overvalued, but aging is trapped in an organic, and melancholy, model.
>
> (p. 68)

In response, he proposes an essential psychology rather than developmental psychology. As in the previous sections, here I offer a diagram of a model of ego states that seeks to represent a different way of thinking about ego states and a resolution to this particular past–present dilemma (Figure 7.7).

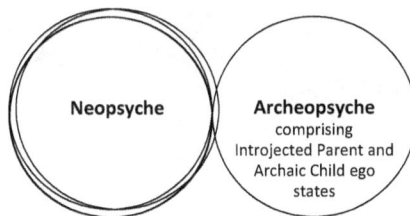

Figure 7.7. The neo-archaeopsyche two ego state model
Source: Developed from Tudor in Tudor & Summers (2014).

Thinking about reading this from left to right, and, in this sense the archaeopsyche being, as it were, in front of a person's neopsychic functioning in the world, Figures 7.7a, 7.7b, 7.7c, and 7.7d offer some variations of this model which represent different experiences and realities of neopsychic function and the influence of the archaeopsyche.

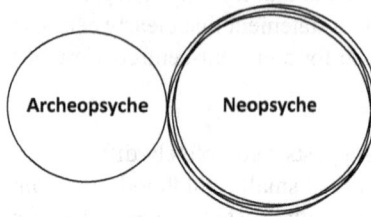

Figure 7.7a

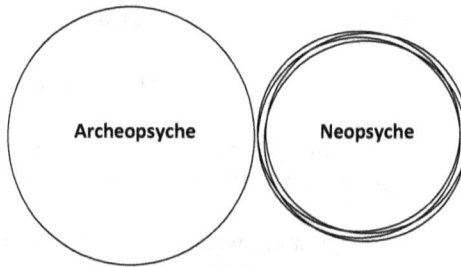

Figure 7.7b

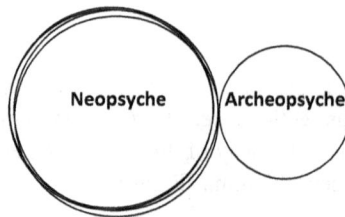

Figure 7.7c

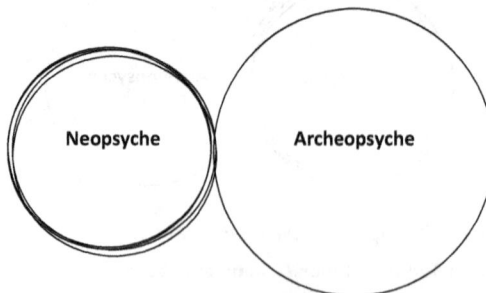

Figure 7.7d

Figures 7.7a–d The neo-archaeopsyche two ego state model (variations)

State—process

If much of this chapter has offered some deconstructivist views of the ego, this final section discusses the problem of the 'state' and, therefore, what I refer to as the state—process dilemma.

For Federn, as Leutner and Piedfort-Marin (2021) remind us, 'ego states were not parallel living entities but rather fluid experiences of the ego' (pp. 2–3). However, the predominant view in TA is that ego states are viewed as a steady state rather than a fluid process. In part, this is due to language (the problem of which is also one of Hillman's themes).

A model is a representation of structure, and, from a constructivist perspective, a structure is representative of a process; thus, we may say that ego state models are representations of the structure of personality as viewed by a number of theorists within ego psychology. However, the names given to the ego states by Berne and others are metaphors, that is a figure of speech in which a name or a descriptive term—in this case, 'Parent', 'Adult', and 'Child'—is transferred to some object (structure or representation) to which it is not always applicable. In the section on the top–down dilemma (pp. 155–156), I gave the example of the problem of certain nomenclature in TA. Following the logic of Gobes' argument (in Novey et al., 1993) that 'a person is actually "born Adult"', elsewhere (Tudor, 2003b) I suggest that we are conceived Adult. However, while I think that this is theoretically consistent, I also think that, at that point, the metaphor breaks down. So, rather than stretching, cutting, or otherwise torturing the metaphor (as Procrustes would have done), I prefer to adapt theory to the clinical situation—and so to use whatever metaphors or images work for the client. Thus, if a client refers to their 'Inner Child', I'm not going to argue with them about their use of the term. It's a handy reference to a way they have of thinking about themselves in a language with which I am familiar. Nevertheless (in my conceptualisation), I am going to be working with them to expand their integrating Adult, rather than to re-Child their Inner Child (Clarkson & Fish, 1988). However, the integrating Adult is also a metaphor for a state of process, that is, an ego *state* that is actually a constant—and, I would say, co-creative—process of neopsychic functioning, which describes a person who is, at best, in a process of fluidity (Rogers, 1961/1967a) or in flow (Csikszentmihalyi, 1975). As Totton (2011) puts it:

> The ego, as it exists in Western culture at least, is functionally identical within a state of muscular tension which aims to control our bodily states and impulses. In fact we can't control our states and impulses, since in many ways we *are* our states and impulses; instead we control their *expression*.
>
> (p. 43)

So, now we are moving beyond ego and beyond state to no ego—and no state. As Sherwood (2019) notes:

> These states, which mystics and meditators over centuries have yearned to attain—the attainment of non-self, dissolution of the ego, merging with the

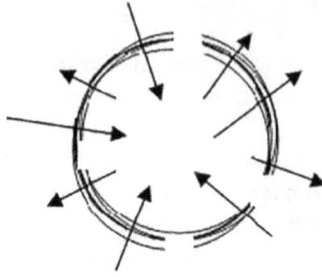

Figure 7.8. The integrating Adult as process

oceanic oneness and the great void or Nothingness—can eventually release into a blissful letting go, a surrender to death or the state of non-being.

(p. 199)

A final diagram represents this process 'state' (Figure 7.8).

Theoretically and visually, this figure represents a link to borderland consciousness (Bernstein, 2005), i.e., that consciousness that is beyond the rational, and found in the borderland, in this case, between no ego—or, at least, a deconstructed ego—and the environment. It is also informed by the concept of wild mind, which Totton (2011) defines and describes as embodied, animal, spontaneous, co-creative, self-balancing, and inherent wisdom; and an organismic, process-oriented, relational perspective on life in which the universe comprises drops of experience and not substances (see Neville & Tudor, 2024). Finally, it reflects a model that is consistent with discussions in TA about non-duality (Wells, 2012); eco states (Marshall, 2021a, 2021b); eco-TA (Barrow & Marshall, 2020, 2023b; Marshall, 2013/2014); the inseparability of self and world (Sedgwick, 2021); non-material consciousness (Heath, 2022), and anthropocentrism (Barrow & Marshall, 2023, Haynes, 2023).[13]

Of course, although this diagram is the final one in this chapter, it's not final. Commenting on this chapter and, specifically, my use of the word process, Hayley Marshall (personal communication, 8 July 2023) writes:

> In fine ecological fashion, I'm reminded that the/my language needs to come from the land, otherwise it's untethered from the very experience we're talking about—and remains of the 'ego-alone'.
>
> So far, and this is what the woodland here tells me today... a word has come as I take your work out to the land here in Derbyshire.
>
> 'They' (our kin) suggest the word 'condition'. It is a word that is also used in Amerta movement practice... and seems to me to express the essence of a supple soft distinctness *in* flow—'the condition of being Adult'.

I particularly like Hayley's suggestion of the word 'condition' as it takes me back to Rogers' (1957a, 1959) use of the word to describe the qualities and factors of the therapeutic relationship, and thus the deconstruction and reconstruction continues...

Conclusion

The state of the world, including/as environment, demands that we attend not only to how we act in and on it but also how we think about it (Key & Tudor, 2023; Neville & Tudor, 2024). Hillman and Ventura (1992) challenge us to pay more attention to the world and to be less concerned with ourselves—and I suggest that this extends to our 'selves' and ego(s), including ego states. In this chapter I have suggested a number of ways in which TA can honour its ancestry with regard to American ego psychology (not least with regard to autonomy, adaptation, and integration), while, at the same time, demystify the self and deconstruct the ego (and models of ego states). This is in order that we can more accurately represent our being and the multiplicities of our being in and as part of the world and the life of things, and think differently about the theories and models that inform our thinking.

Notes

1 Until recently, I thought that we both did this, though it turns out that I feel more strongly about this than Graeme does!
2 We further clarify this in our diagram of contaminations (Figure 7.9).

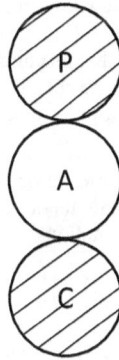

Figure 7.9. Contaminations (integrating Adult model)

Source: Tudor & Summers (2014).

3 Wallerstein (2000) identifies the most salient conceptions of the structure of the ego psychology paradigm as:

> the undifferentiated phase of development; the growth of the conflict-free sphere of the ego; primary and secondary ego autonomy (with attendant change of function); inborn ego apparatuses and autonomous ego development; the synthesizing and integrating functions of the ego; ego interests and *intra*systemic (as distinct from *inter*systemic) conflict; the separation of the ego concept from the self concept; the opposition of self- and object representations; the equal status of the aggressive drives alongside the libidinal; the transformation of the concept of sublimation into deinstinctualization and neutralization; the principle of multiple appeal; and the concepts of social compliance (analogous to Freud's somatic compliance) and the average expectable environment.
>
> (p. 138).

—a list which could (and perhaps should) form the basis of a review of the structure of TA as an ego psychology.

4 In his work Berne does not refer to Hartmann. Hartmann (1939/1958) does refer to Federn and cites Weiss (1937[/1942]). Federn (1928, 1932) refers to Hartmann, and (1929/1952) to Glover. In his own work, Weiss (1950) refers to Glover but not to Hartmann, although he does refer to Hartmann in his introduction to Federn's papers (Weiss, 1952).

5 Elsewhere (Tudor, 2003b), I discuss the nature of metaphor in TA, specifically with regard to ego states, regarding which I particularly like Allen's (2006) question:

> Do you think of ego states as psychic actualities, as metaphors, or as the expressions of neural network activations? Or more than one of these? This question is basically an extension of the old and vexing problem of the relationship between mind and brain.
>
> (p. 4)

6 The discrepancy in dates is due to the fact that the majority of Federn's early work was published in German (see Chapter 6).

7 This chapter is based on a paper read before the Vienna Psychoanalytic Society in 1928.

8 Porter-Steele's article is a response to one by van Beekum and Lammers (1990) in which they extend script theory to account for past-life experiences and reincarnation.

9 These gaps remind me of the theological perspective of and debates about God of the gaps, that is, that gaps in scientific knowledge are seen to be evidence of God's existence, for discussion of which, see Nietzsche (1892/2022), Drummond (1904), Barnes (1933), and Bonhoeffer (1944/1997).

10 In some recent correspondence I had with Robert (Bob) Schwebel, he wrote: 'I do remember walking down the street once with Claude in the early days of RP and him referring to "Ain't it awful" and he mentioned that this didn't take into account that many people had pretty awful life experiences' (R. Schwebel, personal communication, 2 February 2023).

11 Berne's (1961/1975a) full justification is as follows:

> The Parent is the guide for ethical aspirations and empyrean esuriences; the Adult is concerned with the earthly realities of objective living; and the Child is a purgatory, and sometimes a hell, for archaic tendencies. This is a way of thinking, which has come naturally in all times and nations.
>
> (p. 60)

12 Claude gave me a copy of his booklet, *TA Made Simple* (Steiner, 1971d), with the following inscription (dated June 2008): 'Dear Keith, 1971, [the] state of the art. Three ego states. What can I say? This is for you. Claude.'

13 This process state of the ego, with its representation of a merger with the environment also raises a question of whether physis continues after death: in other words, whether the fact that the organism tends to actualise, that is to maintain, reproduce, and enhance itself as an experiencing organism (see Rogers, 1963), ends with death, or whether death might be a fourth aspect or quality of the experiencing organism (see Tudor, 2010a). This theoretical addition or question has significant clinical implications with regard to how we might think about and work with clients who are dying and with suicidal clients.

Chapter 8

Shame, shaming, and 'shame'

A transactional analysis (1995)

Shame... is... a trance which enchants us, just like a hypnotist. So to end shame is to come out of the trance. When someone shames you and your head falls down and you can't reply—that's a trance. And our parents often put us into a trance because we are easier to handle in trance... and [we] have no protection.
(Bly & Meade, 1991)

In this chapter, I review Erikson's (1951/1965) psycho-social description of shame and, with examples from clinical practice, illustrate a transactional analysis (TA) perspective on shame and shaming with specific reference to TA proper, script analysis, and impasse theory. The use of the (almost obsolete) active, intransitive verb 'to shame' (oneself) is suggested as representing and reflecting the decisional aspect of shame. The clinical examples used in this article are of male clients. This is due to my own history and interest and the balance of my practice, rather than any developed gender-specific views about shame, although Steiner (1966) comments on the development of masculinity in the face of a non-masculinity script and others, notably Bly and Meade (1991), in their work with men, focus on the shame and shaming of men.[1]

In an assertion which forms a philosophical and clinical cornerstone of TA, Berne (1964/1968a) states that 'the attainment of autonomy is manifested by the release or recovery of three capacities: awareness, spontaneity and intimacy' (p. 158). Shame (the noun), shaming, and what I define as 'shame' (the intransitive verb), all inhibit autonomy: 'remembrance of past shames and fear of future shame become a straightjacket against spontaneity and knowledge of self-worth' (M. M. Goulding & R. L. Goulding 1979, p. 157).

Shame, defined in many different ways, has been the object of much psychological consideration since Freud (1905/1977). Object relations, interpersonal theory, affect theory, in particular the work of Tompkins (1962, 1963), and, more recently, self psychology, have all contributed to the debates about the nature, dynamics, manifestations, and transmission of shame. Amongst others, Kaufman's (1993) contribution reconnected shame to the individual's psyche as a phenomenological experience: shame is not merely a metaphor. The fact that that the theme of the conference jointly hosted by the International Transactional Analysis Association and

DOI: 10.4324/9780429398223-11

the USA Transactional Analysis Association in Minneapolis in 1993, and a special themed issue of the *Transactional Analysis Journal* (edited by O'Reilly-Knapp, 1994) were both on shame are examples of an increasing interest in TA in this emotion—and perhaps psychology's own enchantment with the subject. Erikson (1951/1965) observes that 'shame is an emotion insufficiently studied, because in our civilization it is so early and easily absorbed by guilt' (p. 244). In the 1990s, shame appears less hidden.

A psycho-social perspective

As far as the psychological aspect of his psycho-social perspective is concerned, in describing growth and crises in the cycle of human development Erikson (1951/1965) poses shame and doubt versus autonomy and recognises this developmental stage as 'decisive for... freedom of self-expression and its suppression' (pp. 245–246). He describes the crisis in this second age of human development as that between the muscular and emotional development of holding on and of letting go. He argues that shame is visual: it is most commonly communicated with a look. As a controlling mechanism on the part of the culture of adults, it leads 'not to genuine propriety, but to a secret determination to try to get away with things, unseen' (Erikson, 1951/1965, p. 245). It precedes guilt which, the Gouldings believe, is a judgement rather than an emotion (M. M. Goulding & R. L. Goulding, 1979). In his consideration of personality development, Kaufman (1993) links the affect of shame directly and crucially to the sense of identity. He does this, classically, by highlighting the phenomenology of shame through its facial signs and then by identifying examples of shame through the life cycle, transmitted through affective statements such as 'Shame on you', 'You are embarrassing me', 'I am disappointed in you', and, later, through disparagement, contempt, and humiliation.

Being seen, being visible and yet not ready to be visible, and hiding are the principal features of shame to which many commonplace phrases attest: for example, being 'covered with shame'; wishing 'the ground could have swallowed me up'; having 'a loss of face'; being 'caught with your pants down'. Children not resolving this crisis will tend to become withdrawn, passive, anxious and over-adapted, and seeking to please or, at the other extreme, may show little control, for example biting, hitting, and having excessive temper tantrums (Schaeffer, 1981). The irresolution of this crisis will be expressed similarly in adult life. Over time, self-consciousness or self-effacement may be turned inwards and somatised, for example in tight sphincters, seizures, stiff neck, intestinal problems (Schaeffer, 1981), or turned outwards and manifested, for instance, in the excessive use of passive language, regularly turning up late or not appearing, or agreeing to do something and then sabotaging it.

Turning to the social aspect of the psycho-sociology of shame, the controlling mechanism of the dominant culture expressed through adults has been well illustrated within psychoanalysis by Erikson and others and within TA by English (1975c, 1994). 'Shame eats the soul. It pushes you to become other than what you are, and it creates its own ring of constant fear. It is a powerful form of social control' (Seidler, 1989, p. 102). In my clinical practice, one client realised the extent of his internalisation of shame about his sexuality and particularly his sexual fantasies, the extent of his own 'ring of fear' and how he maintained that. As a result of deconfusion work with his Child and the establishment of an internal Nurturing Parent he was subsequently able to challenge the personal and social control he had internalised from his parents and his church which he had subsequently projected onto others. Shame—and guilt—are also activated, experienced, and manifested differently according to gender, sexuality, race, and culture, see, for instance, White and White (1975), and Hiremath (1995).

Erikson (1951/1965) describes doubt as 'the brother of shame. Where shame is dependent on the consciousness of being upright and exposed, doubt... has much to do with a consciousness of having a front and a back' (p. 245). One client with whom I worked was acutely aware of how he felt ashamed, by, as Yeats (1933/1962) puts it, 'the mirror of malicious eyes' (p. 144). My client often sat hunched and curled up during sessions with his back to the wall, and came to realise that he doubted and feared me only when he was concerned that a third person would enter the room. He feared exposure (of his neck and back) and that I would *see* something which could then not be unseen. Erikson (1951/1965) describes the back and 'behind' for a child as an area of the body which can be 'magically dominated and effectively invaded by those who would attack one's power of autonomy' (p. 245).

TA perspectives

In order to understand theoretically and to confront clinically such magical thinking and to support clients' autonomy in working with issues of shame, three aspects of TA theory are briefly developed: TA proper, script analysis, and impasse theory.

Transactional analysis proper

Such was I, such by nature still I am;
Be Thine the glory, and be mine the shame!

John Dryden (1687/1990),
The Hind and the Panther (lines 76–77, p. 11)

The stimulus of a shaming transaction originates in the Parent ego state, e.g., 'You should be ashamed of yourself', although it may not always be as literal, verbal, or explicit as this. If the object of such a stimulus accepts the shame and is ashamed (in the Child ego state) then this is a complementary transaction (see Figure 8.1).

In the context of group psychotherapy, one client initially hid from and thereby accepted what he saw to be Parental 'malicious eyes'. I understood this behaviour and social operation historically, in terms of his internalisation of shame as a result of many shaming transactions; and phenomenologically, in terms of Moiso's (1985)

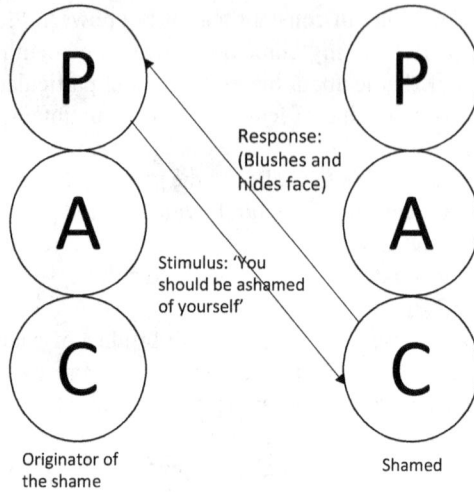

Figure 8.1. Shaming: A complementary transaction

analysis of the transference relationship whereby the client '*in order to reexperience parent-child or primitive object relationships projects onto the therapist* [and, in this case, other group members] *his own Parental Ego States*' (p. 194). I encouraged the client to make and maintain eye contact, initially with me and gradually with other group members. By cathecting Adult in this way and by checking out with other group members what they had actually been thinking or had said, he learnt to cross this projected shaming transaction effectively. Cathecting Adult is generally useful both in breaking the hypnotic quality of a shaming transaction and in decontaminating such notions that qualities and judgements (such as the 'thoughtless youth', misled manhood and pride referred to in Dryden's poem) are part of an inevitable and unchangeable 'human nature'. Such analysis of shaming transactions is essential to any TA study of shame. Curiously, Nathanson's (1994) article on shame transactions misses this opportunity, because he offers no analysis of the transactions.

The acceptance of shame by the object or victim of shaming needs some illumination. It is one thing (stimulus) to shame someone (transitive verb, active voice); it is the other side of the transaction (the response) to be shamed (passive voice). It is another to accept the shame—which is why I propose revitalising the more or less obsolete intransitive verb 'to shame' (oneself) to describe this process, one which acknowledges the decisional quality of accepting or taking on shame. In the tradition of emotional literacy, this verb confronts the passivity of the common literal and psychological 'make feel' construction (as in 'You make me feel') in everyday transactions. Thus, the acceptance of the shaming transaction is 'I shame (myself)'. In order to develop this further I turn to script analysis and impasse theory.

Script analysis

'What, must I hold a candle to my shames?'
William Shakespeare (1597/2018), *The Merchant of Venice*
(Act II, scene 6, line 41)

In order to understand both the origins of internal dialogues as well as the impact of wider social and cultural pressures, I turn to script analysis in general and the script matrix in particular (Steiner, 1966). Indeed, Steiner's own example of a script matrix with its messages about being a man serve as an illustration of how shame about being a man may be internalised (in C_2) as a part of a boy's developing psyche. Script analysis and the concept of cultural scripting (Roberts, 1975; White & White, 1975) also provides a means of analysis of the social and cultural mechanisms of shame and shaming.

As regards individual scripting, Figure 8.2 shows the partial script matrix of a particular client—partial in having no developed P_2. This follows Erikson (1951/1965, 1968) in placing this crisis chronologically as between 18 months to 3 years old, and Steiner (1966) in maintaining that developmentally the Parental injunctions (from C_2) are given earlier than the counterscript (counter-injunctions) (from P_2). Figure 8.2 represents some of the common injunctions identified by R. Goulding and M. Goulding (1976) as well as typical programmes involved in the process of shaming. In structural ego state terms, the Parental injunctions are given from the Child of the parent (C_2) to the Parent of the child (P_1) whilst the programme messages about how to act ashamed are stored and processed in the Adult of the child (A_1). Thus, Figure 8.2 shows the partial script matrix (based on Steiner, 1966), incorporating second order structural analysis (as developed by White & White, 1975). As regards the internalisation of shame, this is also consistent with Steiner's (1966) point that the script is determined by P_1 and is 'pre-Oedipal, non-verbal, preconscious, [and] visceral' (p. 18).

Freud (1905/1977) views shame (along with disgust and morality) as necessary in the repression of sexual drives. Following Freud, Erikson (1951/1965) implies that shame is necessary in order to develop an ego, 'strong enough to integrate the timetable of the organism with the structure of social institutions' (p. 238). Script analysis in general, and the script matrix in particular, is useful in *understanding* and *countering* this perspective in identifying that the acceptance of shame is a life script decision (Berne, 1972/1975b)—the intransitive verb 'to shame' represents this decision. I emphasise *understanding* and as well as countering the script as I seek to understand the advantage of the script, i.e., the child's best strategy for surviving, as much as the strategies for countering the script.

Thus, whilst Erikson (1951/1965) proposes that shame 'is essentially rage turned against the self' (p. 244), I consider the decision to accept shame, i.e., 'to shame' oneself, to be an early, pre-verbal script decision. Shame, therefore, may be analysed in terms of impasse theory.

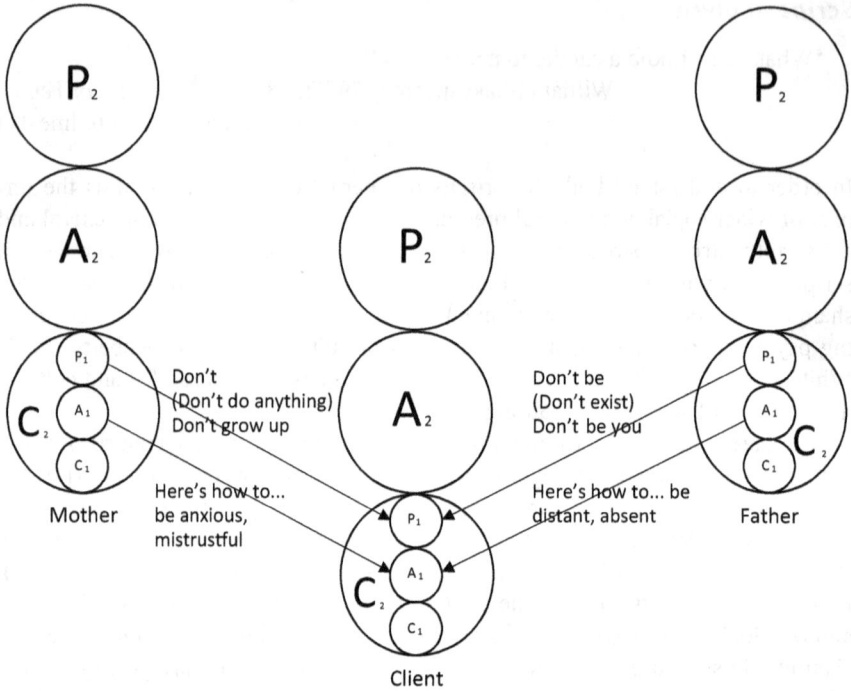

Figure 8.2. Partial script matrix showing second order structural analysis
Developed from Steiner (1966) and White & White (1975).

Impasse theory

> The ignominy of boyhood; the distress
> Of boyhood changing into man
>   W. B. Yeats (1933/1962), *A Dialogue of Self and Soul* (p. 144)

The significance of this application of TA proper and script analysis for clinical practice may be understood in terms of impasses.

In the first example (analysed in terms of transactions), the impasse (Type I) is between the client's P_2 and C_2. In the second example (analysed in terms of script analysis), the internalisation and location of shame is both in P_1 and in A_1. Thus, any redecision on the part of the client will be the result of a resolution in A_1 of a Type II impasse between P_1 and C_1 (Mellor, 1980). Following the deconfusion work with one of the clients referred to earlier, he was able to nurture his internal Somatic Child (C_1) to the extent that he came into more conflict with his largely negative and harsh Magical Parent (P_1) (Stewart & Joines, 1987). The fact that the eventual resolution of this impasse was located in A_1 was evidenced by his quick and smart ('Little Professor') thinking in subsequently interrupting injunctions about his capacity to change, to be himself, to stand his ground, and to 'face' the world.

As Clarkson (1992) points out, in linking impasse theory to the psychology of the self in TA, Type I and Type II impasses 'involve conflict between the self and an internalised other (the Parent introjected at later and earlier stages of development, respectively)' (p. 192), whereas the Type III impasse represents a conflict between two selves, the split self (good and bad, true or false, 'me/not me'). This conflict and impasse is represented differently in the TA literature as between the Free Child and Adapted Child (R. Goulding & M. Goulding, 1976), between P_0 and C_0 (Mellor, 1980), and between A_1 and C_1 (Clarkson, 1989). Clarkson (1992) gives emphasis to C_1 'as the biologically and temperamentally earliest self' (p. 192). This is developmentally and phenomenologically consistent with Stern's (1985) exciting work, identifying senses of self, in particular the first three: the sense of an emergent self, the sense of a core self, and the sense of a subjective self—all of which have emerged by 15 months (Stern, 1985). In my experience, A_1 resolution of shame, shaming, and 'shame' requires psychotherapeutic work in respect of C_1, the client's Somatic Child, specifically in helping the client literally and symbolically to remember (re-member) their body sensations—which are pre-verbal—and to re-decide 'to be myself', i.e. my whole self. The phrasings are important as they represent different impasses. The redecision 'to be me', for example, implies the resolution of a Type II impasse in response to a 'Don't be you' injunction.

By integrating the Type III impasse with Stern's (1985) domains of relatedness, we can be more specific about whether this impasse is developmentally essentially one about the client's sense of emergence (from birth), their sense of core self (from two–three months), or their sense of subjective self (from seven–nine months).

Summary

In this chapter, the emotion of shame (as distinct from the judgement of guilt) has been discussed and the process of shaming developed in relation to three aspects of TA theory. In analysing transactions and scripts and fundamental conflicts about the self I have found it useful to distinguish between shame as the Parental stimulus, shaming as the process, and 'shame' (as distinct from 'being ashamed') as the Child response. Finally, I have indicated a future direction for the integration of TA child development theory with views from developmental psychology.

Note

1 See also Bryant and Tudor (2022).

Chapter 9

Growth

Old scripts, new narratives

This chapter discusses growth and the challenge of growth. In the human potential movement, of which, since the 1960s, psychotherapy (at least in its humanistic form), and, more broadly, transactional analysis in all its fields of application, has been a part, personal growth is viewed as a good thing. At the same time, and, notwithstanding some of the early thinking in humanistic psychology, constant personal growth is, arguably, unrealistic. Moreover, we know that, in other areas of human society, such as economics and population, constant growth is unsustainable. In this chapter, I suggest that 'growth', as we have come to understand it, is part of the script of TA itself, as well as of other forms of psychotherapy, and the broader human potential or growth movement itself. The chapter begins by contextualising this discussion in terms of the two approaches to script in TA, before secondly, defining growth,[1] and thirdly, offering a review of the relatively limited literature in TA on the subject. In the fourth and final part of the chapter, I discuss some challenges of and to the concept of growth, informed by theoretical, political/ ecological, and cultural concerns, and argue that we can—and need to—develop new narratives about both script theory, and growth. As a counterpoint to the previous chapter, which was written from the perspective that scripts are self-limiting, this chapter develops the theory that scripts are also self-defining and not only problematically so.

Script in TA

Traditionally in TA, scripts have been viewed as negative and undesirable, and as something to change. In its reference to personal therapy and/or continuing professional development in its *Certification and Examinations Handbook* (the *Handbook*), the International Transactional Analysis Association's (ITAA) International Board of Certification (IBoC) notes that, while there is no prescribed number of hours of such therapy and/or development for candidates seeking certification, it 'recommends personal therapy over the period of training in order to experience the application of TA and to ensure that the trainee can apply TA *from a largely script-free stance* [emphasis added]' (ITAA IBoC, 2022, Section 7, p. 5), a phrase ('script-free') Berne (1963) himself uses in his book on organisations

DOI: 10.4324/9780429398223-12

and groups. This is despite the fact that Berne's first and last definitions of script (Berne, 1958/1977i, 1972/1975b) are neutral rather than negative, and, indeed, that he suggests that script can be positive, referring in his paper on 'Ego states in psychotherapy' to 'a practical and constructive script' (Berne, 1958/1977i, p. 156); in *The Structure and Dynamics of Organizations and Groups*, to a 'a more constructive example' of a script (Berne, 1963, p. 229); and, in *Games People Play*, to 'constructive scripts' alongside their corresponding constructive games (Berne, 1964/1968a, pp. 62, 71). For a similar analysis of game theory, see Tudor and Summers (2014), and Chapter 11.

In this context, it is worth reviewing Berne's various definitions of and references to script.

- 'A script is an attempt to repeat in a derivative form not a transference reaction or transference situation, but a transference drama, often split into acts, exactly like the theatrical scripts which are intuitive artistic derivatives of these primal dramas of childhood' (Berne, 1958/1977i, pp. 155–156)
- 'This unconscious plan, which is a strong determinant of the individual's destiny' (p. 158).
- 'An extensive unconscious life plan… after the theatrical scripts which are intuitive derivatives of these psychological dramas' (Berne, 1961/1975a, p. 23), by which dramas Berne is referring to pastimes and games.
- 'The script calls for the manipulation of other people' (Berne, 1963, p. 219).
- A script having four destiny choices, including one that corresponds to the 'I'm OK, You're OK' life position (in a co-authored paper on 'Destiny and script choices' by Haiberg et al. (1963), including Berne.
- 'These feelings become rackets when the patient learns to exploit them and collect them in his games and script' (Berne, 1964c, p. 127).
- In terms of a patient 'giving up' her script (Berne, 1965a, p. 49).
- That script is not autonomous:
  - 'the script analyst does not feel satisfied until he has decided whether the patient has actually abandoned his script to live an autonomous life' (Berne, 1966a, p. 303).
  - 'Nearly all human activity is programmed by an ongoing script dating from early childhood, so that the feeling of autonomy is nearly always an illusion' (p. 310).
  - 'A script-free person is prepared for game-free candid intimacy' (p. 310).

    In a further development or perhaps a clarification of this, in response to the question as to whether everyone has a script, Berne (1972/1975b) suggests the human race forms a curve with, at one end, those who become autonomous, and, at the other end, those who are 'script-bound' (p. 132).

- 'It is important to note that the script is not "unconscious" and can be easily unearthed by a skilful questioner or by careful self-questioning' (Berne, 1970/1973, p. 148).

- Having winners (and winning scripts) and losers (and losing scripts) (Berne, 1970/1973).
- 'An ongoing programme, developed in early childhood under parental influence, which directs the individual's behavior in the most important aspects of his life' (Berne, 1972/1975b, p. 418).

From this alone, we can see that see that there are differences and contradictions in Berne's own thinking about script, perspectives which, if anything, have expanded in the 50 years since his death in 1970—see English (1977), Erskine (1980), Levin (1985), Friedlander (1988), Cornell (1988), Erskine (2010), and Erskine et al. (2011).

Some models of script, such as the script system (formerly the racket system [Erskine & Zalcman, 1979]) tend to note the negative messages about the drama and the acts of the person's life story. Indeed, in the introduction to their article, Erskine and Zalcman (1979) refer to the racket system as being 'self-reinforcing and distorted' (p. 51). Other models, such as the script matrix (Steiner, 1966) allow for positive messages from the parents to the child (subject) in the form of permissions (parallel to injunctions), program messages (which can be either positive or negative), and allowers (as parallel to the counter-injunctions or drivers). Nevertheless, and notwithstanding the diversity in Berne's own thinking, in TA, script has been largely viewed as something negative, determining, and restrictive, and from which to be free or unbound.

Of the early transactional analysts, Fanita English most clearly develops a positive perspective on script, viewing them as 'valuable assets' (English, 1979, p. 288): 'Our scripts *enable* us to blossom, rather than preventing us from doing so, even though they may contain certain "conclusions" out of early childhood that can be dysfunctional or downright dangerous' (p. 288). As Cornell (1988) comments, in his excellent, critical review of life script theory, in her development of our understanding of script, 'more than any other TA theorist, English captures the essence of "meaning-making" which is fundamental in much of the current developmental literature' (p. 280). This 'meaning-making' view of script has been taken forward by Cornell himself as well as others within the constructivist tradition or approach in TA, i.e., Allen and Allen (1995, 1997), Summers and Tudor (2000), and some colleagues in Erskine et al. (2011). Concluding his review, Cornell (1988) offers the following definition of script:

> Life script is the ongoing process of a self-defining and sometimes self-limiting psychological construction of reality. Script formation is the process by which the individual attempts to make sense of family and social environments, to establish meaning in life, and to predict and manage life's problems in the hope of realizing one's dreams and desires.
>
> (p. 281)

Cornell's distinction between self-definition and self-limitation is enormously helpful, not only in challenging the over-determined view of script within TA (and in bringing script theory into line with more contemporary views from developmental psychology), but also in navigating our way through the different and contradictory views of script in TA from Berne onwards.[2] However, while different authors and colleagues have their preferences with regard to definitions of script, and whether script is self-limiting or self-defining, these two traditions don't have to be polarised. As Paul Robinson puts it:

> I see it that script may have been self-limiting, but it got us here. And, now we're here, we can challenge the limiting aspects of it, by recognising that we have the power now that we didn't have when we had to survive in order to get to where we are. Now we can make the most of being here!
>
> (personal communication, 6 July 2023)

It is in this context that I explore the issue—and challenge—of growth, and do so by firstly offering some initial thoughts about growth.

Growth

Growth refers to an increase in some quantity over time. The quantity can be physical, such as growth in height or an amount of money, or abstract, such as an organism becoming more mature or a system becoming more complex. Biology studies cell growth, bacterial growth, and fungal growth as well as human development in terms of growth hormones and growth spurts which, whilst commonly associated with puberty, also occur at other stages of human development. Social science deals with human development, personal development or personal growth, individual growth and population growth. Economics is concerned with economic growth, financial growth, and growth investing. Mathematics has concepts of linear growth, logistic growth, exponential growth, and hyperbolic growth. Ecology considers growth in terms of recycling, and renewal,[3] and as such, offers a different paradigm: one that challenges growth as increase, a point which I develop later in this part (pp. 174–175 below) and to which I return (in the last part of the chapter, pp. 180–185 below).

Moreover, it is not just quantity that matters, and, indeed, one of the challenges of growth is to consider the *quality* of growth, a challenge that is encapsulated in concerns about the quality of life. When people talk about having or wanting to have 'quality time', I suggest that this represents a desire or hunger for a balance between endless growth, often measured in terms of success, achievement, and material wellbeing; and, in the words of the poet, W. H. Davies (1911), 'time to stand and stare'.[4] In this sense Berne's (1970/1973) human hungers—for stimulus, recognition, contact, sex, structure, *and incident*—may be viewed as hunger for regulation: both the 'up regulation' of the sympathetic nervous system and the 'down regulation' of the parasympathetic system. We need both for growth. Similarly, games fulfil a regulatory role (see Chapter 11).

From conception onwards, we grow. Whether we like it or not, we grow. In this sense, growth is constant and inevitable. As human organisms, we are in a state—or, more accurately, a process—of constant growth or change: our gut lining is replaced every five days; the skin's outer layer every two weeks; red blood cells every 120 days; bones every ten years; and so on. Research in neuroscience provides us with evidence of the plasticity of the brain: we are hard-wired for growth and change, so we *can* teach old dogs new tricks, and change *is* as good as a rest. Even when we consider our deoxyribonucleic acid (DNA), which one might think is more fixed, it turns out that only 10 per cent of the DNA present in our bodies belongs to our own cells; the rest resides within the ten to one hundred trillion bacteria and other organisms which inhabit our bodies. Thus, we are growing, changing, and, biologically and metaphorically, diverse human beings. We are not only *in* process, we *are* process (see Chapter 7). As Fox (2007) puts it: 'a person should be understood as an active process, not a thing—not even a thing that undergoes change and self-replacement during its lifetime' (p. 11). In this sense, it's not that we need permission to grow—'it's OK to grow', as Boyce (1978) suggests; it's that growth is ubiquitous and inevitable. Indeed, from an ecological perspective, if a permission were needed, it would be 'It's OK not to grow/develop/build/expand/take, etc.' In a rare article in the *Transactional Analysis Journal* that refers to human beings as organisms, Rinzler (1984) reflects that: 'we display a callous and grandiose ingratitude towards the millions of microscopic organisms that make up what we call "my body", which function collectively, cooperatively, and with breath-taking efficiency, to get us from here to there' (p. 231). Writing about human disconnection—from ourselves as organisms and the organism Earth—Rinzler argues for greater connection with our sensory, physical selves, and a commitment to the somatic level or aspect of connection and attention informs much of Marshall's eco-therapeutic work (see Marshall, 2021; Marshall in Enari et al., 2023).

With regard to what this perspective on growth means for how we think about human beings and how to nurture and work with them, Rogers puts it well:

> Too many therapists think they can make something happen. Personally, I like much better the approach of an agriculturalist or a farmer or a gardener: I can't make corn grow, but I can provide the right soil and plant it in the right area and see that it gets enough water; I can nurture it so exciting things happen. I think that's the nature of therapy. It's so unfortunate that we've so long followed a medical model and not a growth model. A growth model is much more appropriate to most people, to most situations.
>
> (Rogers & Russell, 2002, p. 259)

So, like other organisms, human beings, grow—the experiencing organism maintains, enhances, and reproduces itself (Rogers, 1963)—and dies (Tudor, 2010/2021a). If we want to think about this in terms of script, we could consider that growth is part of the self-definition of what it means to be a human being—and, therefore, that we don't have to force that. Following Rogers—and, arguably, Berne and/or other transactional analysts (see pp. 179–180 below)—we might focus on analysing, providing, or co-creating the conditions under which that growth is enhanced for the client,[5] as well as reflecting on the ways in, by, or under which their organismic growth was or is limited (by abuse, oppression, trauma, and so on).[6] This is also consistent with the argument made in Chapter 7.

However, there's a difference between natural, organismic growth, and that growth which is unnatural in the sense that it is manufactured, often supported by an oppressive ideology, and unsustainable, and, therefore, ultimately, self-limiting—for individuals, often for specific oppressed groups, for societies, and, ultimately, for the whole world and all species. Here, I am referring to political and economic growth. Industrialisation, capitalism, colonialism, the expansion and invasion of other countries by force, and the exploitation of the Earth's resources: all are examples of ways in which 'growth', in terms of products, money, territory, borders, and human life and lifestyle, respectively, is viewed as a good thing and used to justify certain actions and policies—as well as inactions, which we can understand in terms of discounting, passivity, and passive behaviours (Schiff et al., 1975).[7]

TA offers some ideas that support critical thinking about growth. The first is to consider such growth as examples and aspects of self-limiting scripts. One aspect of this is the 'Take It' driver (Tudor, 2008c),[8] which both offers a developmental understanding of narcissism, and is informed by a social psychological process which 'in terms of human development and later socialization, encourages greed, competition, and power seeking (i.e., power 'over' people and adversarial transactions)' (p. 47). The negative, 'Grab It' aspects of this counterscript driver include a person getting something at someone else's expense, and taking according to want rather than need; justify overconsumption, addiction, and alienation; and are 'associated with a defensive (and aggressive) position of "I'm OK, You're not OK"' (p. 49). If we consider the I subject as human beings and the other/object/You as the Earth, this driver also describes the human exploitation of the Earth's resources in the service of endless growth. In one of his articles about education, written in a similar spirit and analysis, Barrow (2018) argues that 'much [of] education contributes significantly to the problem of unsustainable consumption, growth at all costs, and cultivating a sense in individuals that the world is theirs to own and objectify' (p. 333). He concludes that:

> Better education, more sustainable and resilient education, is about creating an experiential space in which the student is free to create a renewing story about how the world—this world—might continue to be a home in which a good life might be lived.

> (p. 333)

In a subsequent article, Barrow (2020) challenges the 'assumed virtue…[of] growth' (p. 181), with regard to both personal/individual and economic growth. Arguing robustly that 'In light of so much awareness of climate collapse, pushing toward growth is at best naive and, at worst, irresponsible' (p. 184). Finally, writing about principles of EcoTA, Barrow and Marshall (2020) refer to the 'indoor mind' which sets human beings apart from the environment and the Earth and justifies mindless growth and consumption, as distinct from an 'outdoor mind' which is more at one with or a part of the environment, Earth, and, ultimately, the cosmos (see Neville & Tudor, 2024).

Before I consider certain challenges posed by this analysis of growth, I turn to the concept of growth in TA.

Growth in TA

There is comparatively little in the TA literature specifically on the subject of growth as such. Berne discusses growth in one chapter in *The Mind in Action* (Berne, 1947), in which he generally uses the word synonymously with development. In the updated, second edition of this book, published as *The Layman's Guide to Psychiatry* (Berne, 1969/1971), he makes two comments on growth:

1. That 'since the primitive creative and destructive urges themselves cannot be basically changed, growth or change in the human personality takes place by changing the manner in which these tensions are relieved' (p. 88).
2. That changes in natural development and in the object of gratifications 'are greatly influenced by the Ego, usually in accordance with the Reality Principle' (p. 89)—and that this Ego becomes more efficient in accomplishing its task of relieving libido, mortido, and reducing the threat of the outside world.

In these two points we can see the influence of Berne's psychoanalytic thinking, the implications of which regarding growth are:

1. That, as human urges are given, clinicians need to help clients focus on relieving the tensions caused by these urges—for instance, by encouraging the quality of their thinking, their use of inner resources, and their independent, adaptive patterns: all qualities of the Adult, according to Berne (1963).
2. That, as the 'reality principle' is also given, the second task of the clinician is to help the client develop a more efficient ego/Ego in order to relieve the urges of the Id and reduce the threat of the Superego—which echoes Berne's (1963) view of the Adult ego state as 'not affected by Parental prejudices or archaic attitudes left over from childhood' (p. 186).

Few authors since Berne have referred specifically to growth. In an early article, Campos (1970) refers to 'autonomous growth' (pp. 51, 57). In a short article, Vago and Knapp (1977) write about adequate (P_2) parenting as offering protection for growth. Levin-Landheer (1982) writes about human growth in terms of stages or cycles of development, i.e., being, doing, thinking, identity, being skilful, regeneration, and recycling, a concept and taxonomy that Keepers and Babcock (1986) later develop in their book *Raising Kids OK: Human Growth and Development Throughout the Life Span.* Exploring TA and conflict management, de Graaf and Rosseau (2015) write about embracing conflict as an opportunity for growth and learning but don't develop their argument as far as growth is concerned. Only Massey (1985), in an article on family systems therapy, says anything substantial about growth, which, in the context of growth-promoting families (and systems), he defines as:

- Interconnected, and flexible;
- Having clear and permeable boundaries between ego states, with resultant free-flowing energy, and independent functioning;
- Having ego states that are 'more internally programmed or probability-oriented and spontaneously manifest personal autonomy' (p. 123);
- In terms of time structuring, are 'more involved in creative and reflective withdrawal, productive activity, intimacy, and play' (p. 123); and
- In which children are more differentiated than the(ir) parents.

This is a useful list of descriptors which are, in effect, process outcomes for growth (see Rogers, 1958/1967b).

The apparent lack of interest in TA in growth is reflected in the very few references to the subject in the ITAA IBoC's (2022) *Handbook.* References to growth appear in only two places:

- In the CTA written exam—in one of the questions in the organisation's written examination (Section 8.4.4, Question 5).
- In the Training Proposal Outline (TPO) (Section 10.12)—in which candidates are asked to write about their own experience of personal growth, and, with regard to their own trainees, how they will encourage their personal growth, and to comment on any criteria and requirements they would have for such personal growth.

Although there is little in the TA literature on growth, and it may be that it is viewed as synonymous with development or change, I suggest that all transactional analysts have a view about growth, even if it is implicit. Different ways of thinking about growth in TA include:

- Working through the original protocol and later palimpsest by means of deconfusion, and analysis of the transference to effect transference cure and script cure.
- Helping to effect social control and symptomatic relief by means of ego state, transactional, script, game and racket analysis, and change in cognition and behaviour.
- Challenging the alienation caused by tensions, oppression, mystification, and isolation by means of awareness, contact, and action, principally in groups.
- Freeing the cathexis bound in such tensions by means of regression, reparenting, and rechilding.

- Resolving the impasse between such givens and tensions by means of impasse, Parent resolution, and redecision.
- Working with disowned, unaware, and unresolved aspects of the self, by means of enquiry, attunement, and involvement.
- Evolving different constructions of reality and meanings by means of dialogue, and co-creative transactional relating with a view to expanding the integrating Adult.

From my use of language in these statements, the reader may well have spotted that they represent, respectively, the Classical (psychodynamic), Classical (cognitive behavioural), radical psychiatry, Cathexis, Redecision, integrative, and constructivist/co-creative traditions or approaches within TA (see Tudor & Hobbes, 2007). For a more comprehensive list of traditions, approaches, or sensibilities within TA, see Chapter 12.

If we accept the proposition that growth is inherent and inevitable, then the principal clinical challenge of growth is to identify, accept, and support this growth. As the elaboration of the theme of the 2011 World TA Conference (The challenge of growth) suggests:

> The challenge of growth goes hand in hand with the challenge to support and accept the growth of the people we care for, and of the people we work with....
> Throughout life we will find, sometimes very clearly, many other times more softly, this endless opportunity and need for learning: the constancy of growth as an opportunity and fact.
>
> (ITAA Bilbao Conference Organising Committee, 2011)

I suggest that we do this in a number of ways:

1. That we understand, accept, and support growth by identifying and working with physis, the 'force of Nature, which eternally strives to make things grow and to make growing things more perfect' (Berne, 1947/1971, p. 98).

   Berne referred to physis or phusis in several of his books and, as a concept, this has been picked up by others in TA: P. Clarkson (1992), Piccinino (2018), Milnes (2019), Koopmans (2020), and B. Clarkson (2021), and, indeed, there are a number of TA centres and training institutes called Physis.[9] I suggest that this evolutionary fact and concept supports a clinical leaning or attitude and practice of being alongside, even behind our clients, rather than ahead of them, and a humility that is encapsulated in Berne's (1966) therapeutic slogans: '*Je le pensay, e Dieu le guarit*' (p. 63) (I treat them, and God cures them).

2. That our acceptance, understanding, and support of growth and change is explicit in the contractual method by which we seek to clarify the client's view of both the end(s) and means of therapy (see Chapter 2).

   This is implicit in Berne's (1972/1975b) concept of four stages of cure— social control, symptomatic relief, transference cure, and script cure—by which we (hopefully) understand not but the limits but also the benefits of the client's stage or process of and engagement with change or growth.

3. That we understand, accept, and support both growth and defences by the way we transact or operate with our clients.

   In this regard, Berne's (1966) therapeutic operations, the original techniques of TA, may be viewed as interventions or interpositions which challenge the client to grow and, specifically, to grow or expand their (integrating) Adult. Of course, we will have our own ways of doing and thinking about this. M. Goulding (1975/1978) puts this somewhat robustly when, in a brief article entitled 'To my clients' she said:

   I am bored with pathology. I am excited by health. And growth.

   Tell me your troubles, confusions, mistakes, hates, and I'll listen for as short a time as possible; therefore, I'll treat you as fast as I can. Tell me of your triumphs and I'll hear you out....

   I am not interested in your sucking in my protection, permission or potency. My potency is: I give me to be with you in health, in growth, so that you, too, will discard in boredom your pathology and celebrate yourself in health.

   (p. 15)

   Whilst I have every sympathy with Goulding's focus on health, and am excited by her obvious excitement about and commitment to growth, I think it is also important to understand the meaning of the client's confusions, mistakes, hates, and boredom and what we may think of as 'pathology'—and to transact and interact from and in a more acceptant and empathic frame of reference.

4. That our acceptance of growth and change means that interruptions and ruptures in the way that client and therapist relate can be opportunities for exploring defences, stuck points, and 'bent pennies' (Berne, 1961/1975a) as a particular point of growth.

   This may represent what Hinshelwood (1991) refers to as 'the point of maximum pain' (p. 171), but which we might reframe as the point of maximum change and growth (see Tudor, 2023).

5. That, just as growth is nurtured and fostered by environment conditions, so, we as therapist will pay attention to the past—and present—conditions of the client.

   The idea that there are certain 'conditions' of therapy which facilitate growth and personality change was developed by Rogers in two major formulations (Rogers, 1957a, 1959). What is significant about these for our current interest is that they are, in effect environmental conditions of therapy, and, moreover, co-created by *both* therapist and client (for further discussion of which, see Tudor, 2011d). Within TA, attention to such environmental conditions appears in:

   • Aspects of script theory that focus on the original environmental (family) conditions in response to which the script was informed.

- Aspects of TA as a group treatment that consider the group as the environment.
- Therapeutic communities informed by the Cathexis School/approach, which sought to provide a different Parental environment.
- The TA Asklepieion programme run at the maximum security federal penitentiary at Marion, Illinois, in the USA (1968–1978) (see Corsover, 1979; Groder, 1972, 1977).
- The radical psychiatry tradition (see The Radical Therapy Collective, 1971; Steiner et al., 1975; Wyckoff, 1970, 1976b).
- Aspects of relational TA, especially those that embody a 'two-person-plus' psychology (Tudor, 2011b).
- EcoTA (see Barrow & Marshall, 2023b; Marshall, 2021a, 2021b).

6. That, in doing all of this, we are essentially working with clients to create new narratives about their old, self-limiting scripts.

   In this, I see a link between growth as personal development *that is sustainable*, i.e., in terms of a person's personal and social relationships, and social and economic context, and our ability to make meaning of old, reviewed, and new narratives.[10] Following on from his previous comment (p. 173, above), Paul Robinson suggests that this process may be understood in terms of 'enabling our frame of reference to change, so that our script is also constantly (re)emerging, adjusting, and enabling new possibilities.' (personal communication, 6 July 2023).

Challenges of—and to—growth

From the above, it is clear that the concept of growth is underdeveloped in TA. However, and not surprisingly, given that it has provided the theoretical basis of the human potential movement for more than 60 years, humanistic psychology offers much more on this subject—see especially Rogers (1954/1967c), Cohen (1961), Clark (1963), Rossi (1967, 1971), Sutich (1967), Frick (1990), and Pfaffenberger (2005). So, the first challenge to and in TA is a theoretical one: that of developing a theory of growth, perhaps informed by some of the extensive literature in humanistic psychology, and, not least, so that transactional analysts preparing their TPOs have a greater sense of what personal growth might mean.

However, like TA, humanistic psychology was founded in the United States of America just after the Second World War, and, similarly, focused on individual growth and development also in terms of autonomy (e.g., Lee, 1963; see also Chapter 7), but more in terms of self-actualisation (Maslow, 1954). In one of the early papers on growth, Sutich (1967) writes about the importance of the 'growth-experience' and 'continuous emotional growth' (p. 156) and asserts that 'the desirability of continuous growth ("unlimited" this side of a hypothetical perfection level) goes without saying' (p. 157)—though he does note that this a value judgement. Given that that we are in a different era, with different challenges, not least regarding the value of continuous growth, a second challenge is a philosophical and political/ecological one: that of questioning whether we can have too much growth.

Finally, given that growth is predominantly viewed as personal, and linked with concepts such as self-actualisation and autonomy, it sounds somewhat individual and individualistic (see Barrow, 2020). Given the climate crisis, and the fact that TA is practiced in many different countries and cultures, a third challenge is an ecological and cultural one: that of questioning whether 'growth' is the right metaphor.

In this final part of the chapter, I explore these challenges within the framework of the four fundamental theoretical pillars of TA.

Scripts

Summarising English's (1977) conceptualisation of script, Cornell (1988) writes that: 'script formation is *determining* rather than *determined*, formative rather than acquiescent, unpredictable and creative rather than reductionistic, focused on the future rather than embedded (mired) in the past' (p. 281). I think this is a useful way to think—and ask questions—about growth in TA. What is my history with regard to growth and/or personal development? Is it determined or determining? Is the concept of being 'script-free' determined or determining? What games do I and others play (negative or positive) that foster such scripts? Is my engagement with personal growth and therapy formative or acquiescent? If trainees and training institutes acquiesce to the personal therapy requirements of accrediting bodies, does this compromise the therapy and its formative quality?[11] How can I maintain an unpredictable and creative relationship with growth? Would seeing a spiritual advisor or having singing lessons 'count' as hours of personal and/or continuing professional development,[12] or are such hours determined (by type, form, duration, and so on) and, thereby, reductionistic? To what extent are my experiences of and thinking about growth embedded in the past (as introjects, or unintegrated archaic experiences) and enacted in games, or are they present-centred and future-focused? All these questions are deigned to provoke new frames of reference, and possibilities.

I consider that one of the biggest theoretical challenges of growth in TA is to develop TA as a robust health psychology.[13] As Cornell (1988) put it: 'development studies of healthy individuals and longitudinal studies of human growth and psychological formation challenge some of the basic assumptions and attitudes underlying transactional analysis' (p. 281). These challenges include the clarification—or, at least, the elaboration—of physis as a 'growth force' (Berne, 1947/1971, pp. 142, 216, 228) or 'growth urge' (p. 114), originating in the integrating Adult (see Chapter 7). Clearly, how transactional analysts view the origin of growth, depends on their definition of and perspective on ego states (see Chapter 6).

Part of this involves reconceptualising 'defences' as growth. Traditionally, defences have been viewed as problematic and wrong, and deserving of analysis and/or breach, as in breaking them down. A more humanistic approach is epitomised by the slogan 'Defences are there for protection', and, arguably, TA has been at the forefront of humanistic therapeutic thinking about protection (Crossman, 1966). Taking this a little further we may consider that we 'grow' defences—and may also grow them in psychotherapy. In this context I agree with Speierer's (1990) point that '"resistance" is an error of empathy on the therapist's side' (p. 343). This not only challenges us to be empathic; it also reminds us to be attuned to when we are not so empathic—and, as therapists, to work with the client's reception and perception of our acceptance and empathy (Rogers, 1958/1967b).

All of this points to a meta-theoretical challenge that emerges from this analysis. If, as Cornell (1988) suggests, human growth is 'an interactive, creative, ever-changing process' (p. 273), it follows that human growth theory also needs to be interactive, creative, and changing. Thus, we need to move away from fixed, closed, and universalist theories and towards those that are fluid, open, local as well as generalisable, and, thereby, amenable to development, change—and sustainable growth.

Games

Writing about game(as) as repetitive patterns of maladaptive behaviour, Rossi (1967) examines the 'game–growth dichotomy' (p. 139) in psychotherapy. He summarises this as follows:

> In the game dimension one is generally concerned with the individual's relation to the outside world and his ways of coping with it.... In the growth dimension, on the other hand, one is more concerned with the individual's experience of his inner world and his relation to it.
>
> (p. 139)

He offers a heuristic dichotomy in which, under the game dimension he includes Freud, Sullivan, Wolpe, Skinner, Ellis, Berne, and others, and under the growth dimension, Jung, Rank, Adler, Frankl, and other existential and humanistic thinkers. He goes on to argue that 'all forms of psychotherapy that focus on outer behavior and interpersonal relationships... contain a strong game component' (p. 141)—Freud's mental mechanisms and analysis of defence, Sullivan's interpersonal theory, Skinner's behaviour therapy, and so on, and acknowledges that the 'classic example of this is transactional analysis as described by Berne' (p. 141). It's a very interesting article with regard to the history of psychology, and one which highlights the dichotomy in TA between game and growth.

Thinking about growth in terms of games and game analysis requires us to be able not only to analyse games that deter or inhibit personal growth, but also to acknowledge positive games (see Chapter 11) or games and play that enhance growth. For this, I suggest drawing on:

- The concept of good or constructive games (Berne, 1964/1968a) with gratificatory functions. (Berne, 1961/1975a), for examples of which, see Groder (1971), Wallace (1973), and Zechnich (1973).

- The Winner's triangle (Choy, 1990).
- The reframing of games as 'co-creative confirmations' (Summers & Tudor, 2000; see also Tudor & Summers, 2014).
- Using the criteria advanced by Massey (1985) for growth to assess whether such games, or confirmation help people to be interconnected, flexible, and, in terms of time structuring, 'more involved in creative and reflective withdrawal, productive activity, intimacy, and play' (p. 123).

Transactions

Considering transactions from this view of growth suggests that we need to identify growthful transactions and/or reframe TA proper with regard to growth. These could be complementary (perhaps even complimentary?!), and certainly co-operative, for which we can draw on the radical psychiatry tradition and, specifically, Steiner's (1974, 1976, 1978, 1980, 2003) work on co-operation. They should certainly be aimed at enhancing relationships and life. It's also important to have or develop the emotional literacy to be able to cross transactions—with care—as in that encounter with the other is often where psychological and emotional growth lies. Again, thinking about this from a meta-perspective, Steiner's (1974) point about the political consequences of a transaction is useful here. What are the messages I am receiving—and giving—about growth; are they sustainable; and, what, if any, are the ulterior (commanding) messages?

For example, in terms of global energy, a report on the *World Energy Outlook 2021* shows that, with regard to natural gas and oil demand, the demand predicted from actual stated policies is, in both cases, higher than the scenario predicted from announced pledges (International Energy Agency, 2021). Although both these scenarios are based on figures that are available, the announced pledges appear more like the social level transaction, while the stated policies are more hidden (ulterior)—and, as we know, 'the behavioral outcome of an ulterior transaction is determined at the psychological level and not at the social level' (Berne, 1966a, p. 227).

Ego states

Reparenting (re-Parenting) (Schiff et al., 1975) and rechilding (sic, as technically it's re-Childing) (Clarkson & Fish, 1988) are based on the notion of replacing and growing or regrowing those respective ego states, and thus represent a three ego state model of health, i.e., one in which the fully functioning person has—and the end goal of therapy is that they have—a complete complement of ego states. The model of growth in the co-creative one ego state model of heath is the integrating Adult, an ego state in a constant process of integrating—and, arguably, in a process of not being an ego (see Chapter 7). Either way, I suggest that it's important that transactional analysts have an ego state analysis of growth, for which Massey's (1985) work (noted on p. 177) offers a good basis.

In economics, the concept of an overheated economy describes the situation in which there is too much of some quantity or too many of some products, the main signs of which are rising rates of inflation and an unemployment rate that is below the normal rate for that economy. Energy consumption is the total amount of energy required for a given process; global energy consumption has increased nearly every year for more than half a century (Ritchie et al., 2022). In psychological terms, are we, analogously, in danger of producing or encouraging 'over-heated' personalities whose demand and consumption outstrip their supply or contribution? We have only to think in terms of narcissistic and anti-social personalities to conclude that we may well be doing so (see Tudor, 2008c). Does a psychotherapy with a focus on the self, self-development, and self-actualisation produce a selfish self? Does 'one-person psychology' (Stark, 1999) result in a person who focuses more on the 'one' than the other, i.e., 'you', 'they', 'we', and 'it'? In this context, there may be a danger that empathy encourages clients to develop more of an understanding of themselves than of others, society, the environment, and the planet. Psychotherapy, at least in its individual form and its 'one person' focus, can promote an unhealthy individualism that is no longer sustainable in our interconnected and interdependent world, especially as we face interconnected, complex, and wicked problems.

In this sense it may be less useful to think of ourselves, others, and personalities as changing and growing, and more useful to think in terms of evolving—and devolving.

On the basis of this analysis—with regard to scripts, games, transactions, and ego states—it may be possible to change scripts about growth, whether personal, interpersonal, social, cultural, economic, or theoretical.

Conclusion

Finally, picking up the political thread of this chapter with regard to sustainability, I suggest that the ecological challenge of—and to—growth includes:

- Reclaiming TA as a group psychotherapy—which would make it more accessible and viable.[14]
- Balancing TA's value and goal of autonomy with homonomy (Angyal, 1941) or a sense of belonging (see Cook, 2022; Tudor, 2023)—which would make it more relevant to many people from different cultures.
- Developing TA as a 'two-person psychology' (Stark, 1999), and, further, as a 'two-person-plus psychology' (Tudor, 2011g)—which accounts for the client's context, as well as the impact of the social/political world on the client, and of the client on their world.
- Changing the ecology of TA in all its fields of application and our practice, for instance, with regard to ethics (Salters, 2021), online exams, and travel (de Graaf & Tigchelaar, 2021a, 2021b).

Responding to the challenge of growth is challenging and so we also need to grow, develop, or evolve our ability to challenge—and to be challenged—which will keep TA responsive and relevant to the needs of changing, challenged, challenging, and complex clients in our ever-changing, challenging, and increasingly complex world.

Notes

1 This section of the chapter is developed from a keynote speech I was invited to give on 'Challenges of growth' (Tudor, 2011a).
2 Cornell's (1988) review and views about script theory were also highly influential on the co-creative development of script theory (see Summers & Tudor, 2000).
3 In referencing the concept of renewal, I acknowledge the work of Barrow (2014) on natality.
4 In the spirit of standing or pausing:

> Leisure
>
> What is this life if, full of care,
> We have no time to stand and stare.
>
> No time to stand beneath the boughs
> And stare as long as sheep or cows.
>
> No time to see, when woods we pass,
> Where squirrels hide their nuts in grass.
>
> No time to see, in broad daylight,
> Streams full of stars, like skies at night.
>
> No time to turn at Beauty's glance,
> And watch her feet, how they can dance.
>
> No time to wait till her mouth can
> Enrich that smile her eyes began.
>
> A poor life this if, full of care,
> We have no time to stand and stare.
>
> William Henry Davies (1911)

5 Actions which represent the three modes of Stark's (1999) modes of therapeutic action: one-person psychology, one-and-a-half person psychology, and two-person psychology, respectively.
6 I am aware that not many transactional analysts refer to the organism, either as a biological and social reality or as a metaphor for the human being, for a discussion of which, see Tudor (2003b) and also Chapter 7. In a rare reference to the concept, Steiner (1967), writing about hermetic scripts states: 'Thus, the infant who is biologically a self-preserving organism can be trans-formed into an organism that ignores self-preservation to obtain Parental protection' (p. 70).
7 Interestingly, Hillman and Ventura (1992) associate the decline in politics and an insensitivity to the real issues in life to passivity—and to (an over-indulgence in) therapy.
8 I am grateful to Giles Barrow for his encouragement to include this material in this chapter.

9 Physis, Bangalore, India (https://physis.co.in/), Physis, Rome, Italy (https://www.physis.org/), The Physis Institute, Dunedin, Aotearoa New Zealand (https://www.jostuthridge.co.nz/transactional-analysis-psychotherapy-training), and Physis Scotland (https://www.physisscotland.co.uk/).
10 I am grateful to Paul Robinson for encouraging me to make this point.
11 For discussion of this, see Tudor (2018b).
12 Yes, they could—and have been.
13 For discussion of TA as a positive psychology, see Allen (2006a), Barrow (2007), and Napper (2009).
14 In his last public workshop, Steiner expressed his view that group therapy was one of the most radical contributions of TA (Steiner & Tudor, 2014, 55:04f).

Chapter 10

Regulation and registration

Protection or protectionism? A plea for pluralism (2010)

Preface—Evan Sherrard[1]

Friends in the TA world—I highly commend Keith's article for your careful consideration. I wish I had been as aware of the contents some years ago. I would have changed my stance on statutory registration of psychotherapists. I was a strong supporter of state registration and helped to promote its introduction. I still believe in the need for registration but not by a state agency such as the [New Zealand] Ministry of Health which employs the medical model of health care to psychotherapy and is managed by bureaucrats. We only have to look at how the Accident Compensation Corporation (ACC) in New Zealand has managed sensitive claims to see how bureaucrats work and how resistant they are to making corrections.

I am embarrassed to have to admit how naive and uncritical I was in supporting the move to state regulation through registration of psychotherapists. I have friends and associates who are members of the Psychotherapists Board of Aotearoa New Zealand and supported their appointment to the position. One recently chided me for complaining about how they were functioning by telling me I had not done my homework of studying the legislation under which registration was being set up.[2] If I had, it was suggested, I would not have been surprised by what has come about. It is all there in black and white in the Act of Parliament setting up how the Board has to behave.[3] I am told they are powerless to do anything different. I am distressed to know how inadequately I did my necessary homework, but, in this article, Keith has clearly set it all out; I commend it to your attention.

Sadly, it seems, any modification or changes to the current situation will not come about by reason. It looks as though some campaigning will be necessary, just as it was to secure any alteration to ACC's approach to their recent new regulations of sensitive claims for past sexual abuse. This recourse to campaigning always seems to set up conflictual, adversarial conditions amongst friends and associates, rather than strong, robust debate with goodwill. We can avoid the worst of this pain in the TA community by being fully informed about the issue, and I thank Keith for providing the information which will allow for cool debate about the issues rather than the heat of disputation and disagreement.

Evan M. Sherrard—Once a psychotherapist, still a transactional analyst.

DOI: 10.4324/9780429398223-13

Introduction

There has been a lot of talk both here in Aotearoa New Zealand and in a number of other countries about the statutory regulation of psychotherapy and the state registration of psychotherapists. In most of the world governments do not require psychotherapists to be regulated or registered in this way, although in a number of countries professional associations have established systems of self-regulation and voluntary registers which are maintained and administered by the profession—mechanisms which are acknowledged in a recent New Zealand Ministry of Health (2010b) discussion document:

> Occupational regulation can occur through a range of mechanisms. Statutory regulation is one option, but other industry-led mechanisms are also effective... *Self-regulation allows these groups to assure the public of quality and promote the good standing of their professions.* [emphasis added][4]
>
> (p. 6)

In Aotearoa New Zealand, the term 'psychotherapist' has, since 2007, become a protected title under the *Health Practitioners Competence Assurance Act 2003* (hereafter 'the *Act*') with the result that clinicians who wish to refer to themselves as a psychotherapist have to register with the Psychotherapists Board of Aotearoa New Zealand ('the Board' or PBANZ) which, in effect, administers the *Act* on behalf of the Ministry of Health [MoH] and the government.

I am aware that a number—even the majority—of transactional analysts here [in Aotearoa New Zealand] are, have been, or were in favour of this form of regulation and registration. I am also aware, however, that there was very little debate about this move; almost no reference to the literature or research which was and is critical of such organisation—see Hogan (1979), Dawes (1994), Mowbray (1995), House and Totton (1997), Wampold (2001), Postle (2007), Parker and Revelli (2008), Postle and House (2009); and that very few psychotherapists appear to have read the *Act* prior to or even after voting for this move [see Dillon, 2011/2020; Tudor, 2011/2020e]. Given the zeitgeist of 'evidence-based practice' it seems somewhat ironic that there was little or no critical analysis of the general lack of evidence base for this particular practice and form of regulation.

Objections

The controversies about and objections to statutory regulation and state regulation fall into four main areas:

1. **In principle objections to the statutory regulation of psychotherapy and the state registration of psychotherapists**
   There is significant literature concerning the objections to and problems with the statutory regulation of professions (Dawes, 1994; Hogan, 1979) and specifically the regulation of psychotherapy—Hogan (1979), Mowbray (1995), House

and Totton (1997), Wampold (2001), Postle (2007), Parker and Revelli (2008), and Postle and House (2009)—none of which was referred to in discussions about the move to regulation and registration in Aotearoa. These objections are based on arguments in favour of freedom of association (and free association), of assembly, of trade, and of practice, and against any restriction of these rights and activities. Observing the impact on human babies when their freedom is restricted simply by having their arms held by their sides, Panksepp (1998) suggests that: 'throughout life anything which limits our freedom will be viewed as an irritant deserving our anger, contempt and revolutionary intent' (p. 189). In TA we might think about this objection in terms of autonomy.

2. **Objections to the fact that the *Act* makes no reference to *Te Tiriti o Waitangi | The Treaty of Waitangi***

   For some, this would be sufficient reason to oppose any form of regulation and registration under this particular *Act*. The lack of reference to the Treaty was justified at the time the then *Health Practitioners Competence Assurance* [HPCA] *Bill* was in progress through parliament by the Ministry of Health (2003) which issued a three-page statement in which it asserted (p. 2) that:

   > The Treaty of Waitangi provisions in the *NZPHD* [*New Zealand Public Health and Disability*] *Act* [2000] convey what the Crown, itself and through its DHBs,[5] have done, is doing, and will do under the Treaty for Maori health. The *HPCA Bill* establishes a regime for the registration and discipline of health practitioners. No additional or new Treaty interests are put in issue under the... Bill.

   Whilst this may have been true for the 13 medical professions included in the original *Act* (although I suspect it was and is not), it was clearly inaccurate as far as the profession of psychotherapy was and is concerned, and given the partnership relationship between the New Zealand Association of Psychotherapy (NZAP) and tangata whenua [the first people of the land] in the form of Waka Oranga, the only Māori rōpū [group/organisation] of Māori psychotherapists. In TA we might think about this objection in terms of the ethical principle of respect.

3. **Concerns that the *Act* assumes that the regulation of health practitioners protects the public**

   The *Act*, as the MoH (2010a[/2018]) puts it, 'provides a framework for the regulation of health practitioners in order to protect the public where there is a risk of harm from the practice of the profession'. The argument that the public is in need of protection from harmful practice is *the* rationale for the *Act*, and is often presented as the main justification for statutory regulation. Unfortunately for proponents of statutory regulation and state registration, there is no evidence to support what is, in effect, simply an assertion and, moreover, a lot of evidence that challenges it (see, for example, Gross, 1978; Hogan, 1979; Mowbray, 1995, 1997). I and many others have been challenging this assertion for many years; I know members of the current Board who acknowledge that this rationale is not a strong one; and last month I was relieved and reassured to hear Seán Manning, a TA colleague and currently President of the New Zealand Association of Psychotherapists (NZAP), acknowledge this when he said (at an NZAP Northern Branch meeting) that he accepted that there was not much evidence that statutory regulation protects anyone. From a TA perspective, claiming that potential clients are so vulnerable that they have to be protected against the consequences of their decisions appears to run counter to our basic philosophy that people are OK, have the capacity to think, and can decide their own destiny.

The arguments that statutory regulation benefits *the profession* (in terms of greater respect, respectability, and employment) are debatable points and gains. Moreover, whatever the merits of such claims, what is more interesting is the fact that, in a document on statutory regulation and the health professions, the MoH (2010b/2018) makes clear its disapproval of this line of argument coming from professions seeking statutory regulation (when their motivation should be concerned with the protection of the public).[6]

So, from a TA perspective, we might think about this objection in terms of autonomy (and not Rescuing people), and the ethical principle of integrity.

4. **Concerns that the *Act* and the move to statutory regulation and state registration assumes that psychotherapy is best viewed, positioned, and promoted as a health profession**

Under the *Act* a 'health practitioner' or 'practitioner' means a person who is registered with an authority (i.e., the Board) as a practitioner of a particular health profession (see Section [§] (1)). The fact that psychotherapy is regulated under this *Act* brings it into line with other health professions. Indeed, one of the purposes of the *Act* is to provide (§(2)(a)): 'for a consistent accountability regime for all health professions'—and, indeed, the original professions encompassed by the *Act* were all health professions closely allied to medicine.[7]

More recently, the Ministry of Health (2010b/2018) has asserted that: 'Having one legislative framework allows for consistent procedures and terminology across the professions now regulated by the Act'. Clearly, the idea was that psychotherapy be viewed as a health profession and adopt 'accountability regimes' (in itself an interesting term) and 'procedures', terminology which reflects a medical paradigm (for a critique of which see Postle & House, 2009). One example of this paradigm, and the difference between it and a psychotherapeutic perspective, is the definition of supervision as: 'the monitoring of, and reporting on, the performance of a health practitioner by a professional peer' (see §7(1)). Many supervisors, including TA supervisors, would not agree with this definition of supervision. Whilst some psychotherapists do clearly identify as health professionals both in terms of the paradigm and of the *Act*, the notion that psychotherapy is a health profession is debatable and, indeed, highly disputed (see Postle & House, 2009); and there are many clinical as well as other certified transactional analysts working in other sectors such as education (for example, school and university counsellors), community and youth work, and in organisations and industry who are, in effect, discounted by registration under a *health Act.*

So, finally, from a TA perspective, we might think about this objection also in terms of autonomy, that is, the autonomy of the practice and profession to define itself.

The Psychotherapists' Board

In addition to these points, there are particular concerns about how the PBANZ has operated since its establishment in 2007. In many ways these concerns reflect broader problems inherent in the role of registration boards, although there have been particular concerns with how this particular Board has acted with regard to the definition of psychotherapy; the lack of a code or framework of ethics;[8] and its reneging on agreements with Waka Oranga regarding the development of a Māori scope of practice and a kaupapa Māori pathway to registration [that is a pathway based on principles drawn from a Māori world view], and the development of cultural competencies.[9] Two years ago, the Board, with little or no consultation, decided to extend the definition of the term 'practice' such that it 'encompasses all roles that a psychotherapist may assume such as client care, research, and policy making, educating and consulting' (PBANZ, 2008, p. 3647). Apart from being a misuse of language, this unwarranted and unnecessary extension was out of step with a number of other related professions, such as clinical psychology whose registration Board does not require educators or trainers to be registered practitioners (except those on accredited training programmes and who are supervising clinical practice); it also represented a threat to the freedom, independence, autonomy, and livelihood of educators, trainers, researchers, consultants, and policy-makers, let alone the concept of academic freedom, which is enshrined in the *Education Act 1989*. As Freud (1926/1959) commented some 80 years ago: 'Thus once again in our country a line of intellectual activity would be suppressed which is allowed to develop elsewhere' (p. 234).

Resisting statutory regulation and state registration and promoting pluralism

In the light of these concerns, a number of psychotherapists, registered and unregistered, have come together this year to form a group both to resist and challenge the apparent inevitability of regulation under the present legislation, system, and regime, and to promote a pluralistic approach to regulation of psychotherapy— and, by implication, other helping activities/professions, such as counselling and music therapy (whose practitioners are currently debating the question of registration). We ourselves are a pluralistic group, inspired by different traditions, different theoretical approaches, and different politics, and have different emphases in our concerns. What unites, however, is an objection—and it is a conscientious one—to the imposition by the state and, in effect, a few professionals of a system of regulation and one approach to registration:

a. Which was under-theorised, poorly argued (see Ministry of Health, 2003), over-promoted, and insufficiently discussed (see Bailey, 2004).
b. Which did not consider other models of regulation whereby practitioners could choose whether to be state registered or not, as can social workers under the *Social Workers' Registration Act 2003*.
c. Which addressed neither the context or nature of psychotherapy.
d. Which makes no sense in terms of what we know about human regulation, in terms of the importance of self- and co-regulation—see House and Totton (1997), and Embleton Tudor (2011/2020).
e. Which currently operates as a closed system, governed by a non-elected Board, appointed by a politician, i.e., the Minister of Health.

Of course, in the Alice in Wonderland world of statutory registration and state regulation whereby, like Humpty Dumpty, the Board can choose what a word means, there is no such thing as an unregistered psychotherapist because, if you are not registered, by definition, you are not a psychotherapist and may not hold yourself to be one. Significantly, when Alice challenged Humpty Dumpty and asked, 'whether you *can* make words mean so many different things', he replied: 'The question is... which is to be master—that's all' (Carroll, 1872/2021).

In response, in order to support colleagues who are not registered, not registering, or not paying for their annual practising certificate, and to encourage informed debate, we, the Independently Registered Psychotherapy Practitioners, have, to date:

1. Established a national network, the Independently Registered Psychotherapists, which will shortly have a website (see Fay, 2011).
2. Held one public meeting in Auckland called 'Stopping to Think: Psychotherapy and Its Discontents', which attracted around 40 people and was very successful in promoting pluralistic approaches to and strategies about regulation and registration.
3. Presented this perspective to the Northern Branch of the NZAP.
4. Planned a book on the subject of regulation and registration, which contains a number of different voices in favour of freedom, diversity, and pluralism, and which we are planning to launch in February 2011, hopefully at the NZAP Conference in Dunedin.[10]

I emphasise *informed* debate as, in discussions about regulation and registration, I have heard, and have heard of, a certain degree of scare-mongering such as: 'You've got to be registered to practise'. This is not true. You have to be registered if you want to refer to yourself as a *psychotherapist*. Whilst the term psychotherapist is currently a protected term—indeed, that is the logic of statutory regulation—other terms, including 'transactional analyst' are not. Thus, qualified transactional analysts can say and state that, whilst not holding themselves to be a psychotherapist. On a personal note, in the UK and most of the rest of the world I may say and state that I am a 'UKCP [United Kingdom Council for Psychotherapy] registered psychotherapist' (a voluntary, professional voluntary registration). Here I have been advised that I cannot state that as, according to the Board, using the words 'registered' and 'psychotherapist' in the same sentence, even if this includes a clear reference to the UK, is misleading and could be confusing to members of the public. I disagree, but then I give more credit to the general public in Aotearoa New Zealand than does the Board. This is professional protectionism under the guise of protection and, from a TA perspective, we have an analysis of such protection as a racket—and a game. In response, another strategy in the resistance to state regulation is the creative reclaiming of title: of counsellors, therapists, analysts, psychodramatists, and traumatologists who are doing psychotherapy but who are not holding themselves to be psychotherapists. Some of us have been challenged on this. One colleague of mine said: 'Yes, but, if something looks like a duck, walks like a duck, and smells like a duck, it's a duck!' My rejoinder is: 'Of course it's a duck, but if the government says that it can't call itself a duck, then it's not a duck!'

I have also heard that transactional analysts are being told that they can't practice—or supervise or teach TA—if they are not registered practitioners on the grounds that the ITAA requires us to observe 'local requirements' or 'national laws'. Again, not true. In its *Training and Examination Handbook*, with regard to 'National and regional requirements for psychotherapy and/or counselling', the Training & Certification Council of Transactional Analysis (2009) states that:

> The practice of psychotherapy and/or counselling is officially or semi-officially recognised in some countries and regulated in others. A trainee may therefore need to meet specific national requirements for training and accreditation as well as the requirements for TA training before becoming a recognised practitioner in her or his country. The trainee's national TA organisation(s) should be aware of what these requirements are, and trainees and their supervisors should familiarise themselves with them.

(p. 5)

So, trainees, supervisors, and trainers should *familiarise themselves* with specific national requirements for training and accreditation. No more, no less.[11]

It is clear that many in the field of psychotherapy are in favour of statutory regulation. I have talked to a number of colleagues, for instance, working in the health services, who are keen to be and to remain registered. They feel that, as registered practitioners, they are more respected by other health practitioners and that they now have a place at the table where they can promote psychotherapy in this part of the public sector. Whilst I think that these arguments bear further examination (see Tudor, in press[/2011f]), I support their right to be registered in this way. I simply don't want the way of the state to be the only way, and I don't want to lose my right to call myself a psychotherapist. Exclusive state regulation of psychotherapists is a power play which discounts and excludes people, and encourages over-adaptation and a powerless script. As transactional analysts we are more than capable of analysing the transactions and games involved, for instance, of the government and the Board; and in making an ego state and script analysis of the personalities and organisations involved.

In the UK, psychotherapists have turned back from statutory regulation of the profession and voted for a twin track approach which would mean that a practitioner could be a 'psychotherapist' or a state 'registered psychotherapist'.

TA is a broad church, and, as with any church, holds people with many different beliefs, traditions, theological and political inclinations (see Tudor, 2010d). I would hope that, on the basis of certain common values such as autonomy, respect, and integrity, TA colleagues in Aotearoa New Zealand would and will support pluralism and the freedom to practise.

Notes

1 Evan Sherrard was a New Zealand transactional analyst (CTA and TSTA), a good colleague, and dear friend. Although, for various reasons, he had initially been a supporter of the statutory regulation of psychotherapy, he quickly became disillusioned by the process, and a supporter of pluralism (see Sherrard, 2011; 2017/2020). I wrote this article as I was putting together a book on the history and critique of the statutory regulation of psychotherapy and state registration of psychotherapists (Tudor, 2011f) and, as I knew TA colleagues in Aotearoa New Zealand respected Evan, I asked him if he would write a brief introduction to it—to which he readily agreed. For those interested in knowing more about Evan, see Sherrard (2017/2020).
2 The *Health Practitioners Competence Assurance Act 2003* ('the *Act*', 'the *HPCA Act*').
3 See Tudor (2017/2020f, Appendix 3). This comment is interesting in the light of the fact that another colleague who was appointed to the Board, openly boasted that she hadn't read the *Act*.
4 In Aotearoa New Zealand, counsellors have chosen the path of self-regulation (see New Zealand Association of Counsellors [NZAC], 2016a; Smith & Tudor, 2015). In 2021, the Ministry of Health (MoH) published a document which includes various options for allied health professionals not currently covered by the *Act* (MoH, 2021). In 2022, in the context of the international coronavirus pandemic and the national mental health crisis, the New Zealand government in conjunction with the NZAC published an "opt-in accreditation pathway" for counsellors (Little, 2022; NZAC, 2022).
5 District Health Boards.
6 For a profession to know this, and then to apply for regulation on the basis that it would enhance the profession is a clear Con—or, depending on one's analysis of when this game started, a Gimmick.
7 They were chiropractors; dentists, including dental technicians, clinical dental technicians, dental therapists, and dental hygienists; dieticians; optometrists and dispensing opticians; medical practitioners such as GPs, psychiatrists, surgeons, and other specialists; medical auxiliaries including medical laboratory technologists and medical radiation technologists; midwives; nurses; occupational therapists; pharmacists; physiotherapists; podiatrists; and psychologists.
8 The Board formulated ethical standards in 2013 (PBANZ, 2013).

9 The Board formulated cultural competences in 2019 (PBANZ, 2019).
10 Which we did, selling over 100 copies, i.e., to a third of the attendees. This was subsequently published in an extensively revised edition (Tudor, 2017b), which, in turn, was republished as an open access e-Book in 2020 (Tudor, 2017/2020f).
11 One TA colleague decided not to come to a training event at which Evan and I were training and supervising on the basis that, if they did, they would have to report us to the Board. In fact, at the time, the Board had no policy regarding the status of trainers and supervisors. Indeed, the Board only produced its policy of accreditation of training programmes in 2021 (PBANZ, 2021), i.e., some 10 years after this particular event—a policy which does not preclude non registered practitioners (i.e., clinicians) from teaching or supervising psychotherapy trainees/students.

Chapter 11

Gaming and playing

Re-reading *Games People Play*

In some ways this was, at least initially, the most difficult of the new chapters to write for this Part of the book because, of the four fundamental pillars/pillows of transactional analysis (TA) theory, game theory as a whole has been my least favourite. This was due to a number of reasons:

- That I found *Games People Play* (Berne, 1964/1968a) the least readable of Berne's books, notwithstanding that it was a bestseller—and was even made into a board game (Figure 11.1).[1]
- That I found a number of aspects of game theory contradictory and confusing—and felt somewhat bad about that until (after my training) I read the critiques of it offered by Zalcman (1990) and Hine (1990).
- That I found some of the original names of games both very culturally specific to a place and time, i.e., California in the United States of America in the mid-1960s, and, in some cases, offensive.[2]
- That I experienced game theory, more than other TA theory, used in a Parental fashion and against people, as in 'That's a game' or 'You're playing a game', rather than to facilitate awareness, understanding, and change possibilities, including co-operation. Of course, simply telling someone that they're playing a game is itself the beginning (or continuation) of a game.
- That, for me at least, it most represents the 'pop psychology' aspect of TA, and its inherent oversimplification of transactions and the dynamics of relationships.

So, as part of my project of writing four new chapters to pair with previously published material on transactions (i.e., Chapter 5), ego states (Chapter 7), scripts (Chapter 9), and games (this chapter), respectively, I decided to re-read *Games People Play* to see either what I hadn't previously understood or appreciated about it—or whether such a review would confirm my original critique. As a result of this re-reading, I identified three themes—context, definitions (including, more broadly, the scope of game theory), and play—which structure this present discussion of game theory, in which I also include more contemporary views of this particular pillar of TA theory.

DOI: 10.4324/9780429398223-14

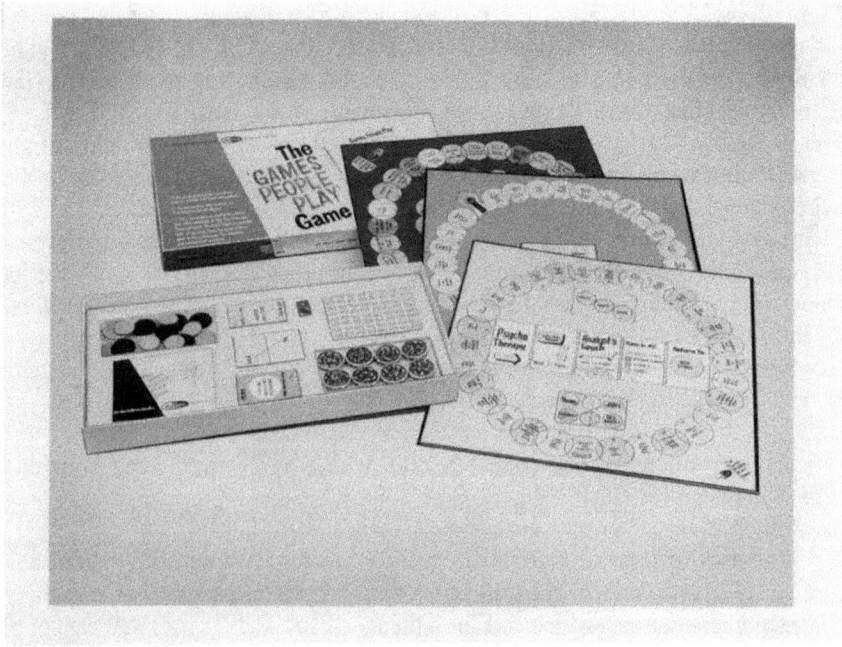

Figure 11.1. The Games People Play board game
(Berne, 1967).

Context

The first thing I noticed in revisiting *Games People Play* was its subtitle: 'the psychology of human relationships' (p. 3). Berne goes on to explain:

> Theories of internal individual psychodynamics have so far not been able to solve satisfactorily the problems of human relationships. There are transactional situations which call for a theory of social dynamics cannot be derived solely from consideration of individual motivations.
>
> (p. 59)

Thus, games, as a theory of social dynamics, link directly to social psychiatry and, thereby, to *Transactional Analysis in Psychotherapy*, the subtitle of which is 'A systematic individual and social psychiatry' (Berne, 1961/1975a, p. 3). Indeed, in *Games People Play*, Berne (1964/1968a) acknowledges that 'the present approach is one aspect of social psychiatry' (p. 51). However, as I note elsewhere (Tudor, 2020g; see also Chapter 12), Berne's view of social psychiatry was little more than 'the study of the psychiatric aspects of specific transactions or sets of transactions which take place between two or more particular individuals at a given time and place' (Berne, 1961/1975a, p. 12), or the analysis of 'the inner causes and motives that result in specific transactional stimuli and responses [which] are the individual's private concern' (Berne 1963, p. 176). For discussion of Berne's limited view of social psychiatry, see Baute (1979), Zalcman (1990), Barnes (2003), Massey (2007), Steiner (2010), and Tudor (2020g). Indeed, in her overview and critique of game analysis and racket analysis, Zalcman suggests that: 'game analysis and racket analysis need to be recognized as separate and distinct areas of TA, with the primary distinction being that game analysis deals with transactional events, whereas racket analysis deals with intrapsychic processes' (p. 4), a distinction which would make game theory and game analysis more clearly a *transactional* understanding of social dynamics.

Berne (1964/1968a) also refers to three other social aspects of games (and game theory):

- Social dynamics—a 'large field' (p. 51), which he contrasts with individual psychodynamics:

  Theories of internal individual psychodynamics have so far not been able to solve satisfactorily the problems of human relationships. These are transactional situations which call for a theory of social dynamics that cannot be derived from consideration of individual motivations.

  (p. 59)

  In his earlier work on *The Structure and Dynamics of Organizations and Groups*, Berne (1963) refers to such dynamics as 'the science which treats of the forces acting on or within any social aggregation of between social aggregations' (p. 318). Thus, as well as being interested in why two or more people are playing a game, we might also be interested in the forces in the field of that relationship (see Lewin, 1952) that drive, help, and enable, or restrain, discourage, and limit us from playing games. Summerton (1993) sees social dynamics as concerned with intragroup and intergroup game analysis or 'the cultural matrices that support group games' (p. 102). Some years earlier, Summerton (1985) had developed the game pentagon, in which he identified the game roles of stage manager, spectator,[3] sniper, scapegoat, and saviour—and which is the only game theory in TA that explicitly references social dynamics (Summerton, 1992). So, whenever and wherever two or more people are playing a game, there is a social matrix that supports that game—a perspective that immediately widens our field of game analysis.

- Social contact—which Berne (1964/1968a) defines as having an opportunity for people to communicate with each other, and, thereby, to be a social aggregation (as distinct from a social dis-aggregation). In *Transactional Analysis in Psychotherapy*, Berne (1961/1975a) introduces the Part of the book in which he outlines social psychiatry and transactional analysis with a few pages on a theory of social contact. In this, and drawing on the work of Spitz (1944) on emotional deprivation, Berne advances the importance of sensory stimulation, 'the most essential and effective forms... [of which] are provided by social handling and physical intimacy' (p. 83). This then sets the scene for his development of his theory of human hungers, which, at this stage, he presents as deriving from stimulus hunger with 'its first order sublimation into *recognition-hunger*' (p. 84)—and (on the same level as this): social contact (whence contact hunger [Berne, 1970/1973]) and structure hunger (whence the structuring of time [Berne, 1961/1975a]). Later (in *Games People Play*), Berne (1964/1968a) identifies a number of advantages to such contact, which (consistent with his earlier work) 'revolve around somatic and psychic equilibrium' (p. 19) (see below, pp. 201–202). In his work on games, play, and intimacy, Cornell (2015) acknowledges Berne's understanding of games as an aspect of 'structuring time through patterns of social contact' (p. 79), and of games and intimacy as the most gratifying forms of social contact.

- Social action—which Berne (1964/1968a) defines as the influence people exert on each other's behaviours and responses. While Berne acknowledges that different disciplines investigate social action from different points of view, he himself emphasises his concern with and focus on 'the personal histories and psychodynamics of the individuals involved' (p. 51). Berne's clarity is helpful, as it suggests that those who have different concerns or foci—who, if you like, investigate social action from a different discipline, point of view, or approach *within* TA—need to articulate that. Thus, for instance, radical psychiatrists have a view of action as a prerequisite for liberation (Wyckoff, 1976a) and social action as necessary for social change. In her work on dependency, Symor (1977) describes 'social action interventions' (p. 41) at each stage of therapy, which includes:

  - In response to dependency, 'analysis of shortages' and the 'selection of specific issue for successful action' (p. 41).
  - With regard to counter-dependence, 'identification and expression of anger about specific issues' (p. 41).
  - With regard to independence, 'exploration... [and] expression of chosen alternatives' (p. 41).
  - In order to consolidate interdependence, the 'identification of where cooperation is possible as equals', and the resumption of contact with the 'power group' (p. 41).

While such therapeutic work does involve the awareness and exploration of personal history and 'psychodynamics'—which Symor explores through the analysis of Victim passivity, Persecutor passive aggression, Rescuer superiority, and the reversal of symbiosis—it is clear that this point of view focuses more on interpersonal and social dynamics than does Berne's transactional aspect of social psychiatry.[4]

Already, I am more excited about *Games People Play*—and I'm only on p. 51!

Definitions and scope

In what is perhaps his most recognised definition, Berne (1964/1968a) describes a game as 'an ongoing series of complimentary ulterior transactions progressing to a well-defined, predictable outcome' (p. 48). Elsewhere, Summers and I observe that this provides a neutral definition of games and, indeed, 'a nonpathological formulation that later definitions restrict' (Summers & Tudor, 2000, p. 37); and, in a later publication, we develop this tripartite analysis of the definitions of games and game theories as negative, neutral, or positive (Tudor & Summers, 2014). While I still agree with that, it is clear from Berne's writing that he viewed games primarily as a way of describing some form or degree of problematic behaviour (see below). Here (and again), we can see that Berne's different definitions create some confusion, a point that is also further analysed and highlighted by others, notably Zalcman (1990), and Hine (1990). Here I offer a summary of different definitions of game(s) and contributions to game theory (in chronological order—and, thus, beginning before *Games People Play*), followed by a note (in parenthesis) as to whether the theory or contribution is neutral, negative, or positive,[5] as well as some comment on them, heavily influenced by the critiques of Zalcman (1990), and Hine (1990), as well as others.[6]

- Games (and pastimes)—'Certain repetitive sets of social maneuvres [which] appear to combine both defensive and gratificatory functions' (Berne, 1961/1975a, p. 23), 'based more on individual than social programming' (p. 86) [**negative and positive**]

  Later in this book (*Transactional Analysis in Psychotherapy*) in his chapter on the 'Analysis of Games', Berne states that:

  > The great bulk of social intercourse is made up of engagements.... [which] are of two types: pastimes and games. A pastime is defined as an engagement in which the transactions are straightforward. When dissimulation enters the situation, the pastime becomes a game.
  >
  > (p. 98)

  Later, in *Sex and Human Loving*, Berne (1970/1973) emphasises his view that what he refers to as human psychological or transactional games are programmed 'to a large degree by the parents' (p. 160), but also genetically.[7]

- Hard game(s) (Berne, 1962) [**negative**]
  A brief note on a group marks the first reference to 'a hard game' (Berne, 1962, p. 8), though it is not defined. In *Games People Play*, Berne writes about 'a flexible, loose, easy game' (p. 64) as a first stage of a game which he equates with a first-degree game, which may progress to an inflexible, tenacious, hard third stage' (p. 64; see also pp. 202–203, below).

- Writing in the context of groups, Berne (1963) suggests that, as members develop more personal relationships with each other [**negative**]:

ulterior transactions begin to creep in. These often occur in chains, with a well-defined goal, and are actually attempts of various people to manipulate each other in a subtle way in order to produce certain desired responses. Such sets of ongoing transactions with an ulterior motive are called games.

(pp. 200–201)

- A game as 'an ongoing series of complementary ulterior transactions progressing to a well-defined, predictable outcome' (Berne, 1964/1968a, p. 48) [**neutral**].

  Eusden and Pierini (2015) consider this definition limited 'because it suggests more emphasis on verbal, symbolic forms of relating, which is more focused on adult relating' (p. 129).

- 'It is a recurring set of transactions, often repetitious, superficially plausible, with a concealed motivation; or, more colloquially, a series of moves with a snare, or "gimmick"... Every game, on the other hand, is basically dishonest, and the outcome has a dramatic, as distinct from merely exciting, quality' (Berne, 1964/1968a, p. 48) [**negative**]

  As these sentences immediately follow Berne's initial definition, this immediately sets up the contradiction and tensions in game theory—almost as if Berne himself is playing a game with us about games: 'Now you see it; now you don't'![8] In response to my categorisation of this quotation, P. Robinson (personal communication, 5 July 2023) argues that 'being dishonest is not, in my view, necessarily negative'. He continues:

  > We could be in protection mode, thus 'Good to see you!' could be 'dishonest' because we're really excited and happy to see you, but we're protecting ourselves in case the other person has forgotten who we are. So, we're being dishonest in the sense that we're not telling the whole truth, rather than telling a 'lie', for instance, saying it's good to see you when, actually, it's not!

- The advantages of games (Berne, 1964/1968a) [**neutral**].

  Berne states that 'the general advantages of a game consist in its stablizing (homeostatic) functions' (p. 56), and goes on to identify six advantages to games:

  - *Biological advantage*, the advantages of which may be expressed in tactile terms, both examples of which Berne gives (i.e., slapping and kicking) are forms of violence.
  - *Existential advantage*, which refers to 'what anxiety-arousing situations of intimacies are being avoided' (p. 70).
  - *Internal psychological advantage*, which can be assessed by 'its direct effect on the psychic economy (libido)' (p. 57).
  - *External psychological advantage*, for example, 'the avoidance of the feared situation by playing the game' (p. 57).
  - *Internal social advantage*, which 'is designated by the name of the game as it is played in the individual's intimate circle' (p. 57), which, by definition, is, at some level, socially acceptable (and thus a first-degree game).

- *External social advantage*, which 'is designated by the use made of the situation in outside social contacts' (p. 57) (which is also more likely to be at a first-degree game).

To this taxonomy, Bary and Hufford (1997) add:

- *Physiological advantage*, which involves 'the body armoring that a person develops to adapt to the psychological-emotional-physical environment [originally] of childhood' (p. 39).

Zalcman (1990) considers the terms used in Berne's analysis as variable, including everyday languages, TA terms, psychoanalytic terms, and so on.

- Games are constructive or destructive (Berne, 1964/1968a) [**positive** and **negative**]
  Following on from the 'both…, and…' perspective he advances in *Transactional Analysis in Psychotherapy*, in *Games People Play* Berne (1964/1968a) states that 'depending on whether the script is constructive or destructive, the corresponding games are accordingly constructive or destructive' (p. 62), acknowledging that 'People who play destructive games will come to see the therapist far more frequently than people who play constructive games.' (p. 71) While this last point may appear obvious, its significance is that here Berne is clearly acknowledging games as both positive/constructive and negative/destructive. In his article on transformation learning, Robinson (2020) refers to positive games as one way to break out of script.

- The formal game analysis of psychological games (Berne, 1964/1968a) [**negative**]
  Zalcman (1990) views Berne's scheme as 'a tool for practical, *not* theoretical game analysis' (p. 6), and his categories for the elements of the scheme analysis (title, thesis, antithesis, etc.) as 'a mixture of clinical descriptions and conceptual hypotheses' (p. 6). She also critiques the fact that, despite the view of games being a transactional event between two or more people, many of the identified games are noted and analysed from the point of view of only one player. Hine (1990) also critiques game theory which does not acknowledge the bilateral nature of games and offers her own model which emphasises this. She also observes that 'By inviting the use of pejorative labels for games, the theory actually furthers games while pretending to offer a solution to a painful process' (p. 28). Eusden and Pierini (2015) acknowledge that, while Berne's identification of games is helpful, it is also reductionistic, and also comment on the fact that Berne 'did not expand his theories into the two-person realm' (p. 129).

- Degrees of games (Berne, 1964/1968a) [**neutral** (in description) but **negative** (in outcome)]. Berne identifies three stages in or degrees of a game:

  - A first-degree game is 'one which is socially acceptable in the agent's circle';
  - A second-degree game is 'one from which no permanent, irredeemable damage arises, but which people would rather conceal from the public'; and
  - A third-degree game is 'one which is played for keeps, and which ends in the surgery, the courtroom or the morgue' (p. 64).

In an article applying this theory to the understanding of domestic violence, Bicehouse and Hawker (1993) compare this taxonomy to levels of controlling behaviour shown by male perpetrators of such violence, as well as the stages of victimisation experienced by abused women; and point out 'the lack of mutuality in games in which violence is a factor' (p. 195). In a more recent article about games and enactments, Stuthridge (2015) considers countertransference in relation to each degree of games.

- Consulting room games (Berne, 1964/1968a) **[negative]**

    I include this reference to a category of games as, in discussing them, Berne acknowledges that they can be played by therapists and caseworkers and, in doing so, in effect, points to the need for professionals to know ourselves. However, in re-reading this chapter, Berne actually only analyses two games played by the professional in the consulting room: 'I'm Only Trying to Help You', which, he comments, 'is found most commonly and its most florid form among social workers with a certain type of training' (p. 143); and 'Psychiatry', in the explanation of which Berne manages to put down non-medical therapists. This subject is much better treated in Samuels' (1971) discussion of games therapists play (see also Graff, 1976; Park, 1971), and more thoroughly and usefully by Stuthridge (2012), Eusden and Pierini (2015), and Novak (2015).[9]

- A good game: 'one whose social contribution outweighs the complexity of its motivations... one which contributes to the well-being of the other players and to the unfolding of the one who is "it"' (Berne, 1964/1968a, p. 186) **[positive]**

    This concept (noted in Chapter 9) has hardly been picked up in TA, the exceptions being Groder (1971), Wallace (1973), and Zechnich (1973), and it is not insignificant that all these date back to the 1970s. Steiner didn't like this concept and, in a conversation we had about this, told me that Berne only added the chapter in *Games People Play* on good games at the request/insistence of his publisher (C. Steiner, personal communication, 21 July 2016). Herein lies another contradiction as, elsewhere, Berne (1964/1968a) writes: 'the significant point is that for every game (played by Parent or Child) and its pathology, there is a healthy (Adult) equivalent' (p. 160)—which supports a psychology of health based on the integrating Adult, but contradicts the idea of a good game, played in Adult, which, for internal consistency, might be better termed play.

- Games are pathological (Berne, 1964/1968a) **[negative]**

    In an article on games published in the same year (but after *Games People Play*),[10] Berne (1964b) states clearly that: 'because of the morbid nature of the payoff for the player (confirming his own unhappiness) it is evident that these games, *like others* [emphasis added], are pathological' (p. 160). This is supported by an article written about Berne by Langguth (published in *The New York Times* on 17 July 1966) in which he directly addresses this issue:

    In the last few months [thus April–June 1966] Dr. Berne has come to believe that games are always harmful because they involve emotional deception – the con. To keep his games theory unmuddied, the doctor would now remove all harmless 'games' from his book and label them 'pastimes.'

(p. 41)

- 'A series of ulterior transactions with a gimmick, leading to a well-defined pay-off' (Berne, 1964/1968a, p. 364) [**negative**]
  Zalcman (1990) argues that this definition of a game does 'not adequately distinguish games from other transactional sequences' (p. 6), such as pastimes.

- Four responses to games (Dusay, 1966) [**negative**]
  In a short article on the therapist's transactional response to a patient's game invitation, Dusay (1966) identifies four types of response: to expose the game; to ignore the game; to offer an alternative; and/or to play the game, options which Zalcman (1990) considers 'are limited in comparison to what is actually done in practice to confront games' (p. 7).

- The Drama triangle (Karpman, 1968), and the concept of the switch (in roles) [**negative**]
  Zalcman (1990) regards Karpman's (1968) concept of the 'switch' crucial to the development of game theory and analysis, while Hine (1990) suggests that the Drama triangle shows the bilateral nature of games better (than Formula G).[11]

- 'A game has three specific parts:... an orderly series of transactions... a gimmick (which means that the transactions are double-levelled and one level is hidden from the other)... and... a payoff' (Berne, 1969/1971, p. 306) [**negative**]
  This definition prefigures formula G (below).

- The game formula, i.e., C (Con) + G (Gimmick) = R (Response) → S (Switch) → P (Payoff) (Berne, 1970/1973) [**negative**]
  English (1977) argues that games are not played to achieve a payoff but, rather that the payoff is the 'consolation prize' (p. 325). She also contributes the view that it is a switch in ego states that is a distinguishing feature of games. Both Hine (1990) and Eusden and Pierini (2015) view this formula as too linear, and propose that such transactions are better conceptualised as superimposed and/or circular dynamics, and Hine offers a new diagram that represents the two-handed nature of this conceptualisation of a game. Hine's (1990) overall presentation of an ongoing game—which includes script milestones, escala-tions, a circular conception of games, and a game episode or segment framed in terms of a bilateral version of Formula G—also acknowledges that the genesis of a game may often be found or traced back to long before what it usually presented as the initial stimulus or start of a game. Of course, 'They started it' or 'It began when...' may well signal not the beginning of a game but, rather a milestone in an ongoing game. Finally (on this), Eusden and Pierini (2015) take issue with Berne's statement 'whatever fits this formula is a game and whatever does not fit it is not a game' (p. 44), which they regard as 'a very narrow view of game dynamics' (Eusden & Pierini, 2015, p. 129).

- 'A game is a repetitively carried out series of transactions' (Ernst, 1971b, p. 257) **[neutral]**

  Zalcman (1990) argues that this definition of a game does 'not adequately distinguish games from other transactional sequences' (p. 6), such as pastimes.

- *Transactional Game Analysis: A Review of TA Literature* (Stuntz, 1971) **[negative]**

  ... which, for Zalcman (1990) illustrates the problem of 'too many examples of games and not enough basic conceptual principles for defining and differentiating games or for identifying basic game prototypes or patterns' (pp. 9–10). Fortunately (for those of us, like Zalcman, who are critical of the obsession, if not compulsion, of the drive, in the early days of TA, to identify and name new games), this has declined over subsequent decades (see Figure 11.2).[12] The peak of interest in game theory in 2015 was the result of a special issue of the *Transactional Analysis Journal* on 'Psychological Games and Enactments' (Deaconu & Stuthridge, 2015).

- The game formula (revised), i.e., $C + G = R \rightarrow S \rightarrow X$ (Crossup) $\rightarrow P$ (Berne, 1972/1975b) **[negative]**

- Solitaire, a game carried out alone (Berne, 1972/1975b) **[negative]**

  Zalcman (1990) critiques this, and other 'one-handed games' (M. M. Goulding & R. L. Goulding, 1979) as (again) representing an intrapsychic process rather than a transactional games, and suggests that they are better understood by racket analysis.

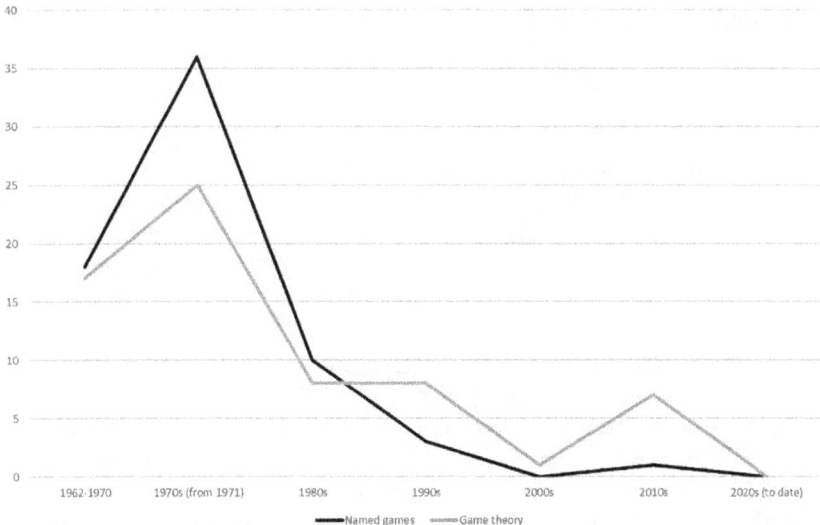

Figure 11.2. Articles on named games and on game theory in the *Transactional Analysis Bulletin* (1962–1970) and the *Transactional Analysis Journal* (1971–2023)

- 'A game has a seemingly plausible and innocent surface statement, or opening move, which is aimed at getting a sympathetic response from a listener. If this response is given, the game goes into more detailed maneuvers, with two or more players engaged' (Ernst, 1972, p. 9) [**negative**]

  Given his reference to manoeuvres, Ernst's subsequent reference to players choosing specific rules of/to the game appears contradictory: 'The players choose specific rules which are interchangeable, and the play is conducted in a way ranging from passive to aggressive—that is, to a soft, medium, or hard degree' (p. 9).

- Goulding–Kupfer game diagram (R. Goulding, 1972) [**negative**]

  This took an individual, psychiatric approach to games, and although Goulding and Kupfer viewed this as related to social dynamics, Berne refused to publish it in the *Transactional Analysis Bulletin* because it was not, in Berne's view, a transactional diagram. Summerton (1992), who observes that Berne himself did not always restrict himself to the interpersonal level in his analysis of games, rehabilitates this model by considering it as offering another (individual or intrapsychic) plane to Berne's game theory on the social psychiatric or interpersonal plane.

- Game plan (James, 1973) [**neutral**, though based on a view of games as **negative**]

  James introduces his plan as a way of discovering *specific* game patterns 'quickly and in a non-threatening way' (p. 194) and, whereas Berne's analysis was more generalised, which focuses on predictable patterns and payoffs. James frames this in a series of questions:

  - What keeps happening over and over again?
  - How does it start?
  - What happens next?
  - And then what happens?
  - How does it end?
  - How do you feel after it ends? (p. 195)

On the basis that James' last question is clearly neutral, P. Robinson (personal communication, 5 July 2023) argues that this theory is neutral rather than negative; and, indeed, Summers and Tudor (2000) apply this to positive patterns or confirmations. The reason I argue that James' view of games is negative is because all the vignettes he includes in his original article illustrate the negative payoff of games.

- Power plays as a game (Steiner, 1974) [**negative**]

  Steiner and other radical psychiatrists brought their analysis of power to TA because, as Steiner (2020) comments: 'the concept of games did not adequately consider the additional payoff of the power struggles that occur between people' (p. 149).[13] In a similar vein, and inspired by the radical psychiatry tradition, Chinnock and Minikin (2015) offer some political perspectives on games.

- The redefining hexagon model (Mellor & Schiff, 1975) [**negative**]

  This model links the theory developed by practitioners within the Cathexis school/tradition on passivity (Schiff & Schiff, 1971) and passive behaviours (Schiff et al., 1975), with the cause and effect of symbiosis, and its manifestation in re-defining transactions (Schiff et al., 1975), and identifies redefining relationships as manifested in six redefining roles: Caretaker, Hard Worker, Angry Righteous, Angry Wrongdoer, Woeful Righteous, and Woeful Wrongdoer. Mellor and Schiff present these as a hexagon, together with their associated game positions, described in terms of the roles of the Drama triangle, on both social and psychological levels.

- Games result 'from unresolved symbiosis... [and are] a desperate attempt on the part of a struggling individual to recreate an environment in which archaic problems can be reenacted and resolved' (Schiff, 1977, p. 71) [**negative**]

  Zalcman (1990) critiques this description as, embedded in it, 'are several as-sumptions that depart significantly from other TA theory' (p. 9), most particu-larly the understanding of symbiosis, and the motivation for human behaviour.

- 'A game is a way in which people can exchanges strokes according to certain rules and with points being awarded to the persons who are in communication with each other' (Summerton, 1979, p. 121) [**neutral**]

- A detailed summary of analysing games according to seven models (Summer-ton, 1979), including the pentagon model [**negative**]

  Zalcman (1990) takes issue with Summerton's emphasis on the intrapsychic aspect of games.

- A game is 'a well-defined series of transactions in which at least one person offers a con (a stimulus with an ulterior message) and eventually pulls a switch and collects a payoff' (Zalcman, 1990, p. 12) [**negative**]

- Games as co-creative confirmations (Summers & Tudor, 2000) [**neutral**]

  As part of our re-reading of TA, and in the spirit of re-naming old concepts in a way that provides new and non-pathological ways of understanding them, we describe games as 'co-creative confirmations'. Jackson and Summers (2010) have followed this up with a definition of games as 'repetitive patterns of inter-action that lead to negative or positive outcomes depending on the implicit and explicit exchanges between people' (p. 2).

- Undersure and oversure character types as the basis of game analysis (English, 2005) [**neutral** in its humanistic orientation, but based on a view of games and racketeers as **negative**]:

  In my opinion, it is not necessary to struggle with details about games. The...
  descriptions of Undersure and Oversure third-degree racketeers and how
  frustration about not receiving the desired strokes for their rackets may lead
  to a switch of ego state and, thereby, to a final crossed transaction (possibly
  with violence) adequately describes the process. Different games are simply
  variations on the Oversure and Undersure kinds of complementary transactions ending with a crossed transaction.

  (p. 85)

I love English's directness about games—as, by now, with regard to this chapter, I was beginning to wonder! I also like her description of sureness as a way of understanding personality.[14]

- Game(s) as medium of co-regulation (Tudor & Summers, 2007, 2014) (neutral), and as affect regulation and dysregulation (Eusden & Pierini, 2015) [**neutral**] In a chapter introducing TA, written from a co-creative perspective, Summers and Tudor (2008) write that: 'People play positive and negative games to regulate feelings, structure time, confirm beliefs about self and others, get recognition, and maintain connected to other people.' (p. 8) This is line with what (little) Berne (1964/1968a) writes about play, 'the essential character of [which]', he notes, 'is not that emotions are spurious, but that they are regulated' (p. 18).

- Games as enactments, relational events, and transferential dramas (Stuthridge, 2012, 2015; see also Eusden & Pierini, 2015, and Novak, 2015) [**neutral**]

Whilst an analysis of these 36 pieces of game theory reflects the dominant view within TA that games are negative and destructive (represented by just over 72% of the theory), it also reveals, perhaps surprising that 20% of TA game theory reflects a positive view of games.

In concluding her critique of game analysis, Zalcman (1990) offers her own definitions (including the one noted on p. 207 above), and, calling for conceptual consistency, parsimony, and logical consistency, offers a final, new (meta-)definition, which, she argues, would redefine game analysis as a major division of TA to include: 'not just the analysis of games, but also *the analysis of all repetitive, stereotyped sequences of interactions, more complex than single transactions and identifiable across cultures as typical patterns of behavior that occur in social situations*' (p. 11). On this basis, concepts currently assigned to or understood as within other areas of TA would be reassigned to game theory, such as time structuring and passivity, theories which currently sit in TA proper. While I like Zalcman's radicalism, I can see a problem with her definition in that it is a neutral one, and thus, while it would encompass, for instance, both positive and negative aspects of time structuring, such a new major division would still suffer from contradictory definitions of games (and, no doubt, other theory) as the previous part of this chapter demonstrates. What I do agree with is her call for:

- A limited number of basic paradigms for different types of games.
- A classification scheme base on these paradigms.
- Differentiating game analysis from other areas of TA.
- Reviewing 'the concepts we have for understanding and describing nonpathological transactional patterns of interactions and develop new concepts where the theory is inadequate' (Zalcman, 1990, p. 12)—a suggestion to which much of my own work in TA, especially that with Graeme Summers, responds.
- Research and clinical observations that helps us to describe the predictable patterns of games.
- Comparative literature reviews and research which helps us maintain consistency—and, I suggest, relevance.

(Almost) concluding this chapter myself, I can say that I have enjoyed writing it, but the more so as I have strayed away from *Games People Play*. In effect, I have used Berne's Introduction (pp. 13–20) and one page in his chapter on Games (p. 51) to consider the more social elements of games (dynamics, action, and psychiatry) of game theory—which, of course, is congruent with my own philosophy (see Chapter 2)—to research and write the first part of the chapter. When I wrote earlier that, then at page 51, I was enjoying re-reading *Games People Play*, I meant it, but didn't anticipate that, 15 pages later, I would be reminded of why I didn't— and still don't—like it. In Part II 'A Thesaurus of Games' (pp. 69–168), which comprises the bulk of the original book, I only have two post-its: one to remind me to say something about consulting room games, and the other, the same about good games (which I have). My last three post-its, in Part III 'Beyond Games', which contains interesting material on the significance of games and autonomy, are placeholders for points of reference for other writing, not about games. So, it is with great pleasure that, I turn from games to—and actually to conclude with—play.

Play—and playing

One of Berne's great strengths was to translate complex ideas, specifically from psychiatry and psychoanalysis, into ordinary language. In his preface to *Games People Play*, he writes: 'this book is primarily designed to be a sequel to my book *Transactional Analysis in Psychotherapy*, but has been planned so that it can be read and understood independently' (Berne, 1964/1968a, p. 11). This endeavour is evident in the title of *A Layman's Guide to Psychiatry and Psychoanalysis* (Berne, 1947/1971), and in the style of his last book, *What Do You Say After You Say Hello?* (Berne, 1972/1975b), in the preface of which, while noting that it is intended as an advanced textbook, he also acknowledges nonprofessional readers for whom he has tried to make it accessible, commenting that: 'it may demand thinking, but I hope it will not require deciphering' (p. xv). However, in making things simple, TA can be viewed as (and accused of) being simplistic, and, in becoming popular (primarily through *Games People Play*), as and of (only) being a 'pop psychology'. Those of us in TA would refute these arguments, not least by pointing to the development of TA over the past 50 years, including a vast literature (which ranges from the simple to the complex); to its appeal to many people in different countries across the world; and to the effectiveness of its practitioners in four fields of application. Nevertheless, and as I have been commenting on elsewhere and especially in this Part of the book, Berne and his immediate colleagues have left us with contradictions and tensions. One of these is that, in popularising games as (predominantly) negative patterns and in pathologising playing games, Berne has created a problem with play and playing.

In *Games People Play*, Berne (1964/1968a) begins his explanation of the genesis of games by stating that: 'from the present point of view, child-rearing may be regarded as an educational process in which the child is taught what games to play and how to play them' (p. 58). Given that Berne frames psychological games as predominantly negative, this appears a somewhat pessimistic view of child-rearing. Lest the reader think this is my particular bias, Berne clarifies this in the next sentence when he acknowledges that: 'he [the child] is also taught procedures, rituals and pastimes appropriate to his position in the local social situation, but these are less significant' (p. 58). Berne explains this by distinguishing between procedures, rituals, and pastimes as determining the availability of opportunities (the what), from games as determining the use the child will make of those opportunities (the how). This is consistent with Berne's (1966) third rule of communication, that 'the behavioral outcome of an ulterior transaction is determined at the psychological and not at the social level' (p. 227). It is also consistent with Berne's (1972/1975b) view of the relative safety of the time structuring of withdrawal, ritual, pastimes, activity, and (some) games, compared with intimacy.

Offering some criticism of the original intimacy experiment (Berne, 1964/1968a), and what they regard as a certain anomaly in Berne's positioning of games in the time structure sequence, Cowles-Boyd and Boyd (1980) suggest the inclusion of play. They place play between games and intimacy, in terms of stroke intensity; and between activities and intimacy, in terms of risk, a seventh form of time structuring which Cornell (2015) explores further. Cowles-Boyd and Boyd also compare play and games with regard to Berne's (1964/1968a) advantages of games, a structure and analysis which includes viewing play as a source of positive strokes; confirming OK positions; allowing new options to be tested, including those for trust, intimacy, autonomy, and awareness; providing dramatic and authentic excitement; and much more. In a subsequent, related article, Cowles-Boyd and Boyd (1980) present a game/play shift, based on Formula G (Berne, 1972/1975b). In their scheme, following the point (S) at which the client offers a standard game switch, Cowles-Boyd and Boyd (1980) propose a therapist switch (S_{th}) which takes the form of an ulterior transaction that conveys the message 'We don't have to believe what we're saying'. Cowles-Boyd and Boyd frame this as both a permission and a confrontation, following which there is a Crossup and then (an additional stage of) Play, often accompanied by genuine laughter. In terms of ego states, these authors (operating in the three ego state model of health), view play as a function of the Child and, specifically, the Free Child. In their article on the ludic third, King and Temple (2018) make the case that play workers play in the here-and-now, i.e., in their integrating Adult.

Other than references to play in articles on working with children, and on play therapy, it was 35 years until another colleague (in the *Transactional Analysis Journal*) explored the concept of play in the context of games. Just before that, and citing Winnicott's (1967/1971) work on play, Summers (2014) writes that he 'emphasises "playing" as both a way of being with clients and a way of working and exploring themes together without getting overly anxious about being right or wrong' (p. xxxvii). In his article, 'Play at your own risk: Games, play, and intimacy', Cornell (2015) also draws on Winnicott's thesis that play is (in Cornell's words) 'both a developmental achievement and an essential aspect of the therapeutic process' (p. 79). While acknowledging Cowles-Boyd and Boyd's work on the function (and structure) of play in the interpersonal realm or field that is the focus of Berne's theory of time structuring, Cornell (2015) focuses on the intrapsychic realm of development, creativity, subjectivity, and selfhood, which is the focus of Winnicott's theory of play. As he (Cornell) puts it: 'games can be seen as the arena for mutual enactment; play, as described by Winnicott, is the terrain of mutual exploration and unconscious communication' (p. 82). Cornell also refers to Winnicott's (1967/1971) concept of interplay:

> The thing about playing is always the precariousness of the interplay of personal psychic reality and the experience of the control of actual objects. This is the precariousness of magic itself, magic that arises in intimacy, in a relationship that is being found to be reliable.
>
> (Cornell, 2015, p. 47)

In quoting this passage from Winnicott, Cornell emphasises that play is as precarious as it is pleasant, and observes that, unlike Berne, Winnicott links play and intimacy. Cornell also references multiple meanings of play, including 'sex play, foreplay, playboy, playing with yourself, being a player, making a play for, playing around, and playing the field', commenting that 'as one sees in these common phrases, sex is not inherently loving, tender, or intimate; it can be an impersonal or tricky pursuit' (p. 84).

Finally, in his article, and again drawing on Winnicott, Cornell (2015) addresses play in psychotherapy, from which I identify a number of themes:

- Play as the primary form of unconscious communication
  While Winnicott (1967/1971) views psychoanalysis as 'a highly specialized form of playing in the service of communication with oneself and others' (p. 41), not many transactional analysts (other than Cornell) talk or write about playing as fostering such communication.

- The importance of mutual play
  Winnicott asserted that this has to be '*spontaneous and not compliant or acquiescent*' (p. 51), a point Cornell emphasises, and elaborates in terms of what it takes for the therapist to allow and to facilitate this.

- The importance of the therapeutic space in which to play
  Following on from the previous point, Winnicott—and Cornell—emphasise the importance of the space in which to play. Cornell (2015) picks this up with regard to TA and cautions that:

> Likewise, in classical transactional analysis, the predominantly interpretative/analytic approach to the treatment of games and script risks a complete foreclosure of the potential space for play. It is important to note that therapeutic styles overly invested in empathy and the provision of corrective experiences also may foreclose the freedom of the therapeutic play space.
>
> (p. 86)

I agree—and extend this to having the space to play with theory and having the theoretical and intellectual space to do so, at all levels of knowledge, exploration, and training.[15]

Cornell goes on to observe that Winnicott 'was not offering his patients a relationship so much as a space, an environment, within which they could begin to find and articulate themselves' (p. 86). Re-reading this, I feel some affinity between what I mean by relating (as distinct from the relationship) and playing, and that perhaps playing catches more of the sense of what we as therapists are doing and being or aspire to do and to be.

• The importance of language
  Cornell reminds of us of Winnicott's idiosyncratic use of language and suggests that, in being vague, evocative, and elusive, Winnicott is creating a space: 'in Winnicott the writer there is a glimpse of Winnicott the therapist creating a play space between his mind and that of the reader' (Cornell, 2015, p. 86).

In this last part of the chapter, I have used the words gaming and playing. I have done so in the same way I tend to use the word relating rather than relationship (see Chapters 4 and 5). I suggest that this is important with regard to game theory in order to emphasise the present-centred nature of gaming; and with regard to play, partly for the same reason, and partly in order to reclaim playing and play, and not in the same way that we might play a psychological game or even as the antithesis of a game, after all, 'The play's the thing' (Shakespeare, 1603/2019, Act II, scene 2, l. 557). Towards the end of *Games People Play*, in a short chapter on autonomy, Berne (1964/1968a) writes: 'spontaneity means option, the freedom to choose and express one's feelings from the assortment available.... It means liberation, liberation from the compulsion to play games and have only the feelings one was taught to have' (p. 180). So let's play—or continue playing, interplaying, and risk(ing)—and hav(e)ing the feelings we have.

Notes

1 I am not alone in this. Writing in 2005, English (2005) says boldly: 'I do not recommend this book (except for the introductory chapter, which summarizes transactional analysis theory) because I think it trivialises behavior and does not distinguish between racketeering and games' (p. 85).
2 Notably, 'Now I've Got You, You Son of a Bitch', 'Frigid Woman', and 'Rapo' (Berne, 1964/1968, pp. 74, 85, 110).
3 Summerton identified this role a couple of years before Clarkson's (1987) work on the Bystander role in which she adds to the original three roles of Karpman's (1968) the Drama triangle the role of 'Audience or Bystanders' (p. 84), though does not acknowledge Summerton's work.
4 For a summary of the extent of social action that various transactional analysts have taken in TA, see Tudor (2020g).
5 Where this is not applicable, I have simply not entered an assessment.
6 I have not noted specific games which have been added to the canon over the years since *Games People Play*, with the exception of 'Solitaire' (Berne, 1972/1975b) as that added something conceptually different to the theory of games.
7 Berne's cynicism about life is revealed in his elaboration of this point:

  Man is the freest of all animals, but the life script and the games that go with it still make him the victim of a mighty joke played by the ineluctable forces of evolution.

Despite our aspirations and our illusion of awareness, we are not much better off than a poet marching with upturned gaze and outstretched arms towards a rainbow, and slipping on an unseen banana peel or worse beneath his feet.

(Berne, 1970/1973, pp. 160–161)

8 It is perhaps no accident that the Jorgensens sub-titled their biography of Berne '*Master Gamesman*' (Jorgensen & Jorgensen, 1984).

9 In the same vein, Ernst (1972) considers games teachers play.

10 The book was published in July 1964, the article in October of that year—which adds verisimilitude to Steiner's comment about good games (see p. 203 above), though, in an article Berne wrote about his experience of writing the book, which appeared in three parts over two years (Berne, 1965b, 1966b, 1966c), including dealing with the publisher, he didn't take the opportunity to say anything about the chapter on good games—and so the discission continues...

11 With its roles of Assertive, Caring, and Vulnerable, the winner's triangle (Choy, 1990) offers an antithesis to Karpman's (1968) Drama triangle and its Persecutor, Rescuer, and Victim roles. Whilst some may view these as positive game roles, Choy herself describes them as 'specific skill[s] for game-free relating' (p. 40).

12 This review was based on electronic searches of both the *Transactional Analysis Bulletin* (1962–1970) and the *Transactional Analysis Journal* (1971–2023).

13 See the report of the conversation Robert (Bob) Schwebel had with Claude Steiner (in Chapter 7, p. 162, n10).

14 I have a similar appreciation for Clarkson's (1992) re-framing of Kahler and Caper's (1974) counterscript drivers, i.e., Hurry Up, Be Perfect, Try Hard, Please me (others), and Be Strong, as, respectively, Speed, Excellence, Experimentation, Agreeableness, and Endurance, which, elsewhere (Tudor, 2022a), I have described as virtues—to which I would add sureness, though this might involve identifying a seventh driver!

15 This, of course, also requires the freedom to choose where to train; with whom to engage in supervision; and if, how, and by whom to be regulated (see also Chapter 10).

Part III

Looking back, looking forwards

There is a Māori whakataukī or proverb 'ka mua, ka muri', the interpretation of which is 'looking back in order to move forward'. I think that is a useful way of summarising what we do as transactional analysts, i.e., analysing present trans-actions (transacting) and games (gaming) to ascertain past, self-defining and/or self-limiting scripts and scripting, in order to develop different present, relational possibilities, in turn, in order to shape the future. Based on the argument developed in the first half of Chapter 2, I argue that this is equally true with regard to how we may look at our traditions and teach TA, i.e., from the present, looking back, in order to move forward. This final part comprises two chapters which does this in two ways.

In the first, which is a much-expanded version of a keynote speech I gave to the Singapore Transactional Analysis Association's Conference 'Honouring our Tradi-tions, Securing our Future' in 2018, I consider our various traditions in TA, firstly by reviewing how we identify them. In this chapter (12), I begin by discussing the nature of honouring, and, after a review of the different schools, traditions, approaches, and sensibilities in TA, I present some ideas about meta-theory and meta-analysis in order to be able to reflect on and take an overview of these tradi-tions, and TA theory.

Finally, inspired by Berne's concept of Martian thinking, in the last chapter of the book, I take a Vulcan view of TA and comment on how TA might live long and prosper.

DOI: 10.4324/9780429398223-15

Chapter 12

Honouring our tradition(s), developing personal praxis

In this chapter, I review different traditions of and approaches in transactional analysis (TA), beginning with the three, original 'schools' of TA: the Classical School, the Cathexis School, and the Redecision School (see Chapter 4). It has always been part of the requirement for examination as a certified transactional analyst (CTA) to have a certain knowledge of TA theory, and, indeed, a part of the stated purpose of the written examination for CTA is that the candidate 'works effectively and ethically as a theoretically based transactional analyst' (International Transactional Analysis Association [ITAA] International Board of Certification [IBoC], 2022, Section 8.1.2). Moreover, when it comes to the CTA oral exam, one of the criteria refers to the capacity to conceptualise the particular application or field of TA (i.e., counselling, education, organisational, or psychotherapy) in terms of different TA theoretical concepts/models, with reference to approaches:

- In counselling—'understanding and application of a wide range of TA theory including different trends and approaches' (ITAA IBoC, 2022, Section 12, Form 12.7.9, scale 3).
- In education—'understanding and application of a wide range of TA concepts including different approaches' (Section 12, Form 12.7.10, scale 8).
- In psychotherapy—'discussion of TA theory including different trends and approaches as well as recent developments' (Section 12, Form 12.7.12, scale 3).[1]

Thus, in this chapter, I discuss the significance of different terms used, i.e., 'Schools', 'traditions', 'approaches', and 'sensibilities'—the last a term I first heard Hayley Marshall use in an interview after a keynote speech (Marshall, 2021a). I do so in order to clarify some confusion within TA, both about the different approaches and about how these are categorised by various authors, and also to honour the richness and diversity within TA, and thus I begin with some discussion of honouring. The second purpose of the chapter is to encourage the reader to develop their own integration of theory and practice, and hence the use of the words 'personal praxis', which I foster through a final discussion (in the third part of the chapter) of meta-theory and meta-analysis. As Allen (2006b) puts it:

DOI: 10.4324/9780429398223-16

We are now surely ready for extended reflections on the diversity of our method-ologies and theories. In this, there are two major issues that we need to consider: (1) When and with whom or at what stage of relationship might a particular framework or strategy be most relevant? and (2) What are the assumptions, con-notations, and the contextual and developmental histories that come with each approach, including what is left unsaid?

(p. 5)

As the chapter is based on a keynote I gave to the Singapore Transactional Analysis Association's Conference 'Honouring our Traditions, Securing our Future', held in Singapore in November 2018 (Tudor, 2018c), although I have considerably ex-panded and updated it, in some parts I have retained some of the direct style of the original form.

Honouring

From the Latin words *honos* and *honor*, the English word honour connotes dignity, office, reputation, distinction, position, and respect. Later, it also became associ-ated with victory and triumph; with splendour, beauty, and excellence; and with (usually feminine) purity and chastity—though I would argue that the fact that pu-rity and chastity were or are associated with the feminine is a patriarchal perspec-tive on honour. In this first part of the chapter, I briefly discuss three of these ideas: dignity, respect, and position, as they all have some resonance in TA—see ITAA IBoC (2022, Section 3), and Tudor, 2016e (Chapter 1), respectively.

Dignity

According to the ITAA IBoC's (2022) *Ethical and Professional Practice Guide-lines*, acknowledging the dignity of human beings is the first of our primary fun-damental values. Drawing on the concept of human rights, and, specifically, the *Universal Declaration of Human Rights* (1948), transactional analysts agree that 'each human being is of worth, regardless of gender, social position, religious creed, ethnic origin, physical or mental health, political beliefs, sexual orientation, and ability' (p. 2)—so, if we don't agree with this, we need to talk about it. Whether or not we agree with such statements is not (simply) a question of signing up to an abstract declaration, as, when things go wrong (for instance, when we lay or receive a complaint) or get difficult (for instance, in times of conflict, social unrest, and war), what we have agreed to and signed becomes subject to greater scrutiny, and, therefore, more important in holding ourselves and others to account. For example, in te Ao Māori (the Māori world), there is a strong emphasis on upholding the mana (dignity, authority) of the guest and, indeed, of the client, two roles that are seen as synonymous in the concept of clinical hospitality as developed by Orange (2011). In TA we refer to this as 'I'm OK, You're OK', but here I am interested in looking beyond the slogan to what we actually *do* in our practice. How do we uphold the dignity of the client? How do we embody our sense of their worth, not so much 'regardless of difference' (as it is sometimes put), but, I would say, *'with regard to difference'*—and how do we do this, when we find some differences challenging and difficult? One of the reasons I'm interested in acknowledging and honouring the client's dignity is because I think that this represents a psychology of health as distinct from a psychology that focuses on psychopathology, which is one feature of the co-creative approach to TA that I have developed with Graeme Summers over the past 25 years (Summers & Tudor, 2000; Tudor & Summers, 2014). Also, 'the right to physical health and mental stability' is another of our primary values (ITAA IBoC, 2022, Section 3.1.2, p. 2).

Respect

Respect means and involves looking at and looking back at and, in this sense, is close to regard or, in TA terms, recognition, which Berne views as a basic human hunger. Our hunger for recognition is met through strokes. In TA, on the whole, I think we do well in being respectful and in giving recognition, not least by acknowledging each other, our contributions, and achievements. One way we do this is by giving awards.[2] Of course, the giving and receiving of recognition doesn't always come easily and we know that this is mediated by certain social, cultural, and familial rules that we internalise, which Steiner (1971c) identifies as forming a restrictive 'stroke economy', the rules of which are:

- Don't give strokes you want to give.
- Don't ask for strokes you want.
- Don't accept strokes you want.
- Don't reject strokes you don't want.
- Don't give yourselves strokes.

In order to challenge this restrictive psycho-social economy, we need to turn these rules around in what we might consider rules for respect:

- Only give strokes/recognition you want to give.
- Only ask for strokes/recognition you want.
- Only accept strokes/recognition you want.
- Reject strokes/recognition you don't want.
- Give yourselves strokes/recognition.

Position

The third aspect of honouring I want to address briefly is that of position—which, in TA, we tend to think about in terms of I, You, They, It, and We. We tend to honour positions of authority we respect, even if we don't respect or like the specific person in that particular position. In the political world, this is often manifested when members of an opposition party stand up when the president of the country (who is from another party) enters the room: in effect they are standing to honour the position, not the person (or the party). I think of this aspect of honouring as knowing the people in position in our history and knowing our lineage, what Traue (1990) refers to as '*Ancestors of the Mind*'. Of course, as transactional analysts, we share a common ancestor, i.e., Eric Leonard Berne (1910–1970) (né Bernstein) and, no doubt, a number of others (to whom I will refer in a moment).

As some of you will know from my writing, I don't always agree with what Berne wrote—and, indeed, with regard to ego state theory, I have pointed out (Tudor, 2003b, 2010c) that some of what he wrote was contradictory—for an analysis of this with regard to contracts, see Chapter 2; to ego states, see Tudor 2010c and Chapter 7; to scripts, see Chapter 9; and to games, see Chapter 11. Nevertheless, in my writing on TA, I always go back to Berne as I take him as the source and my starting point, especially if I'm going to disagree with him, and also seek to afford that respect to other transactional analysts (see, for instance, Tudor, 2008c).

A two-person psychology perspective

Just before I focus on our traditions, I want to say a final word about honouring. It is tempting to think of honouring as a one-way process: I or we uphold the dignity of the other, respect our elders (for instance, here in Singapore, by use of the honorific 'Aunty' and 'Uncle'), and honour the position (if not the person). However, I would argue that this represents what Stark (1999) refers to as a one-person psychology, and that, as a *social* psychiatry, transactional analysis is interested in the analysis of transactions *between* people and, therefore, in a two-person psychology. What this means is that the person we are honouring also needs to be honourable; that elders are not necessarily wise by virtue of their years but may also be foolish (just as young people may be wise); and that the incumbent of a position of a particular office also needs to respect the position of the people who created the office. I think this is particularly important as we get older. Sadly, I have seen too many examples both in and beyond TA of colleagues who stay on too long and who do not retire gracefully,[3] a social dynamic that we could usefully analyse as a social transaction and a game, with a script payoff, perhaps for all concerned.[4]

Schools of TA

While Berne was alive, and although there were clearly major differences between some of the people who attended the San Francisco Social Psychiatry Seminars—and here I'm thinking of Jack Dusay and Steve Karpman, Bob and Mary Goulding, Jacquie Schiff, and Claude Steiner—they all referred to themselves as transactional analysts, and did so in generic terms, not as consultants, counsellors, educationalists, psychotherapists, and so on (primarily as they already had professional identities). It was only after Berne's death in 1970 that particular 'schools' of TA began to be recognised, as a result of which, for many years, TA was seen as comprising: the Classical School (including Berne himself, Jack Dusay, Steve Karpman, and Claude Steiner), the Cathexis School (which referred to the radical reparenting work of Jacquie Schiff and her associates), and the Redecision School (which referred to the work of Bob and Mary Goulding and their integration of gestalt therapy with TA). This tripartite division has been particularly influential in the clinical field of application (counselling and psychotherapy) and in structuring people's thinking about TA (for an example of which, see Chapter 4).

However, in a number of ways, this tripartite division of TA didn't make much sense as, included in the Classical School were people who did not have much in common with each other either theoretically or in practice; the Cathexis tradition was not widely spread and some of its practices were quite quickly discredited (for discussion of which, see Cornell, 2022; Gheorghe et al., 2022; Jacobs, 1994; Mountain, 2022; Robinson, 1998); and Redecision therapy was not exclusive to TA. Moreover, in just over a decade after Berne's death, a number of authors had expanded the original number of schools to include at least eight different ones (Table 12.1).

However, what this table reveals is that there was no consistency about what constituted a school. R. L. Goulding (1976) identifies four schools in TA but offers no criteria by which he defines a school; Karpman, whilst identifying ten 'schools', writes that: '"school" is a misnomer because it suggests divisiveness, whereas in TA many areas are investigated simultaneously and the knowledge is pooled and used eclectically' (p. 73); and Woollams and Brown's (1978) list is, by their own admission, only a partial one. In the following issue of the *Transactional Analysis Journal* (to the one in which Karpman's article appeared), Holloway (1976) comments that:

> Occasionally I hear of 'schools' of TA, yet in my inquiries I cannot find clear evidence of such. There certainly are major contributors, each of whom espouses certain conceptual or clinical views. However, the contrasts among such persons reveal more of their personal style than some marked variance of theory.
>
> (p. 126)

Barnes (1977a) does offer a definition: 'A school of TA is a body of persons under a common personal influence who hold a common theoretical position and follow the same clinical methods. A school can be identified by its unique leadership canon, and group culture' (p. 3). Although this definition informed the excellent book he edited on *Transactional Analysis After Eric Berne* (Barnes, 1977b),[5] unfortunately, it didn't influence others who followed, and so we have so-called schools based on individual or co-authors' preferences, which (as represented in Table 12.1) don't distinguish between:

- A common theoretical position, which is distinct from another, i.e., the Classical School, the Cathexis School, and Radical Psychiatry. Indeed, it is clear from

Table 12.1. Different schools of TA (as identified 1976–1981)

	Schools (R. L. Goulding, 1976)	Schools (Barnes, 1977a)	Schools (Wilson & Kalina, 1978)	Schools (Woollams & Brown 1978)	Schools (Karpman, 1981)
Classical	Eric Berne San Francisco Seminar	San Francisco Group	Bernean		
Cathexis	Schiff 'reparenting'[16]	Schiff family	Symbiosis/Passivity	Cathexis Institute	Reparenting
Redecision	✓	✓	✓	Western Institute for Group and Family Therapy	✓
Asklepieion	✓	(included under Classical)			✓
Radical Psychiatry		(included under Classical)	✓	✓	Radical therapy
Huron Valley Institute				✓	
Miniscript				✓	
Social Transaction			✓	✓	Social level TA (also referred to as Social Transactions TA, the San Francisco School, Bernean TA, or the Social Relationship School)
Action analysis					✓
Bodyscripting					✓
Psychological level TA					✓
Holistic					✓

reading Berne, that the Classical School/tradition/approach comprises different definitions and views of theory (for an analysis of which with regard to ego states, scripts, and games, see Chapters, 6, 9, and 11, respectively).

- Different categories, such that Barnes (1977b) includes Radical Psychiatry under the Classical School, and Karpman (1981) names his own and Dusay's Social level TA both as distinct from and the same as the Classical School. Indeed, there is an argument, as 'Classical' TA theory underpins all TA theory, even that which appears to diverge from it, it should not be regarded as a School of the same status as others but, rather, as an underlying set of theories or trunk (depending on the organising metaphor).
- Integrative or combining approach, i.e., the Redecision School, which combines TA and gestalt therapy; Psychological level TA, which, according to Karpman (1981), combines TA and neurolinguistic programming (NLP) (Lankton et al., 1981); and Bodyscripting (Cassius, 1975, 1980; Childs-Gowell & Kinnaman, 1978), which combines TA scripting and Reichian body armouring.
- A particular programme, i.e., Asklepieion (see Groder, 1972, 1977a; Windes, 1977).
- Specific institutes, i.e., the Huron Valley Institute, and the Western Institute for Group and Family Therapy.
- Specific theories, i.e., the miniscript (Kahler with Capers, 1974).
- Specific techniques, i.e., Action analysis (Mart et al., 1975; Palmer, 1974).
- An approach or direction, such as Holistic (as represented in the work of James, 1981a, 1981b).

Philosophically speaking, this is a clear example of a category error—or, more accurately, eight such errors—whereby people don't compare like with like. Colloquially speaking, it represents a mess of different opinions, ideas, and categories! Whilst, clearly, I am critical of Karpman's (1981) eclectic selection of 'schools', I do agree with the point he makes in an earlier article (Karpman, 1975) about the *clinical* success of a school resting on a number of factors, which he summarises as:

> 1) Resolution: the degree to which it stays creative and solves new problems, 2) Adaptability: the readiness to incorporate ideas from beyond its system, 3) Relevancy: the compatibility with the changing times, and 4) Purging: the extent to which it rids itself of its growth inhibiting traditions
>
> (Karpman, 1981, p. 73)

—and the *popular* success of a school depending on factors such as 'personalities, publicity, proselytizing, and politics' (p. 73). In their comment on the claim of schools, Allen and Allen (2000) state that 'in reality, these "schools" might be compared to rugby, bridge, and scrabble: All are games of sport that share a number of rules, but no two necessarily share the same rules' (p. 189). They go on to observe that: 'the different emphases of the schools seem to reflect several factors, including the personalities and styles of their founders, the kinds of people they tend to treat, and the environments in which they work' (pp. 189–190).

Apart from Barnes (1977a), who offers a definition of a school, only Wilson and Kalina (1978) justify their selection of schools with any reference to definitions or theory, in their case, models of madness as identified by Siegler and Osmond (1974, 1976). Thus, each school of TA represents one of the models of madness (though, for some reason, Wilson and Kalina only considered four of the original eight models identified by Siegler and Osmond):

- The Bernean school—the family interactional and medical models.
- The Social transaction school—the family interactional and decisional models.
- The Radical psychiatry school—the social model
- The Symbiosis/passivity school—the family interaction model, and medical models.
- The Redecision school—the decisional model.[7]

Notwithstanding Wilson and Kalina's partial application of Siegler and Osmond's model, I like their overall thesis as it is the first meta-analysis to invite transactional analysts to take a fundamental Bernean metaphor, that of the splinter in the toe (Berne, 1971) and then to consider it in a comparative analysis (across five schools) that includes how they each view aetiology; how the 'splinter' is understood; how the symptoms/problems are described; what constitutes removing the splinter; and what therapeutic tools can be used to remove the splinter; as well as the result. It is another excellent early article (which I don't think is referred to very much,[8] and I do think deserves more attention). As Wilson and Kalina (1978) themselves state: 'other theoreticians and their views can be compared using a similar schema. Doing so would be valuable for the student of TA interested in developing theoretical consistency, and for the trainee preparing for examination' (p. 201). In their summary of six schools of TA, Woollams and Brown (1978) acknowledge and draw on the work of Wilson and Kalina in comparing the schools according to their perspectives on treatment emphasis, etiology, presenting problems, treatment methods, tools, and goals.[9]

For most of the 1980s and 1990s, most people training in TA were taught that there were three Schools of TA—the Classical, Cathexis, and Redecision—which, as Cornell (2020) notes, 'were in fierce competition with one another during the decade after Berne's death—trainees during that period were faced with demands for loyalty from senior trainers, most of whom were personally (narcissistically) identified with a particular model' (p. 169). In this period, articles that compared theory tended to do so between these three Schools, for example, with reference to script theory (Sills & Salters, 1991), and to the therapeutic relationship (Tudor, 1999b [Chapter 4]). However, as TA continued to develop, a number of publications in the 2000s identified other 'schools' or 'approaches', the latter of which, as noted above, is the word that tends to be used nowadays, though, in their recent publication, Dijkman and Geuze (2021) use the term 'Schools' (see Table 12.2).

What is noticeable about these various contributions (comprising a handout, two articles, a chapter, a book, and a special issue of a magazine, respectively), is that there appears to be more thought behind the selection of approaches and more consistency in the selection (than previously, at least as expressed in those categorisations represented in Table 12.1).

Table 12.2. Different schools, traditions, and approaches in TA (2000–2021)

	Schools (Moiso & Novellino, 2000)	Schools of Change (Lee, 2001)	The tree of TA (Campos, 2003)	Branches (van Beekum, 2006)	Traditions (Tudor & Hobbes, 2007)	Recent approaches (Grégoire, 2009)	Schools (Novellino, 2010)	Schools in TA (Dijkman & Geuze, 2021)
Classical	Psychodynamic (neo Bernean) / Classical	✓	Psychodynamic / Traditional Bernean		Psychodynamic / Cognitive behavioural	Psychoanalytic	✓	✓
Cathexis	Reparenting	✓		✓	✓			✓
Redecision	✓	✓	Redecision therapy	✓	✓		✓	✓
Radical Psychiatry					✓			
Integrative	Integrative-eclectic	✓	Multi-modality integrative	✓	✓	✓	✓	✓
Constructivist	✓	✓	Post-modernist reconstructions	✓	Narrative			
Systemic				✓				
Body	✓	✓				Body-relational		
Personality Adaptations	✓	✓						
Relational	✓	✓		✓		✓		✓
Spiritual	✓	✓	✓					
Educational/ organisational applications								
Co-creative	✓			✓		✓		✓
Cognitive-structuralist							✓	

In her work, which takes the form of a wheel divided into nine segments, Lee (2001) not only identifies certain 'Schools'—Classical Cathexis, Redecision, Constructivist, Body, Personality Adaptations, Integrative, Relational, and Spiritual—but also, like Wilson and Kalina with the metaphor of the splinter, focuses on a specific theme, in this case, change, and examines that in each School. Thus, she notes in each School segment of the wheel, the antecedents of the School, the TA theorists associated with the School, the means of cure, and the outcome of cure. The latter, she summaries as: autonomy (Classical), reactivity (Cathexis), redecision (Redecision), new meaning (Constructivist), release (Body), effective communication (personality adaptations), attunement and involvement (Integrative), healthy relating (Relational), and physis and spirit (Spiritual). While I have some issues with the categories, especially that of personality adaptations (which is a piece of theory, not a school, tradition, or approach), and the ordering of the segments, this model or meta-model is a great summary and useful guide. Some years later, I and Robin Hobbes did something similar, but with regard to different 'traditions' in TA (see Table 12.2, column five), with regard to their focus, key theories and methods, and theorists—and to the presence and influences of these traditions both inside and outside TA. In his summary of the schools of TA, which he divides into approaches from the 1960s to the 1980s (encompassing Steiner, Dusay, Kahler and Capers, Karpman, James and Jongeward, Goulding and Goulding, and Joines), and those from the 1980s to 2014 (encompassing Haykin, Novellino, Moiso, Clarkson, Erskine, Hargaden and Sills, Cornell, Allen and Allen, and Summers and Tudor), Novellino (2014) considers differences in terms of methodological orientation, mental level of intervention, the (working) style of the therapist, advantages and risks, and prevalent clinical indications.

In their contributions, both Campos (2003) and van Beekum (2006) draw on natural metaphors of a tree, its branches, and roots, to describe TA, though they describe quite different trees (Figures 12.1 and 12.2). One of Campos' branches is educational/organisational applications, which acknowledges the development of TA from its initial focus on the clinical to other fields of application (now counselling, education, organisations, and psychotherapy). However, while Campos makes an important, historically accurate, and inclusive point, these fields are not schools, so again, we are not seeing the comparison of like with like.

In his *Dizionaio Didattico di Analisi Transazionale* (Teaching Dictionary of TA), published in 2014, Novellino acknowledges the work of Barnes (1977), Woollams and Brown (1978), Campos (2003), and Grégoire (2009) in defining different schools, and his own work (Novellino, 2010), in which, in addition to the classical, redecision, integrative, and psychodynamic schools, he includes the cognitive-structuralist (though he does not identify any authors with this school).

For ease of comparison between all these contributions, Table 12.3 offers a complete summary of the identified schools, traditions, approaches, and sensibilities.

The reader will note that, in this summary table, I have added a final row 'Ecological' (ecological TA or EcoTA), which, while it hasn't yet been formally recognised in any published review or overview of TA, is an emerging 'sensibility' (Marshall, 2021a), and is the subject of a recent special, themed issue of the *TAJ* (Barrow & Marshall, 2003a).

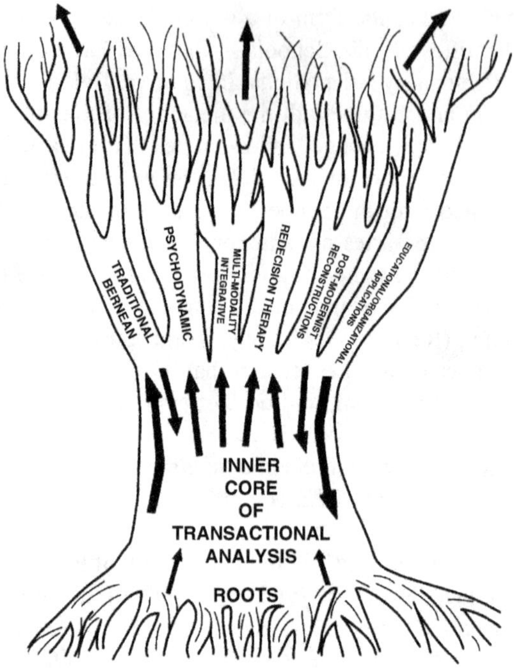

Figure 12.1. The tree of transactional analysis
(Campos, 2003).

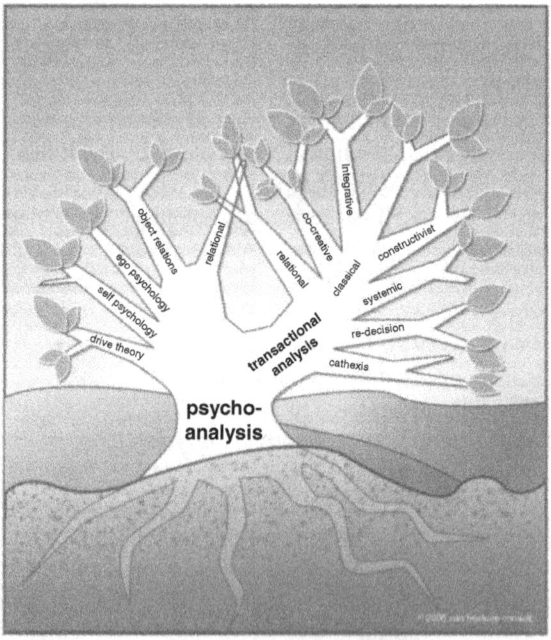

Figure 12.2. Roots and branches (of TA)
(Van Beekum, 2006).

Table 12.3. Different schools, traditions, approaches, and sensibilities in TA

	Schools (R. L. Goulding, 1976)	Schools (Barnes, 1977)	Schools (Wilson & Kalina, 1978)	Schools (Woollams & Brown, 1978)	Schools (Karpman, 1981)	Schools (Moiso & Novellino, 2000)	Schools of Change (Lee, 2001)	The tree of TA (Campos, 2003)	Branches (van Beekum, 2006)	Traditions (Tudor & Hobbes, 2007)	Recent approaches (Grégoire, 2009)	Schools (Novellino, 2010)	Schools in TA (Dijkman & Geuze, 2021)
Classical	Eric Berne San Francisco Seminar	San Francisco Group	Bernean			Psychodynamic (neo Bernean) Classical		Psychodynamic		Psychodynamic	Psychoanalytic	✓	
Cathexis	Schiff 'reparenting'	Schiff family	Symbiosis/ Passivity	Cathexis Institute	Reparenting	Reparenting	✓	Traditional Bernean	✓	Cognitive behavioural		✓	✓
Redecision	✓	✓	✓	Western Institute for Group and Family Therapy	✓	✓	✓	Redecision therapy	✓	✓		✓	✓
Asklepieion	✓	included under Classical			✓								
Radical Psychiatry		included under Classical	✓		Radical therapy					✓			
Huron Valley Institute				✓									
Miniscript		✓		✓	✓								

(Continued)

Table 12.3. (Continued)

	Schools (R. L. Goulding, 1976)	Schools (Barnes, 1977)	Schools (Wilson & Kalina, 1978)	Schools (Woollams & Brown, 1978)	Schools (Karpman, 1981)	Schools (Moiso & Novellino, 2000)	Schools of Change (Lee, 2001)	The tree of TA (Campos, 2003)	Branches (van Beekum, 2006)	Traditions (Tudor & Hobbes, 2007)	Recent approaches (Grégoire, 2009)	Schools (Novellino, 2010)	Schools in TA (Dijkman & Geuze, 2021)
Social													
Transaction			✓	✓	Social level TA[10]								
Action analysis					✓								
Body					Bodyscripting		✓				Body-relational		
Psychological level TA					✓ (with NLP)								
Holistic					✓								
Integrative						Integrative-eclectic	✓	Multi-modality integrative	✓	✓	✓	✓	✓
Constructivist							✓	Post-modernist reconstructions	✓	✓	Narrative		
Systemic									✓				
Personality Adaptations							✓						
Relational							✓		✓		✓		✓
Spiritual							✓						
Educational/ organisational applications								✓					
Co-creative									✓		✓		✓
Cognitive-structuralist												✓	
Ecological													

In concluding this summary of schools, traditions, approaches, and sensibilities, and this part of the chapter, I offer some reflections on Table 12.3.

1. That it's useful in offering an overview of the diversity that is TA, and in helping people locate the theories on which they draw as well as with which they identify—and do not identify.
2. That, clearly, not all of these approaches are practiced, taught, or studied everywhere, and some no longer exist.
3. That, as a list or a tabulation of lists, as noted, it doesn't necessarily compare like with like, and (as I have indicated), different people will have different ideas about where the different schools, traditions, and approaches belong. For example, I don't think that 'the relational' is a school as such, or that it is exclusively psychodynamic. I also think that co-creative TA (a) is part of the relational approach within TA (see Tudor & Summers, 2014); and (b) that it not a school,[11] but, rather, a sensibility that offers a re-reading of TA on the basis of certain principles as outlined in Summers and Tudor (2000).
4. That, as TA does, we should certainly distinguish approaches from fields of applications (see Table 12.4).
5. That not all these approaches are distinct from each other, and that some TA theorists and practitioners are associated with more than one approach; indeed, it could be argued that we are all Classical and, therefore, that this is not—or should not be considered as—a School but, to borrow Campos' and van Beekum's metaphors, rather, the trunk of the TA tree. For example, as I note in the Introduction, Lee's (2001) wheel model chart positions me in both the Classical and Constructivist Schools of TA.
6. That the value of any such analysis or taxonomy is to do what Wilson and Kalina (1978), and Lee (2001) do, which is to develop a scheme by which the different approaches can usefully be compared, which not only offers different options for practice, but also clarifies our thinking about practice.

Meta theory and meta-analysis

Following on from that last point, in the final part of this chapter, I make some comments about thinking about thinking and, in this way—and as I do at various points in this book (pp. 47–48, 170–173, 201)—offer something of a meta-theory, i.e., a theory about theory.

Although there is no mention of the need to demonstrate a meta-perspective in the outline of requirements for the CTA written exam (ITAA IBoC, 2022, Section 8), the 'Rating Scale for [the] Written Examination' (Section 12, Form 12.7.7, scale 4) is concerned with meta-perspective (Table 12.4).

The pass marks of the four sections are: 13, 6.5, 23, and 23, respectively, representing a pass of 65.5%.

Here, as an organising framework for these ideas, I draw on five elements of Bloom's (1956) taxonomy of educational objectives—comprehension, application, analysis, synthesis, and evaluation, as renamed and slightly re-ordered in a revised edition of the original work (Anderson & Krathwohl, 2001), i.e., understand, apply, analyse, evaluate, and create.[12]

Table 12.4. References to meta-perspective in the CTA written exam marking criteria

(Scale 4) descriptors	'Takes meta-perspective and complexity into account'	'Takes many aspects of meta-perspective and complexity into account'	'Takes some aspects of meta-perspective and complexity into account'	'Hardly any awareness of meta-perspective and complexity'	'Does not take any aspects of meta-perspective and complexity into account at all'
Section A	20–17 marks	17–13.5 marks	13.5–9.5 marks	9.5–5 marks	5–0 marks
Section B	10–8.5 marks	8.5–6.75 marks	6.75–4.75 marks	4.75–2.5 marks	2.5–0 marks
Section C	35–30 marks	30–23.5 marks	23.5–17 marks	17–9 marks	9–0 marks
Section D	35–30 marks	30–23.5 marks	23.5–17 marks	17–9 marks	9–0 marks

(ITAA IBoC, 2022, Section 12, Form 12.7.7).

Comprehension (understand)

Once we have gained knowledge or learned something, we can reflect on it and comprehend or understand the meaning of the knowledge. In this context, after some 35 years of training/education, practice, sustaining professional development, and research in TA, I have some knowledge—and some comprehension of that knowledge. So, from my particular summary of approaches to TA (Tudor & Hobbes, 2007; see also Table 12.2), I would say:

- That, from Classical (psychodynamic) TA, i.e., Berne's early work, and its development by colleagues such as Carlo Moiso, Michele Novellino, Petrūska Clarkson, Helena Hargaden, and Charlotte Sills, amongst others—I have an appreciation of intuition, the unconscious, and the different kinds of transference.
- That, from Classical (cognitive-behavioural) TA, which also draws on Berne's work, and its development by Steve Karpman, Claude Steiner, Muriel James, Ian Stewart, and others—I have an appreciation of the radicalism of the concepts of contract and cure, as well as of a certain straightforwardness and direct style of transacting.
- That, from Radical Psychiatry, as developed by Claude Steiner, Hogie Wyckoff, Becky Jenkins, Beth Roy, and others—I have a deep appreciation of psychopathology as representing forms of alienation, of the importance of groupwork, and of the influence of the political in and on the personal.[13]
- That, from the Cathexis School, founded by Jacqui Schiff and others—I have an appreciation that TA can contribute to our understanding and ways of working with severely disturbed and psychotic clients, and of the usefulness of the theories of passivity and discounting.
- That, from Redecision therapy, as practiced by Mary and Robert Goulding, and others—I have an appreciation of the possibilities inherent in the decisional model.
- That, from integrative TA, as developed by Muriel James, Fanita English, Richard Erskine, Janet Moursund, Rebecca Trautmann, Petrūska Clarkson, and others—I have an appreciation of the different conceptualisations of the ego and self, of its emphasis on health, and its holistic and pluralistic view of the person.
- That, from narrative or constructivist TA, as developed by Jim and Barbara Allen—I find a deep resonance in its acknowledgement of the influence of field theory, social constructivism, discourse, and dialogic psychotherapy.

Application (apply)

Practice is the principal application of theory. In this context, and thinking about this at a meta-level, I share the questions I posed in the keynote speech at the conference in Singapore as examples of application, on which I invite the reader to reflect in the context of their context, and to which to add (together with an evaluation of them in terms of Bloom's taxonomy) (Table 12.5).

Table 12.5. The application of TA in Singapore and its evaluation in terms of educational objectives

Questions regarding the application to TA in Singapore	Assessment of the questions in terms of Bloom's taxonomy of education objectives (Bloom et al., 1956)
1. What traditions do you draw on and how do these inform your use of TA?	Comprehension, analysis
2. How relevant is TA to Singaporean culture and cultures?	Evaluation
3. How might you apply TA as a social and/or radical psychiatry to different aspects of life here in Singapore, i.e., the world, others, and yourselves?	Application
4. To what extent are the therapeutic methods of TA, i.e., the contractual method and open communication, relevant to your lives and work here in Singapore?	Evaluation
5. To what extent is the basic philosophy of TA—that people are OK, that everyone has the capacity to think, and that people decide their own destiny—compatible with Singaporean values, culture(s), and society?	Analysis, synthesis, evaluation
6. Does TA help you achieve a balance between the collective and the individual, and between autonomy and homonomy?	Analysis
7. How might TA help the integration of the 'Other' in Singaporean society?	
8. Could the values represented by the five stars of the national flag—of peace, justice, equality, democracy, and progress—be the basis of a Singaporean transactional analysis?	Analysis, synthesis, evaluation
9. What do you need in order to adapt, change, and/or reject elements of TA theory and practice in order to shape your work and future(s)?	Comprehension, analysis, evaluation
10. How do or might you criticise your elders (Aunties and Uncles), including me, in order to help them/ (us), as Bob Dylan (1964) puts it, to get out of the new road if they (we) can't lend a hand?	Application, analysis, evaluation

Analysis (analyse)

Meta comes from the Greek word meta, meaning after or beyond (which, conceptually, can be above or below); also beside, with, among, and adjacent. This gives us the sense of meta referring to a second-level activity, e.g., thinking after, beyond, above, or below first-level thinking. Berne (1966a) gives us an example of this when, in the context of a discussion about selection criteria for groups, he suggests that the question "'What are criteria for the selection of patients?" [has] the underlying assumption "Criteria for selection are good"' (p. 5). Thus, pointing out this underlying assumption and/or asking the question 'Why do you have criteria for the selection of patients for groups?' are examples of thinking and operating at a meta-level.

When combined with some words in English, meta signifies a change or alteration, as in morphic (pertaining to shape or form) and metamorphic (referring to changing shape or form). This gives us the sense that operating at a meta-level changes things. Thus, we might consider Berne's (1966a) definition of confrontation—which 'disconcert[s] the patient's Parent, Child, or contaminated Adult' (p. 235), as a meta-transaction that transforms something. Another example of meta thinking in TA is Steiner's (1981) point that 'every message has a meta-communication, a message about the message' (p. 171), which brings us to the reflexive aspect of meta, which I have attempt to achieve in this present work by offering some transactional analysis of TA; ego state analysis of ego state theory; script analysis of script theory; and game analysis of game theory.

Evaluation (evaluate)

Whenever we integrate something, we evaluate it, consciously or unconsciously. Theoretical integration is based on integrating two or more theories and, therefore, on having some meta-theory by which we do it. It's not a question of simply putting two theories together (which would be additive or combined), or of choosing pieces from different theories (eclectic), but, rather, of having some basis on which we integrate. The model of therapeutic relationships based on the work of Gelso and Carter (1985), Barr (1987), and Clarkson (1990) is an example of this.

Just before the conference in Singapore (the keynote speech for which inspired this chapter), I attended a dinner celebrating students' completion of the clinical training part of the Master of Psychotherapy at Auckland University of Technology (where I work). As I was about to leave, one of the students asked me for some words of advice as she embarked on her work and independent practice. My response was to encourage her to be herself, as I think we can do no other,[14] and I don't think in terms of having a 'toolkit' or specific skills or interventions so much as that we are our own toolkit (Tudor, 2020c).

It is in this sense and context that I think about integration—and evaluation. The developmental psychologist Jean Piaget (1950) describes the difference between accommodation and assimilation with reference to eating an olive: if we eat and swallow the olive, we accommodate both the flesh and the stone, with some discomfort; if we chew and swallow the flesh but spit out the stone, we assimilate or integrate the nutritious part of the olive and reject (and eject) what is not nutritious. So with integration: we integrate the theory that makes sense and that accords with our values, a process I and Mike Worrall refer to as 'philosophical congruence' (Tudor & Worrall, 2006), and we reject the theory that doesn't make sense.

Of course, if—especially if—we have swallowed TA theory whole, we may need to revisit this and reject (and again eject) those parts of the theory that are not or are no longer compatible with who we are and how we practice. Thus, for example, as noted in Chapter 2, I no longer give permissions (as in the traditional permission transaction). Of course, this perspective on integration is based on a particularly free-thinking view of adult (and Adult) education (and I am aware that not everybody supports that perspective). In any case, this requires support, not least from ourselves and others, including trainers, supervisors, and other colleagues.

Synthesis (create)

With regard to the material on schools, traditions, approaches, and sensibilities I have presented in this chapter, Table 12.6 offers a synthesis which, I suggest, makes some helpful distinctions, and resolves some of the problems of categories inherent in previous ways of thinking about these aspects of TA (as noted above). It offers a relationship between philosophy, that is, the philosophical roots of TA as identified by Weinhold (1977) (see also Chapter 2) and Tudor and Hobbes (2007); the different dimensions of life (identified by Groder, 1977a); the approaches in TA (based on Tudor & Hobbes, 2007); interventions (including specific practice and techniques); and the fields of application, to which, I have added social psychology, to acknowledge the application of TA to life beyond the four fields.

This schema provides a map by which we can trace any TA theory and practice. Thus, in concluding this chapter, I offer some examples from the literature, together with my analysis of it with reference to this schema.

Example 1 (from Berne, 1970)

SAM: Dr. Berne, why does a man have to stay in a hospital for 8 weeks when he wants out?
DR. BERNE: What does he have to do to get in?
SAM: I just worked a little harder than the average.
DR. BERNE: What did you do that caused people to say you had to go to the hospital?
SAM: They got uncomfortable with the way I was acting. I thought I was acting pretty good.
DR. BERNE: How Were you acting?
SAM: Working fast all day long. That's all.
DR. BERNE: Sounds all right to me. Why should someone put you in the hospital for that?
SAM: I've asked that question for 3 weeks.
DR. BERNE: What did you do to get in the hospital?

Table 12.6. Philosophical roots, dimensions, approaches, the place of interventions, and fields of application in TA

Philosophical roots (see Tudor & Hobbes, 2002; Weinhold, 1977)		Dimensions (developed from Groder, 1977a)		Approaches (from Tudor & Hobbes, 2007)		Interventions		Fields of application
Existentialism		Affective		Classical (psychodynamic)				Counselling
Phenomenology		Behavioural		Classical (cognitive-behavioural)				Educational
Idealism		Cognitive		Cathexis		Multiple		Organisational
Empiricism (logical positivism, and scientific realism)	><	Ecological	><	Radical psychiatry	><		><	Psychotherapy
Experimentalism		Somatic		Redecision				Social psychology
Humanism		Social/political		Integrative				
		Spiritual		Constructivist (including co-creative)				

SAM:	I asked for help. I said I needed a vacation in some far-off place. The doctor immediately said I had to go to the hospital.
DR. BERNE:	What did you do to get in the hospital?
SAM:	I was working 18 hours a day, sleeping 4—having a grand time.
DR. BERNE:	The reason you're here is because you don't answer questions. I still don't know why you're in the hospital.
SAM:	I was losing control.
DR. BERNE:	What did you do when you lost control?
SAM:	Worked like 2 men.
DR. BERNE:	Okay, that's why you're in the hospital. (pp. 75–76)

Meta-analysis
Field of application: Psychotherapy (group treatment)
Approach: Classical (cognitive-behavioural)
Interventions (primarily): Confrontation (Berne, 1966a)
Dimension: Cognitive
Philosophical roots: Phenomenology and empiricism (logical positivism, scientific realism)

Example 2 (from Fornaro, 2016)

S[ofia]:	My mother used to ask me and I used to withdraw...
T[herapist]:	What did your mother ask you?
S:	'What's the matter?' I'd say, '"I don't know' or "nothing".' 'Come on, what's the matter? I can see you're feeling down.'

T: And you?

S: I didn't know how to say it (cries). And she used to go away. I felt she was defenseless, and I felt guilty because she had gone away and I kept feeling confused in being with myself.

The session ends with my interpretive intervention aimed at understanding the conflict, expressed in the impasse (a need to be with/fear of abandonment):

T: My impression is that today, at the start of our session, you feared you would do with me what you used to do with your mother. What do you think?

S: What? You mean I withdrew? I went away?

T: In your opinion?

S: Well, yes. While I was on my way I was thinking of telling you those things. I was a little afraid you'd get angry.

T: And I realize that you and I have talked and neither of us felt defenseless. (p. 214)

Meta-analysis
Field of application: Psychotherapy (individual)
Approach: Classical (psychodynamic) (relational, intersubjective)
Interventions: Interpretations (co-constructed)
Dimension: Affective
Philosophical roots: Phenomenological[15]

Example 3 Therapy with a hebephrenic patient (from Schiff et al., 1975)

Patient: It scares me when things eat houses.

Therapist: There is nothing about eating you really need to be afraid of.

Patient: But it might eat up the whole world. Then we would all disappear.

Therapist: Eating and disappearing don't really go together, and you aren't at all likely to get eaten up. Very few people get eaten up by anything.

Patient: Jonah got eaten up by the whale.

Therapist: One example of something doesn't make it very likely. Anyway, even in the story, Jonah didn't disappear. If you stop putting together things that scare you and working yourself up, you could probably explain to me what you saw that did really scare you.

Patient: Well, I saw this big machine that was eating up a house, It had a big mouth and was chomping on big boards.

Therapist: Oh, you mean a bulldozer. That isn't a mouth. It's a machine that people use to tear down.... (p. 72)

Meta-analysis
Field of application: Psychotherapy (individual treatment)
Approach: Cathexis
Interventions Reparenting
Dimension: Cognitive
Philosophical roots: Phenomenology

Example 4 (from Morgan, 1988)

> Angela, a sixteen year old Black female was brought to the clinic by her mother, Mary, for truancy. Although Angela had various physical complaints, her doctor could not substantiate them. Mary, who did all the talking during the session, admitted that she enjoyed Angela's company during the day. Mary also stated that she, Mary, had left her husband soon after Angela's birth: 'It was like she was all I really wanted.'
>
> My assessment was that Mary's needs were being partially met by Angela's school problem. I therefore met with them individually, and helped Mary develop outside interests and other support systems. (p. 191)

Morgan goes on to reflect on her work with Mary and Angela in terms of giving permissions, being active (taking Angela to the library), giving 'homework', validating perceptions, understanding internalising fear, and confronting the Pig (Critical) Parent.

Meta-analysis
Field of application: Therapy (psychotherapy, counselling in a public agency)
Approach: Radical psychiatry
Interventions: Demystifying internalised oppression (about race, craziness, and sex)

Dimension: Social, behavioural, cognitive, then affective
Philosophical roots: Experimentalism

Example 5 (from M. M. Goulding & R. L. Goulding, 1979)

Mary Goulding is working with Ned on his primary injunction 'Don't be close'. He is remembering the one happy period in his life, when he lived on a farm with his grandmother before he was forced to join his parents in Chicago.

Mary: Go back to the grade school in Chicago, What do you see?
Ned: A bunch of sadistic boys fighting.
Mary: Look around carefully. Go into the school and walk around.
        Ned reports on the dilapidated, dirty classrooms, the crowded conditions, the crabby teachers, and the boys who are fighting.
Mary: Good for you. You have great ability to put yourself back into the scene. Now go on to the playground. See the boys fighting?
Ned: Yeah. (*He describes the scene*)
Mary: Are all the boys fighting?
Ned: Well, not exactly. Some kids are throwing the ball around.
Mary: Interesting. What is Ned doing?
Ned: Just sitting there on a bench. Sad.
Mary: Are there other kids sitting on benches?
Ned: Yeah.
Mary: I wonder why Ned doesn't make friends with them.
Ned: I don't know. He just doesn't. It's a huge school. I do remember one kid like me... lived in the same building. I didn't play with him much. I don't know. I was sad.
Mary: Be Ned. On the bench. And say, 'I'm going to stay sad until....'
Ned: I'm going to stay sad until... until... until I get back to Grandma's. (*Weeps briefly*) I never got back.
Bob: Yeah. Now see your wife and say, '*I'm going to stay sad with you until I get back to grandmother.*'
Ned: For Christ's sake! (*Laughs*)

Meta-analysis
Field of application: Therapy (psychotherapy) (group treatment)[16]
Approach: Redecision
Interventions: Directive with regard to an early scene
Dimension: Affective, cognitive
Philosophical roots: Phenomenology

In offering these meta-analyses, I am not saying that I am correct; I am suggesting, however, that it's possible and desirable to analyse practice in a way that reveals its underlying assumptions. The reader will notice that I have not included vignettes from either the integrative or constructivist approaches. With regard to the integrative work of Erskine and Moursund (1988), Erskine (1991), Clarkson (1992), and

Erskine et al. (1999), their published case material tends to be long (i.e., complete sessions or demonstrations), and (in my view) the shorter published vignettes do not demonstrate the overall integration these theorists promote. With regard to constructivist TA, we (as I include myself in this category) tend not to publish case material as we don't want one specific way of working with a particular client to be seen as *the* way of working—which we would want to deconstruct. Notwithstanding this point, in their article on script work with a constructivist sensibility, Allen and Allen (1997) offer a number of practical applications of working in this way, and elsewhere (Tudor, 2011b) I offer a description of the method of co-creative TA.[17]

Conclusion

By knowing more about the history of TA and our traditions, and by developing our critical thinking, not least to be able to evaluate, create (and co-create) ways of working and being with others (clients and colleagues), we have more freedom and more options. In this way, I hope it is more possible to develop a robust personal praxis as transactional analysts while knowing more about and, therefore, being able to honour our traditions.[18]

Notes

1 The CTA oral exam in organisations scoring sheet (ITAA IBoC, 2022, Section 12, Form 12.7.11) only refers to different approaches with regard to organisational theory, not TA theory.

2 In the original keynote speech, I acknowledged the fact that Mark Widdowson (who was present at the conference) received the first ITAA Research Award in recognition of his research into the effectiveness of TA (see Gentelet & Widdowson, 2016; Widdowson, 2011; see also Widdowson, 2018).

3 A notable exception to this perspective, if not rule, is James (Jim) Allen who, in 2014, announced his retirement—and did retire. I remember talking with him about this at the 2014 TA World Conference and him telling me about the number of colleagues who assumed that he would still come to conferences, to which his response was a kindly 'No, I'm retiring'—tēnā koe e hoa | my respect.

4 That said, at the Singapore conference, Nicole Lenner spoke about a positive example of gracious retirement, describing a ritual in the German national TA trainers' group whereby colleagues who were retiring were formally farewelled.

5 Barnes (1977a) goes into great detail about what constitutes a school, including an analysis of leadership (charismatic, primal, psychological, effective, and responsible); the canon; group culture (in terms of character, etiquette, and technical); and some comments on autonomy. It is an excellent 11 pages which still warrants close reading—for trainers and trainees alike.

6 The use of different terms in the various cells refers to that author's reference to the school or tradition, thus, Goulding (1976) refers to Cathexis as 'Schifff reparenting', while Barnes (1977a) refers to it as 'Schiff family', and so on.

7 The other models are: the moral, the impaired, the psychoanalytic, and the psychedelic.

8 According to CrossRef (July 2024), it has been cited only once, though viewed 128 times.

9 In a book published in Italian in 1985, Woollams and Brown's comparative summaries were based on: language, ego state and script (theory), contract, decisional model, and I'm OK, You're OK position.

10 Which, as noted in Table 12.1, Karpman also refers to as Social Transactions TA, the San Francisco School, Bernean TA, and the Social Relationship School.

11 I was invited to contribute to an issue of a TA magazine on Schools in TA (Dijkman & Geuze, 2021), in response to which I made my point about co-creative TA not being a school/School, following which the editors (who I like and respect) and I had some discussion, as a result of which, while they retained the concept of School in the issue, I decided still to contribute the article, which was published (Tudor, 2021c), in which I simply stated my position—and left and leave it for the reader to decide.

12 I have not included knowledge (remember) as this is not a meta-activity, but more the ground on which the meta-analysis and processes draw, i.e., comprehension, application, analysis, evaluation, and synthesis/creativity.

13 In one of the guidebooks to Singapore I read before attending the conference, I came across the following statement, that 'Singaporean writers are also increasingly preoccupied with social and political themes. There is a new openness here, a willingness to engage and hear different views, and more topics are being talked about in the open' (Leck, 2016, pp. 85–86). If this statement is also true of Singaporean transactional analysts, then it would echo something of the engagement with the social/political world that was—and is—represented by radical psychiatry.

14 Following the logic of what I have written elsewhere, especially Tudor and Worrall (2006) and Chapter 7, I should have said 'Just be your organism'!

15 In their exploration of the philosophical foundations of what they refer to as the psychodynamic school of TA, Moiso and Novellino (2000) write about an underlying epistemology of uncertainty.

16 Although this form of group treatment is clearly therapy in the group, as distinct from therapy through the group, and therapy of or with the group itself (Roberts, 1982).

17 Interestingly, as I was finishing this book, I had the opportunity to do some workshops in Europe (in March and April, 2023) in which, as usual, I offered a number of demonstrations, and again had requests to record and transcribe them–so perhaps the universe is calling me to do this? (Watch this space!)

18 In her feedback to me about this chapter, Jan Grant (personal communication, 22 May 2023) wrote: 'What I am left with is two things: 1. It is complicated and 2. It is important to develop my own philosophy and approach that fits for me, my clients and my field of practice.'

Chapter 13

Live long and prosper

A Vulcan view of transactional analysis

Nothing exists except atoms and empty space; everything else is opinion.

(Democritus)

Throughout this book I have played with and between the retrospective and the prospective. Publishing previously published material necessitates re-reading it, an activity that inevitably takes the author (in this case me) back, and creates a reflective space in which I have reviewed the old (material that forms Chapters 1, 3, 4, 6, 8, and 10) and been able to create the new (i.e., Chapters 2, 5, 7, 9, 11, 12, and this final chapter).

To my involvement as a TA trainee/student (from 1985), a practitioner/clinician (from 1987), an author (from 1990) and editor (from 2002), and a supervisor and a trainer/educator (from 1997), I have brought a critical perspective—which hasn't always been easy either for me, or for others. Whilst, in many respects, I imagine that, as an experienced practitioner and a relatively senior TSTA, and, certainly, a prolific writer, I am seen as a part of the TA world and, in that and some sense, central, insofar as I am a critic, I am also on the periphery—and perhaps even peripheral. However, as I argue elsewhere (Tudor, 2012; see also Chapter 12), I think that voices from the periphery are important, not least in offering a critique of what is seen as central, core, and mainstream.

I write this is an introduction to the themes of this last, prospective chapter which takes as its starting point the imperative that TA live long and prosper—and I discuss how I think it and we might do that. This catchphrase is spoken by Mr Spock, a character in the TV series *Star Trek* from the planet Vulcan, whose father was Vulcan and whose mother was from Earth. Spock's character is strong on logic and, in this sense, has some similarity to the qualities that Berne associates with Martian thinking. So, I begin this chapter with some consideration of the elements of Martian thinking, and Vulcan being. The rest of this chapter is devoted to my own 'Vulcan view' of the challenges ahead for TA—encompassing the nature and purpose of TA itself, the practice of TA, the nature and purpose of transactional theory, and professional and personal identity as transactional analysts—which also incorporates references to other, closing reflections on TA in books written and/or edited by other TA authors.[1]

DOI: 10.4324/9780429398223-17

Thinking Martian

The first mention of the 'the 'Martian' approach' appears in a brief report by Berne (1962a) of a presentation at one of the San Francisco Social Psychiatry Seminars by Franklin Ernst on 'the multi-problem family and the decision for treatment'. At the meeting Berne had requested a discussion of 'the paper' before discussion of its content in order to illustrate what he refers to as the Martian approach, by which he and others question the motivation of the presenter, both generally ('Why do people write papers?) and specifically ('E [the presenter] should sort out his Adult, Parent, and Child motivations in this respect'), including a game analysis ('See How Hard I'm Trying'); and the redundancy of the title. In this report, 'Martian' appears a way of bringing attention to bear on meta-communication (in this case of presenting a paper) (see also Hostie, 1982).

Another example of this is Berne's comment on the selection of patients for group. Arguing against 'the homogeneity demanded or preferred by some therapists as a matter of policy', Berne (1966a) suggests that 'The real issue in this connection is not the one commonly debated, "What are the criteria for the selection of patients?", but the underlying, usually unstated assumption "Criteria for selection are good"' (p. 5).

In *What Do You Say After You Say Hello?*, Berne (1972/1975b) writes more about what he refers to as 'Thinking Martian', from which I identify a number of elements:

• That it ascertains what is 'real'

   Berne explains this by referring to the situation 'When parents interfere with or try to influence their children's free expression' (p. 100), in response to which he identifies five different viewpoints: '(1) What the parent says he meant. (2) What a naive onlooker thinks he meant. (3) The literal meaning of what was said. (4) What the parent 'really' meant. [and] (5) What the child gets out of it' (p. 100). Berne goes on to name the first two viewpoints as 'square' or 'Earthian' and the last three as 'real' or Martian. It is important to note that (from the example) Martian encompasses the literal and the psychological, i.e., actual as in intentional, and perceived or received. Later, in the same section, Berne explains that thinking Martian is based on an assessment of results and the observation of outcome: 'Martian translates words into the true meanings according to their results, and judges people not according to their apparent intent, but from the "final display"' (p. 101). Berne does this by offering a re-reading of fairy tales, famously (at least within TA), of Little Red Riding Hood, and of myths such as Europa (Berne, 1972/1975b). An example of this in my own work is my critique of the arguments used by some colleagues (and professional organisations) to justify the state registration of psychotherapists and the broader statutory regulation of psychotherapy (see Tudor, 2011d [Chapter 10], 2011e, 2011f, Tudor, 2017/2020d) and, specifically, my attempts to ascertain what is or was 'real' about the motivations of the advocates of such arguments and campaigns (see Bailey & Tudor, 2011/2020).

- That it is innate

  Commenting on another example, Berne (1972/1975b) writes that: 'children think Martian until they are discouraged from doing it by their parents' (p. 101), which suggests that human beings are born with the capacity for free expression, knowing what is real, and, by implication, knowing what we know and that we know it. I relate to this strongly, especially given my own parents' commitment to free thinking, especially theologically. I have, however, come up against strong reactions to and discouragement of such free and critical thinking, notably in the responses to my article on a sixth driver (Tudor, 2008d) from Kahler (2008), Karpman (2008), and Parr (2008), for a discussion of which, see Tudor (2008/2017d).

- That it is uncorrupted

  Berne writes that children's Martian thoughts are uncorrupted and that as such they appear fresh and new. Elsewhere he writes about such thinking as without preconceptions. I think of this as when people put their head on one side as if to see things differently. Berne's use of the word uncorrupted has echoes of the concept of decontamination—of the Adult ego state by either or both Parent and Child ego states—which suggests that this free and fresh thinking is Adult, and, more specifically, integrating Adult (see Tudor, 2003b).

- That it is linked to intuition

  In the following section of the chapter in *What Do You Say After You Say Hello?*, entitled 'The Little Lawyer',[2] Berne (1972/1975b) states that:

  > Martian thinking enables the child to find out what the parents 'really' want, that is, what they will respond most favorably too. By using it effectively, he ensures his survival and expresses his love for them. In this way he builds of the ego state known as the Adaptive Child. (p. 104)

Berne's view here is that Martian thinking develops the Adapted Child in a way (of thinking) that holds the balance between the non-adaptive behaviour and feelings (the Parent in the Child) and the self-expressive or Natural Child (the Child in the Child). Berne refers to the part that holds this balance as the 'Professor' (elsewhere, the 'Little Professor'), i.e., the Adult in the Child. Then, in a short passage that suggests some form of epigenetic development of this part of the human personality, Berne argues that: 'After he has learned Martian thinking... The Professor turns his attention to legal thinking, in order to find more ways for the Natural Child to express himself' (Berne, 1972/1975b, p. 104). Such expression is manifested in quick, clever, and shrewd thinking—and hence Berne's argument that this thinking contributes to the child's adaptation to life.

While Berne's image of the Martian is primarily about *thinking*, there is a sense in which, in operation or practice, Martian is about talking 'straight', with crispness (Berne, 1966a), with frankness and respect (Berne, 1968b); and, as Hostie (1982) puts it, without 'wast[ing] time in introductory comments or in trivialities' (p. 168).

In his article on 'Eric Berne, The Martian', Hostie (1982) focuses on the aspect of the Martian that operates—or aims to operate—without 'preconceived ideas', and on the necessary fitness to maintain this position, including:

a. Paying attention to what is on the back of someone's T-shirt, literally or, more commonly, psychologically.
b. Observing closely—Hostie quotes Berne's prescription for transactional analysts to 'Observe that every moment (of a group meeting) every movement of every muscle of every member' (p. 169).
c. Taking 'the opposite of what is generally said and see[ing] if the result sheds any light on the question' (p. 169).

In an article on focusing and TA, Goodman (2007) links thinking like a Martian to working with the bodily, felt sense within the client as well as within herself as a therapist, and, thereby, arriving at 'fresh new information about the client's situation' (p. 283). As Goodman (2007) herself puts it, in doing so, 'I step outside my own cognitive processing and listen from a more embodied, attuned place within me' (p. 282). This is similar to the concept of negative capability promoted by psychoanalysts such as Bion (1970), who took the term from John Keats (1817/2011) who defined it as: 'when a man is capable of being in uncertainties, mysteries, doubts, without any irritable reaching after fact and reason' (p. 48).

In her article on the phenomenology of thinking Martian, Deaconu (2020) emphasises its usefulness in helping the therapist to remain phenomenological, an approach that includes seeing the other (the client) as a phenomenon; staying fresh (following Berne, and Goodman); and not distorting one's perceptions to the point that it becomes difficult to see the other. Deaconu suggests that Berne's (1972/1975b) concern about what was 'real' (p. 100) or actual, was, in effect, 'calling attention to the importance of mak[ing] space for the somewhat raw level of experience whereby sensorimotor mechanisms of processing information take precedence over abstract reasoning' (p. 194). Following on from this, she refers to the importance of 'embodying a Martian presence' (p. 195), viewing this 'not so much a receptive but rather an active mode of engaging in the therapeutic process [which] has generative effects' (p. 195). Finally, Deaconu writes about the therapist '[g]rowing a Martian skin' as a form of resilience again a certain—and inevitable—discomfort and objectification in therapy.

I appreciate Deaconu's (2020) reframing of Berne's concept of Martian, which does much to shift it from being exclusively focused on thinking to incorporating a sense of being, both as a stance, and engagement. I am less sure about her reference to the necessity that humans need to take a Martian body-mind in order to reclaim aspects of humanity. My own, somewhat playful alternative suggests a being who has—and integrates—aspects of two planets and cultures.

Being Vulcan

In *Star Trek*, Vulcans are a fictional extra-terrestrial humanoid species, noted for their attempt to live by logic and reason and, in this way, they appear akin to Berne's fictional Martian, not least their straightforwardness: as Mr Spock puts it: 'Vulcans never bluff' (Spinrad, 1967). However, in the *Star Trek* universe, Vulcans are portrayed as also being capable of experiencing extremely powerful emotions, including rage, suspicion, admiration, contempt, joy, etc. Apart from the fact that it's not possible not to have preconceived ideas or preconceptions, the reason I am drawing on the image of thinking and being Vulcan (and, specifically, being Mr Spock) is because it/he (a) brings together logic and emotion, thinking and feeling; (b) acknowledges ethics—in *Star Trek* Vulcans have a consistent ethical system akin to utilitarianism ('The needs of the many outweigh the needs of the few' [Coto, 2004]); and (c) brings some fire and passion to review, retrospection, and reflection. In Roman mythology, Vulcan is the God of fire, and was associated with both the destructive (deconstructive) and fertilising power of fire. In his book *The Other Side of Power* Steiner (1981) writes about using TA concepts to help people in the project of 'rebelling against obedience, hierarchies, respect for authority, the leader–follower relationship' (p. 172). Of course, thinking and being Martian and/or Vulcan are playful ways of expanding our repertoire as Earthians or humans. As Hostie (1982) puts it: 'the Martian (who was Eric Berne) never ceased to be human. Therein lies his appeal. And his genius' (p. 170). In a more critical vein, and in the context of writing about EcoTA, Barrow and Marshall (2023b) suggest that Berne's concept of thinking Martian represents a disconnect from the ecological domain, preferring an alternative position 'which is about increasing our capacity to be "earthlings"' (p. 9) I agree and, while drawing on the metaphor of (a) Vulcan being, it is in the spirit of being an earthling[3] that I offer the following reflections on TA, which, broadly, focus on the philosophical/political, the practical, the theoretical, and the professional/personal.

The nature and purpose of transactional analysis

The nature of TA and purpose is the analysis of transactions or, what used to be referred to as 'TA proper'. This book reaffirms this and, indeed, suggests (in Chapter 5) that TA (re)define itself in terms of TA proper rather than ego states.

From its origins in clinical practice (psychiatry, psychoanalysis, and psychotherapy) in the 1950s, TA quickly developed as a post-qualifying (if not always postgraduate) application. Thus, in the 1960s, Berne and his colleagues introduced TA to a range of professionals. These included community workers, medical doctors, ministers, nurses, pastors, psychiatrists, psychologists, social workers, and teachers, who, generally, and at that stage, viewed TA as providing analysis and skills additional to their original professional training and/or formation. In modern parlance, it was a form of continuing professional development. Over time, and as TA become more established, it developed a structure for training, examination, and qualification, initially in the 'clinical' field and later in 'special fields'. TA now has four fields of applications, i.e., counselling, education, organisations, and psychotherapy (see Chapter 12), which suggests that TA views its purpose as analysing transactions—and ego states, scripts, and games—in these fields, and, arguably, as a social psychology, in the wider, social/political world.

Despite the fact that Berne (1961/1975a) refers to TA as a social psychiatry, he defines this simply as denoting: 'the study of the psychiatric aspects of specific transactions or sets of transactions which take place between two or more particular individuals at a given time and place' (p. 12)—and, as Steiner (2010) points out, Berne did not apply this to society at large. A number of transactional analysts have discussed Berne's limited view of social psychiatry, notably Baute (1979), Zalcman (1990), Moiso (1995), Barnes (2003), Massey (2007), and Steiner (2010). Some transactional analysts have also discussed the extent to which TA is a social *psychology*, i.e., a psychology that focuses on human behaviour in a relational and social context, namely, Price (1978), Massey (1996), and Tudor (2020g), and a number of transactional analysts have applied TA as a social psychology to all aspects of the social world, including: social issues (Boulton, 1976); social justice (Barnes, 1977a; Campos, 2010); modern racism (Batts, 1982, 1983); cultural scripts (J. James, 1983b); nuclear disarmament (Trautmann, 1984); power (Jacobs, 1987, 1994); nationalism (Jacobs, 1990); autocracy (Jacobs, 1991); social applications (Novey, 1996); gay and lesbian issues (Cornell & Simerly, 2004); war (Campos, 2014, 2015; Tudor, 2023); intrapsychic, interpersonal, and social conflict (Monin & Cornell, 2015); gender, sexuality, and identity (McLean & Cornell, 2017); social responsibility (Cornell & Monin, 2018); religion, faith, and spirituality (de Graaf & Monin, 2019); TA and politics (Tudor & Cornell, 2020); systematic oppression (Minikin & Rowland, 2022); and ecological TA (Barrow & Marshall, 2023a). Moreover, if we consider the organisation of TA, the International Transactional Analysis Association (ITAA) has had a Women's Caucus (see Levin, 1977); a Social Action Committee (see Levin & Fryer, 1980);[4] and a Committee for Social Engagement; has supported the network of Transactional Analysts for Social Responsibility (TASR) (see Campos, 2011);[5] and Project TA101 (United States of America Transactional Analysis Association, 2023); has held and/or sponsored numerous conferences with social themes (for a summary of which, see Tudor, 2020g); and has published a statement on anti-racism (ITAA, 2020).

I note these citations and examples as there is a clear tension regarding the nature and purpose of TA between those who argue that TA should be neutral and 'apolitical', and those who argue that TA is and should be political. The former position is represented by those who were unhappy about the existence of the Women's Caucus; those (40%) who voted against the establishment of TASR in 2010; those who objected to the ITAA's 2020 statement on anti-racism; and those who are opposed to the ITAA making statements in support of Black Lives Matter, and against the Russian invasion of Ukraine. Writing about the 'Future of Transactional Analysis',

O'Hearne (1977) expresses a number of fears, including that 'TA will gradually become more left-wing' (p. 483). He continues, referring to 'right-wing, conservative, clinically trained people who do not need the credentials of [the] ITAA behind their names' (p. 483), a comment which seems to imply that left-wing people who were not clinically trained were using (or would use) TA as a form of entry to a respectable profession! Those of us who view TA as social and political take inspiration from Berne himself who, writing in 1969, and acknowledging the then establishment of TA—from the reading of the first formal paper on TA in 1956, the San Francisco Social Psychiatry Seminars (from 1958), and the *Transactional Analysis Bulletin* (from 1962)—suggested that: 'We are sufficiently well established to undertake one, or even two crusades, or rather the Editor feels that he can take it upon himself to do so' (Berne, 1969, p. 7). He went on to suggest crusades against infant mortality, war, and oppressive governments: what he summarised as 'the Four Horsemen', that is, war, pestilence, famine, and death. Whilst I wouldn't use the word crusade to describe such challenges, I agree with Berne's vision and exhortation that transactional analysts—and TA itself—could and should be impacting on the social world. In an interview with Bill Cornell, Eric Berne's son, Terry, expressed something similar: 'That brings to mind how TA can be applied to society and culture as a whole as opposed to just the individual… The way TA can be applied to broader societal and political patterns is of particular interest to me' (T. Berne & Cornell, 2004, p. 7). Towards the end of his own *Explorations in Transactional Analysis*, Cornell (2008) makes a couple of forward-looking comments, including the following:

> It seems essential to me to end this volume with a reminder that the work we do is fundamentally social and political and its implications. We have no right to do the work of influencing the course of people's lives if we detach ourselves from the political, cultural, and economic realities in which they struggle to develop and thrive.
>
> (p. 252)

This first reflection and point concerns the philosophy—or philosophies—of TA, as discussed throughout this book, as well as the philosophy of the transactional analyst. Those who view TA primarily as a professional practice (in whatever field of application) may attach great(er) importance to the neutrality of the professional and the apolitical nature of professional organisations. Those of us who come from a background of social service, and even social and political activism, will tend to take a more social and political view of professions and professionals (Shaw & Tudor, 2022; Tudor & Shaw, 2022)—and a more critical view of who is living and prospering in and as a result of TA. Whilst it is unlikely that transactional analysts will agree about the nature and purpose of TA, my point about this is that we can think about it both logically and passionately and draw on elders, past, present, and emerging to support our particular perspective and ensuing action (or inaction).

The practice of transactional analysis

The fact that there are four fields of application of TA means that the practice of TA encompasses: counselling (in various forms and settings); educational practice (including teaching, facilitation, curriculum design, management, and so on); organisational work (coaching, consultancy, development, team-building, etc.); and psychotherapy (also in various forms and settings). Of course, educational practice includes the education or, what is more commonly referred to as the training of TA students/trainees—in all four fields of application.

What this means is that practitioners in each field of TA need to be clear about what they view as the purpose of their practice. With regard to psychotherapy, I particularly like Joines' (2006) perspective of the goal (purpose) of therapists in TA, which, he asserts, 'is to work themselves out of a job, as clients are helped to experience their own autonomy and to learn to take charge of their own lives' (p. 3).

With regard to practice, here I offer two reflections which focus on: clients (i.e., those with whom we work—and don't work), and TA as a group therapy.

Clients

Psychotherapy in all its forms (individual, couple, group) and in its different theoretical modalities may be found in many contexts in the public and private sector, though predominantly in the latter. This gives rise to one of the main criticisms of psychotherapy: that it is it inaccessible to the majority of the population (Albee, 1990). Within TA, Joines (2006) suggests that:

> Of course, the wealthy are still able to receive adequate psychotherapy, but the poor often go without. The less money one has, the poorer the quality of treatment one receives. Is this really the direction we want for the future? I, for one, believe it is not.
>
> (p. 3)

There are complex reasons for this, including the universal position of psychotherapy as a poor relation to psychology, and the public funding of psychology and certain therapies such as cognitive behavioural therapy in preference to forms of psychotherapy. The solution to this is also complex and requires change at the organisational (institutional and governmental) level. Some psychotherapists make a difference by doing voluntary work or offering low-cost therapy, which, whilst undoubtedly significant for the clients who benefit, represents an individual and very partial solution.

Another issue regarding clients concerns their demographics. Nearly 45 years ago, Baute (1979) questioned whether TA was 'a middle-class tranquilizer' (p. 170), and others since, both outside and within TA, have questioned the applicablity of psychotherapy—a therapy founded in a predominately white, Western intellectual tradition—to people, groups, and cultures outside that particular tradition. Just as the notion of universal theory has been questioned, so, too, the applicability of a theory or method founded in one culture to different populations and cultures has come under scrutiny (for examples of which see Rodgers & Tudor, 2020; Tudor & Rodgers, 2023), precisely in order to make it—in this case, TA—relevant and more widely applicable. As his early publications attest, Berne himself was interested in transcultural psychiatry (Berne, 1949, 1956, 1959a, 1959b, 1959c, 1960a, 1960b; Bernstein, 1939); and the more recent social and political discourses about gender, race, sexuality, ability, and intersectionality have found some expression in TA, e.g., Shivanath and Hiremath (2003), Cornell and Simerly (2004), McLean and Cornell (2017), Baskerville (2022), and Dhananjaya (2022).

If we, as transactional analysts, have any ambition for TA as a practice to live long and prosper—and to meet the needs of the many rather than those of the few—this suggests that we need to find ways to engage in ways with clients who, by and large, do not access or, previously, have not accessed our services. This is a project that may well—and, arguably needs to—involve being open to different ways of practicing, as, for instance, many practitioners have done during the coronavirus pandemic; and to explore new worlds and cultures, and to changing and developing theory to embrace different ways different people have of experiencing and looking at the world (as I hope I have indicated throughout this present work, and see below).

TA as a group therapy

One of the features that drew me to TA in the first place was the fact that it was originally a group therapy (Berne, 1966a) and, for many years, a requirement for the certification of TA psychotherapists was that they had to complete a certain number of group clinical hours. This was deregulated due to reports that psychotherapy trainees were finding it hard to establish groups and, especially in the counselling and psychotherapy fields, to obtain permission to record groups, and thus, the requirement to run such groups was placing an undue burden on the trainee/student/candidate. This deregulation led, in turn, to a change in the requirement for the group recording for the CTA oral exam.[6] Whilst I appreciate the responsiveness of the ITAA (and the EATA) to trainees' experience, I question this on a number of counts:

1. How was this feedback gathered and evaluated? How large was the sample and from what contexts (practice, countries, and regions) did these reports originate?
2. Was or is there any evidence that it's any harder to get permission to record a counselling or psychotherapy group than an individual client?
3. If the argument is that it's harder to get the permission of a *group* (than of an individual), how is any easier to get permission to record 'a personal or staff development group' (ITAA IBoC, 2022, p. 7) as distinct from a counselling or psychotherapy group?

4. Given that the current *Handbook*(s) still requires (require) that, in all fields of application/specialisation, one of the recordings 'demonstrate the candidate facilitating group dynamics in an effective way' (ITAA IBoC, 2022, p. 6), is there any evidence that it's easier for a candidate to ask a group (or couple) to be willing to facilitate their dynamics on a one-off basis than to ask this of an ongoing group?

I suggest that the rationalisation for deregulating the requirement for group clinical hours and the recording of a therapy group is more to do with privileging the individual and the zeitgeist of individualism; and that this represents a turn away from the transactional and the relational, at least as far as this is expressed by analysing transactions in groups (Berne, 1966a). This is problematic on various levels:

- The ontological—If we think that the essence of human beings is that we are group animals (see Chapter 1), then it makes sense to work in, through, and with human groups.
- The axiological—There are ethical principles, including protection, respect, and empowerment (ITAA, 2014; ITAA IBoC, 2022) that support the rationale for working with clients in groups.
- The epistemological—If we think about how we know what we know in terms of relationship, then it also makes sense to be able to analyse this with others—in groups.
- The methodological—This lies at the heart of Berne's (1961/1975a) description of group therapy: 'Transactional analysis is offered as a method of group therapy because it is a rational, indigenous approach derived from the group situation itself' (p. 165).
- The practical—As Berne (1961/1975a) describes it, 'The objective of transactional analysis in group therapy is to carry each patient through the progressive stages of structural analysis, transactional analysis proper, game analysis, and script analysis, until he attains social control' (p. 165), so groups provide a practical opportunity to do this.

Also, and following on from the point made in the previous section, as group therapy is generally more affordable for each client, it makes TA more accessible to those who otherwise might not afford it, a point that Steiner made in his last workshop (in Steiner & Tudor, 2014; see p. 186, n14), arguing that this was possibly TA's most radical contribution.

The nature and purpose of transactional theory

Very few founding fathers or mothers of a school of or approach to psychotherapy make the case for theory. By and large, theory is assumed to be a good thing; and, despite his advocacy of Martian thinking, Berne himself didn't ask what is real, innate, uncorrupted, and/or intuitive about TA theory. Elsewhere (Tudor, 2018b), I discuss the inevitability and necessity of theory; and consider the purpose of theory as providing: stimulation for further thinking and research, as advocated by Rogers (1959); communication about practice, a prime example of which is Berne's (1971) comment that 'There's only one paper to write, which is called "How to cure patients"' (p. 12); and a conceptual structure, which Ragnell (1985) considers plays a dynamic part within the therapeutic process.

There is no reference to any theory or theorising about the nature of theory in the *Transactional Analysis Bulletin* (1962–1970), and, in 52 years of the *Transactional Analysis Journal* (1971–2023), there are only two references to a 'theory of theory', in the most relevant of which Barnes (2000) reflects on such a theory which he views as, by definition, a critique. In a recent article, Karpman (2019) presents a list of what he refers to as Berne's five rules for theory-making, which were:

1. Don't say anything that you cannot diagram.
2. Don't say anything that has ever been said before.
3. Always apply Occam's Razor.
4. Always write it up in lay person's language.
5. Always keep inventing. (p. 7)

Whilst I don't agree with these being rules or imperatives, I do think they're (still) interesting as invitations to think about theory-making, as follows:

- The first encourages us to present ideas in different forms, which acknowledges different ways of knowing and learning, and fits well with Gardiner's (1983) theory of multiple intelligences, which includes visual-spatial intelligence.
- The second encourages us to be novel in our thinking, although there's also some wisdom in the view that 'There's nothing new under the sun'; at the same time, each generation needs to re-new and re-create old stories, including our stories about stories (for an example of which, see Chapter 9).
- The third references the principle (from the 14th-century English Franciscan friar) that, all things being equal, explanations that posit fewer entities (or kinds of entities) are preferable to those that posit more, and, thus, encourages to be parsimonious or streamlined. Graeme Summers and I drew on this principle in critiquing Clarkson (et al.)'s[7] theory of therapeutic relationships (see Summers & Tudor, 2000). Equally, and responding to the aspect of things not being equal or sufficient, I suggest that, when adding to existing theory, it's important to justify the addition (for an example of which, see Tudor, 2008c).
- The fourth encourages us also to keep theory accessible; I have included the word 'also' in order to acknowledge the different dialects in which theory may be presented (see Berne, 1972/1975b; and the Introduction).
- The fifth one encourages us to be innovative and inventive, which is particularly important if we're thinking about the application of theory invented in one culture and applying it to other cultures and contexts (for an example of which with regard to the definition of contracting, see Chapter 2).

Others have offered ideas about the criteria for (good) theory, including that it is:

- Improvised (Rank), of whom Kramer (1995) writes that he (Rank) 'improvised a new theory for each client' (p. 78).
- Practical (Lewin, 1951).
- Open (Rogers, 1959), and adaptable (Berne, 1972/1975b).
- Fallible (Rogers, 1959), and/or falsifiable (Riebel, 1996).
- Local (van der Ploeg, 1993), as applied to therapy by Totton (1999).
- Reflexive (Barnes, 1994; Tudor, 2018b), and, therefore, in this context, transactional, which is the approach I have taken in this book.
- Diverse (Allen, 2006b).

These ideas about theory are useful in understanding the purpose of theory and, therefore, in being able to navigate theoretical debates, differences, and disputes. For instance, in December 2006, two articles about TA appeared in *The Script*, one by James Allen, the outgoing president of the ITAA, and the other by Claude Steiner. Both articles make for interesting reading as they not only offer two different views about the (then) state and direction of TA theory, but also, I suggest, are based on different views about an underlying theory of theory or meta-theory. The juxtaposition of the authors' relative perspectives is, moreover, enhanced by the fact that the articles appear alongside each other.[8]

In his article, which is titled 'Transactional analysis as an interpretive community', Allen (2006b) identifies a number of what he refers to as 'flavours' of TA (p. 1), commenting that, 'Although some may disagree, I consider this proliferation of flavors as evidence of a flexibility with exciting intellectual and methodological possibilities' (p. 1), and, throughout, welcomes and advocates 'the diversity of our methodologies and theories' (p. 5). In his article, 'Quo vadis transactional analysis?', Steiner (2006) bemoans what he views as some 'substantial theoretical deviation[s] from Berne's basic views' (p. 6). He goes on to identify these deviations (principally about OKness, ego states, and language), and four different views of TA, namely: 'Eric Berne's original view... post-Bernean views adhering to Berne's basic postulates... post-Bernean views deviating from Berne's basic postulates... [and a] broad view that unites people in the global transactional analysis movement' (p. 6) (which Steiner asserts coalesces around OKness. He offers this analysis as the background to his motivation to establish a committee to compile a set of core concepts on which everyone would agree. The project was completed and published in an article in the *TAJ* (Steiner et al., 2003), a short version of which still appears on the ITAA's website (ITAA, 2023). Steiner also notes his surprise regarding the opposition to this project. Allen acknowledges the variations even within one TA tradition, and views this as a benefit in practice. Steiner's perspective (and that of others who supported the core concepts project) is that it was predicated on the view (belief) that Berne was consistent in his theory—and we know, not least from the examples presented in this book, especially in Chapters 2, 6, 9, and 11, that he wasn't.[9] Allen ends his article with a series of open questions that invite the reader to think about the implications of using a particular framework or strategy, as well as 'the assumptions, connotations, and the contextual and developmental histories that come with each approach' (p. 5). Steiner ends his article by reporting the results of his own review of how many of the core concepts of TA have the substantial support from research in the behavioural sciences, concluding that they are: that strokes are essential to healthy development; the OK existential life position; the importance of life scripts; and of the transactional theory of change. However, again, Steiner implies that there is agreement about these areas and the theory within them.[10]

In order to ascertain the differences between Allen (2006b) and Steiner (2006), in Table 13.1 I apply Berne's five 'rules' for theory-making and the other criteria noted above to their respective views of TA theory (also drawing on their other work in TA).

Table 13.1. A meta-theoretical analysis of Allen (2006b) and Steiner (2006)

	'Transactional analysis as an interpretive community', Allen (2006b)	*'Quo vadis transactional analysis?',* Steiner (2006)
Berne's five rules for theory-making *(Karpman, 2019)*		
	Allen would be less interested in these rules, for instance, he doesn't tend to use diagrams (rule 1), and would take a constructivist position about saying things that have been said before from a different perspective (rule 2). He would take a similar perspective as the one I expounded above with regard to adding to theory, and acknowledging complexity (rules 3 and 4); and, as someone who has always been inventive, would certainly agree with rule 5.	Steiner would say that he would agree with Berne's rules, with the possible exception of the last one (rule 5) or, at least, he would want to put some parameters around the extent of the invention. He would, for example, not like my 'deviation' presented in this book of putting transactions rather than ego states at the heart of TA.
Criteria for theory		
Improvised	Yes	No
Practical	Yes (as evidenced in the article)	Yes; for instance, he referred to himself as a psychomechanic (Steiner, 2008; see Tudor, 2020b)
Open, and adaptable	Yes	No, as he advocates agreed, core concepts (and, therefore, closed or restricted theory)
Fallible and/or falsifiable	No; as a constructivist, I would say that he would not be so interested in this view of scientific validity	Yes
Local	Open to it	No, as he proposes universal theory
Reflexive	Yes	Not so much
Diverse	Yes	No

Whether this particular assessment of these transactional analysts' views about an underlying theory of theory are accurate or not, what's important is that debates and especially differences and disputes about theory are often if not always based on differences about meta-theory—which is why it's important to know on what basis we base our view of theory. I suggest that this approach also helps us to resolve the contradictions in TA theory. The fact is that Berne wrote and said different things about the same theory (for an analysis of which with regard to ego states, scripts, and games, see Chapters 6, 9, and 11, respectively).[11] We can regard this as problematic, or welcome, or, at least, see it as an opportunity to encourage diversity in and of thinking—or both! Either way, whilst it is clear that there are now many approaches in TA (see Chapter 12), what is also clear is that the Classical School/tradition/approach does not represent one unified theory.

Again, a Vulcan perspective is useful here: specifically, the central tenet of Vulcan philosophy, that is, the principle of 'infinite diversity in infinite combinations' (Aroeste, 1968) While this principle appears to be the equivalent of cultural relativism, Barad with Robertson (2001) argues that it 'represents a Vulcan belief that beauty, growth, and progress result from the union of the unlike' (p. 21). This, I suggest, offers a more radical and challenging view of the nature and future of theory.

Professional and personal identity as transactional analysts

> Good morning. I am Claude Steiner and I am a transactional analyst. Why do I make a point of this? Because I am constantly surprised to hear people who have been with transactional analysis for decades, who protest that they are rooted in transactional analysis, and who candidly admit that they hide their allegiance. They do this, they say, because revealing one's transactional analysis roots will lead to an automatic discount.
>
> (Steiner, 2006, p. 1)

In becoming a CTA, all candidates need to describe their identity as a transactional analyst as follows.

In counselling:

- 'The candidate describes the context of their working style and their identity as a transactional analyst counsellor in their field of application' (ITAA IBoC, 2022, Section 8.2.1).
- 'Reflect on important learning experiences, which are significant for the development of your identity as a TA counsellor' (Section 8.2.2).
- 'The description of the process should clearly demonstrate your roles/professional identity in TA counselling' (Section 8.2.3).

The reference to professional identity and ethics in the CTA oral examination (which forms the first scale by which candidates are assessed) is more generalised, i.e., 'Has awareness of own social, ethnic and cultural identity' (Form 12.7.9, Scale 1).

In education:

- 'Choose your case/project study to demonstrate... your identity as an educational TA practitioner' (Section 8.3.3).
- Personal and professional identity as a TA educator—which is the first scale in the oral examination (Form 12.7.10).

In organisations:

- How did these learning experiences influence you in finding your identity when working in your profession and your field of application respectively? (Section 8.4.2).[12]

In psychotherapy:

- Interestingly, and, I think, significantly—even, fascinatingly, as Mr Spock would say[13]—in the application or field of psychotherapy, identity is not linked to transactional analysis, but to being a psychotherapist, i.e., (in the CTA written examination) 'How have these learning experiences influenced you in finding your identity as a *psychotherapist*?' [emphasis added] (Section 8.5.2). With regard to professional and personal identity (in the CTA oral examination), as with counselling, this forms the first scale in which two of the descriptors include references to 'awareness of social, racial and cultural identity and differences in the therapeutic relationship' (Form 12.7.12, Scale 1, descriptor 3), and 'awareness of own social and cultural identity and that of the client, and the possible implications of these on the therapeutic work' (Form 12.7.12, Scale 1, descriptor 1), but not to one's identity as a transactional analyst.

This perhaps explains why a number of certified transactional analysts, especially those whose certification as a CTA in psychotherapy, leads them to seek accreditation or registration with another body (such as the United Kingdom Council for Psychotherapy), and then choose another title, such as that or integrative or relational psychotherapist.

It has also been the case that the different needs of and requirements for practitioners in the four fields, as well the impact of legislation, especially regarding the registration of psychotherapists and the regulation of psychotherapy in different jurisdictions, has, at different times, led to disagreements and splits in TA communities—which means that the identity 'transactional analyst' is not straightforward. Moreover, despite the heat that such differences have generated, it is perhaps surprising that there are no articles on professional identity in either the *TAB* or the *TAJ*, though there is an excellent article on 'Personal identity and moral discourse in psychotherapy' by Tosi (2018), much of which could be applied to professional identity.

Given my interest in multiple narratives and identities (see Chapter 9), and in the context of this reflection on living and prospering as transactional analysts, I suggest that the way forward needs to be based on a genuine understanding of different needs and contexts, and an embracing of diverse identities.

Living and prospering

I believe we are and will continue to be a worldwide movement, a movement with an elegant theory about human interaction and a useful and effective method for bringing about beneficial change. We are also a global organization that seeks to support equality, cooperation, nonviolence, democracy—true, incremental democracy—and yes, dare I say it, we are a movement that seeks to support love as a positive force among people.

(Steiner, 2006, p. 7)

Steiner's belief, assessment, assertion, and dare offer a lovely, aspirational vision for TA. Having spent most of my adult life working as a transactional analyst and engaging in and with TA as a therapeutic, supervisory, and educational practice, and a theory—or theories—of course I want it to live on. At the same time, I think we need to reflect on what constitutes the 'life' in and of TA, and what—and who—prospers in and by it. If TA is not supporting equality, co-operation, non-violence, and/or democracy, and other progressive values, then it doesn't deserve to live or prosper. As Mr Spock puts it: 'Every life comes to an end when time demands it. Loss of life is to be mourned but only if the life was wasted' (Fontana, 1973).

Finally, given that I have drawn on an image from *Star Trek* as a central metaphor in this chapter, it is appropriate that I have dedicated this book to the next generation of transactional analysts as it is they who will boldly go where my generation will not be going, in a future that will bring challenges, some of which we can imagine (and for at least some of which we are responsible), but others of which we cannot imagine. In facing these wicked problems, for which even more wicked solutions will be needed, I can only hope that they/you will be supported by the analysis and the spirit of this book, with its independence, impropriety, and impertinence, which, hopefully, gives rise to further pertinent questions.

Live long and prosper!

Notes

1 As I reflected on my own work as well as that of others, and re-read some TA classics as well as less known work, I became interested in what some authors reflected on about TA. Of course, not every book does this; in fact, relatively few do; nevertheless, I found those that did interesting and, therefore have incorporated them into this chapter.
2 A concept I have never heard presented and has never been cited or referenced in the *Transactional Analysis Journal*.
3 … and, moreover, a Taurean, in that, according to my astrological chart, my moon is in Taurus.

4 Steiner (2006) identifies Denton Roberts, Pearl Drego, Carla Haimowitz, Nancy Porter, Felipe Garcia, Alan Jacobs, and others as the 'small core of devoted social action activists... [who] brought about a number of changes aimed at correcting ITAA's political stance' (p. 6).

5 Campos' work in this area was recognised when he received the 2020 Goulding Social Justice Award.

6 As the ITAA IBoC puts it: 'IBOC has recognized the need for flexibility in the requirement for a group recording for the CTA examination. It is sometimes difficult to obtain permission to record groups, especially in the fields of counselling and psychotherapy. A group recording may therefore be a personal or staff development group, training or experiential group' (ITAA IBoC, 2022, Section 9.3.3.2, p. 7).

7 See Chapter 5, p. 116, n2.

8 Allen's article starts on page 1 and continues on pages 4–5; Steiner's article also starts as a column on page 1 and continues on pages 6 and 7.

9 Whilst much of the brief overview of the key concepts in TA published on the ITAA's website is accurate, the summary of the concepts of games people play and of life script does not reflect the complexity and diversity of Berne's own theory on these subjects, as represented and summarised in Chapters 11 and 9 of this book, respectively, let alone that of other TA theorists.

10 I mention (in Chapter 6) that Steiner and I disagreed about theory, especially about different models of ego states and the nature of integration (see Tudor, 2003b). One of the outcomes of those disagreements was the original article (Tudor, 2010c, which forms Chapter 10), in response to which Steiner said to me 'Well, now I get what you integrationists are on about!' (personal communication, November 2010)—which I took as a positive stroke.

11 Discussing this with Claude Steiner on a number of occasions (and feeling irritated with his assumption that Berne had been theoretically consistent), I once said to Claude, 'Well, you should have edited him', to which he replied (in a somewhat shocked tone), 'I would never edit Eric's work.... I was his disciple', to which I responded: 'Well, that's a problem.'

12 There is no reference to professional or personal identity in the oral examination CTA organisations scoring sheet (Form 12.7.11).

13 As distinguished in the following dialogue:

> *Dr. McCoy*: Ah, there's that magic word again. Does your logic find this fascinating, Mr. Spock? *Mr. Spock*: No, 'fascinating' is a word I use for the unexpected. In this case, I should think 'interesting' would suffice.
>
> (Schneider, 1967)

References

Albee, G. W. (1990). The futility of psychotherapy. *Journal of Mind and Behavior, 11*(3–4), 369–384.

Alexander, F., & French, T. M. (1946). *Psychoanalytic therapy: Principles and application.* Ronald Press.

Allen, J. R. (2006a). Oklahoma City ten years later: Positive psychology, transactional analysis, and the transformation of trauma from a terrorist attack. *Transactional Analysis Journal, 36*(2), 120–133. https://doi.org/10.1177/036215370603600205.

Allen, J. R. (2006b). Transactional analysis as an interpretive community: Identity and destiny in 2007. *The Script, 36*(9), 1, 4–5. https://www.itaaworld.org/sites/default/files/itaa-pdfs/the-script/script-2006/ITAA%20The%20Script%202006-12.pdf.

Allen, J. R. (2009). Constructivist and neuroconstructivist transactional analysis. *Transactional Analysis Journal, 39*(3), 181–192. https://doi.org/10.1177/036215370903900302.

Allen, J. R., & Allen, B. A. (1972). Scripts: The role of permission. *Transactional Analysis Journal, 2*(2), 72–74. https://doi.org/10.1177/036215377200200210.

Allen, J. R., & Allen, B. A. (1995). Narrative theory, redecision therapy, and postmodernism. *Transactional Analysis Journal, 25*(4), 327–334. https://doi.org/10.1177/036215379502500408.

Allen, J. R., & Allen, B. A. (1997). A new type of transactional analysis and one version of script work with a constructionist sensibility. *Transactional Analysis Journal, 27*(2), 89–98. https://doi.org/10.1177/036215379702700204.

Allen, J. R., & Allen, B. A. (2000). Every revolution should have dancing: Biology, community organization, constructionism, and joy. *Transactional Analysis Journal, 30*(3), 188–191. https://doi.org/10.1177/036215370003000303.

Allen, J. R., Allen, B., Barnes, G., Hibner, B., Krausz, R., Moiso, C., Welch, C., & Welch, S. (1996). The role of permission: Two decades later. *Transactional Analysis Journal, 26*(3), 196–205. https://doi.org/10.1177/036215379602600302.

Allen, J. R., Bennett, S., & Kearns, L. (2004). Psychological mindedness: A neglected developmental line in permissions to think. *Transactional Analysis Journal, 34*(1), 3–9. https://doi.org/10.1177/036215370403400102.

Althöfer, L., & Riesenfeld, V. (2020). Radical therapy: The fifth decade. In K. Tudor (Ed.), *Claude Steiner, emotional activist: The life and work of Claude Michel Steiner* (pp. 131–144). Routledge.

Althöfer, L., & Tudor, K. (2020). On power. In K. Tudor (Ed.), *Claude Steiner, emotional activist: The life and work of Claude Michel Steiner* (pp. 155–171). Routledge.

American Counseling Association. (1995). *Code of ethics and standards of practice.* https://www.counseling.org/docs/default-source/library-archives/archived-code-of-ethics/code-of-ethics-1995.pdf.

Anderson, L. W., & Krathwohl, D. R. (2001). *A taxonomy for learning, teaching, and assessing: A revision of Bloom's taxonomy of educational objectives.* Longman.

Angyal, A. (1941). *Foundations for a science of personality.* Commonwealth Fund.

Anthony, P. (2018). Managing the therapeutic relationship: Parental roles. *Transactional Analysis Journal, 48*(4), 365–378. https://doi.org/10.1080/03621537.2018.1505102.

Anzieu, D. (1989). *The skin ego.* Yale University Press.

Aristotle. (2004). *A treatise on government* (W. Ellis, Trans.). Project Gutenberg. https://www.gutenberg.org/cache/epub/6762/pg6762-images.html. (Original work published 350BCE)

Aroeste, J. L. (1968). Is there in truth no beauty? In *Star Trek* (R. Senensky, Director; Series 3, Episode 5). Desilu Productions.

Azzi, L. G. (Ed.). (1998). Regression in psychotherapy [Special issue]. *Transactional Analysis Journal, 28*(1). https://www.tandfonline.com/toc/rtaj20/28/1.

Bader, E. (1994). Dual relationships: Legal and ethical trends. *Transactional Analysis Journal, 24*(1), 64–66. https://doi.org/10.1177/036215379402400112.

Bager-Charleson, S., & McBeath, A. (Eds.). (2020). *Enjoying research in counselling and psychotherapy: Qualitative, quantitative and mixed methods research.* Palgrave Macmillan.

Bager-Charleson, S., & McBeath, A. (Eds.). (2022). *Supporting research in counselling and psychotherapy: Qualitative, quantitative and mixed methods research.* Springer.

Bailey, P. (2004). Towards the statutory registration of psychotherapists in Aotearoa New Zealand: Political and personal reflections. *Ata: Journal of Psychotherapy Aotearoa New Zealand, 10*, 31–37. https://doi.org/10.9791/ajpanz.2004.04.

Bailey, R., & Brake, M. (Eds.). (1975). *Radical social work.* Edward Arnold.

Bailey, P., & Tudor, K. (2020). Letters across "the Ditch": A trans Tasman correspondence about regulation and registration. In K. Tudor (Ed.), *Pluralism in psychotherapy: Critical reflections from a post-regulation landscape.* [E-book edition] Tuwhera Open Access Books. https://ojs.aut.ac.nz/tuwhera-open-monographs/catalog/book/1. (Original work published 2011)

Balint, M. (1968). *The basic fault: Therapeutic aspects of regression.* Tavistock Publications.

Bandura, A. (1969). *Principles of behavior modification.* Holt, Rinehart & Winston.

Barad, J., with Robertson, E. (2001). *The ethics of Star Trek.* Perennial.

Barad, K. (2003). Posthumanist performativity: Toward an understanding of how matter comes to matter. *Signs, 28*(3), 801–831. https://www.jstor.org/stable/10.1086/345321.

Barnes, E. W. (1933). *Scientific theory and religion: The world described by science and its spiritual interpretation.* Cambridge University Press.

Barnes, G. (1977a). Introduction. In G. Barnes (Ed.), *Transactional analysis after Eric Berne: Teachings and practices of three TA schools* (pp. 3–31). Harper & Row.

Barnes, G. (Ed.). (1977b). *Transactional analysis After Eric Berne: Teachings and practices of three TA schools.* Harper & Row.

Barnes, G. (1981). On saying hello: The script drama diamond and character role analysis. *Transactional Analysis Journal, 11*(1), 22–32. https://doi.org/10.1177/036215378101100105.

Barnes, G. (1994). *Justice, love and wisdom: Linking psychotherapy to second-order cybernetics.* Medicinska Naklada.

Barnes, G. (2000). Retrieving a flourishing psychotherapy: A transactional-cybernetic meditation on transactional analysis. *Transactional Analysis Journal, 30*(3), 233–247. https://doi.org/10.1177/036215370003000308.

Barnes, G. (2004). Homosexuality in the first three decades of transactional analysis: A study of theory in the practice of transactional analysis psychotherapy. *Transactional Analysis Journal*, *34*(2), 126–155. https://doi.org/10.1177/036215370403400205.

Barnes, G. (2005). Acceptance speech on receiving the 2005 Eric Berne Memorial Award: Transgressions. *Transactional Analysis Journal*, *35*(3), 221–239. https://doi.org/10.1177/036215370503500303.

Barnes, G. (2007). Not without the couch: Eric Berne on basic differences between transactional analysis and psychoanalysis. *Transactional Analysis Journal*, *37*(1), 41–50. https://doi.org/10.1177/036215370703700108.

Barr, J. (1987). The therapeutic relationship model: Perspectives on the core of the healing process. *Transactional Analysis Journal*, *17*(4), 134–140. https://doi.org/10.1177/036215378701700402.

Barrow, G. (2007). Wonderful world, beautiful people: Reframing transactional analysis as positive psychology. *Transactional Analysis Journal*, *37*(3), 206–209. https://doi.org/10.1177/036215370703700304.

Barrow, G. (2014) Natality: An alternative existential possibility. *Transactional Analysis Journal*, *44*(4), 311–319. https://doi.org/10.1177/0362153714559923.

Barrow, G. (2018). For whom is the teacher and for what is the teaching? An educational reframe of the Parent ego state. *Transactional Analysis Journal*, *48*(4), 322–334. https://doi.org/10.1080/03621537.2018.1505113.

Barrow, G. (2020). Teaching as creative subversion: Education encounter as an antidote to neoliberal exploitation of the educational task. *Transactional Analysis Journal*, 50(3), 179–192. https://doi.org/10.1080/03621537.2020.1771021.

Barrow, G., & Marshall, H. (2020). Introducing eco-TA—A movement of our time. *The Transactional Analyst*, *10*(2), 4.

Barrow, G., & Marshall, H. (Eds.). (2023a). Ecological transactional analysis (Eco-TA) [Special issue]. *Transactional Analysis Journal*, *53*(1). https://www.tandfonline.com/toc/rtaj20/53/1.

Barrow, G., & Marshall, H. (2023b). Revisiting ecological transactional analysis: Emerging perspectives. *Transactional Analysis Journal*, *53*(1), 7–20. https://doi.org/10.1080/03621537.2023.2152528.

Bary, B. B., & Hufford, F. M. (1997). The physiological factor: The "seventh" advantage to games and its use in treatment planning. *Transactional Analysis Journal*, *27*(1), 38–41. https://doi.org/10.1177/036215379702700109.

Baskerville, V. (2022). A transcultural and intersectional ego state model of the self: The influence of transcultural and intersectional identity on self and other. *Transactional Analysis Journal*, *52*(3), 228–243. https://doi.org/10.1080/03621537.2022.2076398.

Baskerville, V. (2023). Deconstructing and reconstructing the curriculum. *The Transactional Analyst*, *13*(2), 19–25.

Batts, V. A. (1982). Modern racism: A TA perspective. *Transactional Analysis Journal*, *12*(3), 207–209. https://doi.org/10.1177/036215378201200309.

Batts, V. A. (1983). Knowing and changing the cultural script component of racism. *Transactional Analysis Journal*, *13*(4), 255–257. https://doi.org/10.1177/036215378301300416.

Baute, P. (1979). Intimacy and autonomy are not enough. (Is TA a middle-class tranquilizer?) *Transactional Analysis Journal*, *9*(3), 170–173. https://doi.org/10.1177/036215377900900303.

Bergmann, M. S. (Ed.). (2000). *The Hartmann era*. Other Press.

Berlin, A. (2019). A stark choice between subjectivity and objectivity in the therapeutic relationship. *Transactional Analysis Journal*, *49*(3), 169–180. https://doi.org/10.1080/03621537.2019.1602414.

Berne, E. (1947). *The mind in action*. Simon & Schuster.

Berne, E. (1949). Some oriental mental hospitals. *American Journal of Psychiatry*, *106*(5), 376–383. https://doi.org/10.1176/ajp.106.5.376.

Berne, E. (1956). Comparative psychiatry and tropical psychiatry. *American Journal of Psychiatry*, *113*(3), 193–200. https://doi.org/10.1176/ajp.113.3.193.

Berne, E. (1959a). Difficulties of comparative psychiatry: The Fiji islands. *American Journal of Psychiatry*, *116*(2), 104–109. https://doi.org/10.1176/ajp.116.2.104.

Berne, E. L. (1959b). Psychiatric epidemiology of the Fiji Islands. In J. H. Masserman & J. L. Moreno (Eds.), *Progress in psychotherapy. Vol. IV: Social psychotherapy* (pp. 310–313). Grune & Stratton.

Berne, E. (1960a). The cultural problem: Psychopathology in Tahiti. *American Journal of Psychiatry*, *116*(12), 1076–1081. https://doi.org/10.1176/ajp.116.12.1076.

Berne, E. (1960b). A psychiatric census of the South Pacific. *American Journal of Psychiatry*, *117*(1), 44–47. https://doi.org/10.1176/ajp.117.1.44.

Berne, E. (1962a). July 17. Franklin Ernst. The multi-problem family and the decision for treatment. *Transactional Analysis Bulletin*, *1*(4), 32.

Berne, E. (1962b). The classifications of positions. *Transactional Analysis Bulletin*, *1*(3), 23.

Berne, E. (1963). *The structure and dynamics of organizations and groups*. Grove Press.

Berne, E. (1964a). The intimacy experiment. *Transactional Analysis Bulletin*, *3*(9), 113.

Berne, E. (1964b). Pathological significance of games. *Transactional Analysis Bulletin*, *3*(12), 160.

Berne, E. (1964c). Trading stamps. *Transactional Analysis Bulletin*, *3*(10), 127.

Berne, E. (1965a). Evolution of a script. *Transactional Analysis Bulletin*, *4*(15), 49.

Berne, E. (1965b). The public eye. *Transactional Analysis Bulletin*, *4*(106), 80.

Berne, E. (1966a). *Principles of group treatment*. Grove Press.

Berne, E. (1966b). The public eye. *Transactional Analysis Bulletin*, *5*(17), 101–102.

Berne, E. (1966c). The public eye. *Transactional Analysis Bulletin*, *5*(18), 132.

Berne, E. (1967). *The games people play game* [Board game]. Adult Leisure Products Corporation.

Berne, E. (1968a). *Games people play: The psychology of human relationships*. Penguin. (Original work published 1964)

Berne, E. (1968b). *The happy valley*.

Berne, E. (1968c). Staff–patient staff conferences. *American Journal of Psychiatry*, *125*(3), 286–293.

Berne, E. (1969). Editor's page. *Transactional Analysis Bulletin*, *8*(29), 7–8.

Berne, E. (1970). Eric Berne as a group therapist. *Transactional Analysis Bulletin*, *9*(35), 75–83.

Berne, E. (1971). *A layman's guide to psychiatry and psychoanalysis* (3rd Ed. rev.). Penguin. (Original work published 1969)

Berne, E. (1973) *Sex in human loving*. Penguin. (Original work published 1970)

Berne, E. (1975a). *Transactional analysis in psychotherapy: A systematic individual and social psychiatry*. Souvenir Press. (Original work published 1961)

Berne, E. (1975b). *What do you say after you say hello? The psychology of human destiny*. Penguin. (Original work published 1972)

Berne, E. (1977a). Concerning the nature of communication. In P. McCormick (Ed.), *Intuition and ego states: The origins of transactional analysis* (pp. 49–65). Harper & Row. (Original work published 1953)

Berne, E. (1977b). Concerning the nature of diagnosis. In P. McCormick (Ed.), *Intuition and ego states: The origins of transactional analysis* (pp. 33–48). Harper & Row. (Original work published 1952)

Berne, E. (1977c). The ego image. In P. McCormick (Ed.), *Intuition and ego states: The origins of transactional analysis* (pp. 99–119). Harper & Row. (Original work published 1957a)

Berne, E. (1977d). Ego states in psychotherapy. In P. McCormick (Ed.), *Intuition and ego states: The origins of transactional analysis* (pp. 121–144). Harper & Row. (Original work published 1957b)

Berne, E. (1977e). *Intuition and ego states: The origins of transactional analysis* (P. McCormick, Ed.). Harper & Row.

Berne, E. (1977f). The nature of intuition. In P. McCormick (Ed.), *Intuition and ego states: The origins of transactional analysis* (pp. 1–31). Harper & Row. (Original work published 1949)

Berne, E. (1977g). Primal images and primal judgment. In P. McCormick (Ed.), *Intuition and ego states: The origins of transactional analysis* (pp. 67–97). Harper & Row. (Original work published 1955)

Berne, E. (1977h). The psychodynamics of intuition. In P. McCormick (Ed.), *Intuition and ego states: The origins of transactional analysis* (pp. 159–166). Harper & Row. (Original work published 1962)

Berne, E. (1977i). Transactional analysis: A new and effective method of group therapy. In P. McCormick (Ed.), *Intuition and ego states: The origins of transactional analysis* (pp. 145–158). Harper & Row. (Original work published 1958)

Berne, E. (2010). *A Montreal childhood*. Editorial Jeder.

Berne, T., & Cornell, B. (2004). Remembering Eric Berne: A conversation with Terry Berne. *The Script, 34*(8), 6–7.

Bernstein, E. L. (1939). Psychiatry in Syria. *American Journal of Psychiatry, 95*, 1415–1419. https://doi.org/10.1176/ajp.95.6.1415.

Bernstein, J. S. (2005). *Living in the borderland: The evolution of consciousness*. Routledge.

Bestazza, R., & Ranci, D. (2015). Using transactional analysis in work with immigrant families. *Transactional Analysis Journal, 45*(1), 23–37. https://doi.org/10.1177/0362153714568804.

Bicehouse, T., & Hawker, L. (1993). Degrees of games: An application to the understanding of domestic violence. *Transactional Analysis Journal, 23*(4), 195–200. https://doi.org/10.1177/036215379302300404.

Bion, W. R. (1968). *Experiences in groups*. Tavistock. (Original work published 1961)

Bion, W. R. (1970). *Attention and interpretation: A scientific approach to insight in psychoanalysis and groups*. Tavistock.

Blake, W. (1958). Augeries of innocence. In W. Blake. *A selection of poems and letters* (pp. 67–71). Oxford University Press. (Original work published 1863)

Blatt, S. J., & Blass, R. B. (1990). Attachment and separateness: A dialectic model of the products and processes of development throughout the life cycle. *The Psychoanalytic Study of the Child, 45*(1), 107–127. https://doi.org/10.1080/00797308.1990.11823513.

Bloom, B. S., Engelhart, M. D., Furst, E. J., Hill, W. H., & Krathwohl, D. R. (Eds.) (1956). *Taxonomy of educational objectives: the classification of educational goals; Handbook I: Cognitive domain*. David McKay.

Bly, R., & Meade, M. (1991). *The shadow and the soul* [Cassette recording, Tapes 1–8]. Open Gate.

Bolten, M., & de Jong, N. (1984). Reparenting, or therapeutic regression. In E. Stern (Ed.), *TA: The state of the art. A European contribution* (pp. 129–142). Foris Publications.

Bond, T. (1993). *Standards and ethics for counselling in action*. Sage.

Bonhoeffer, D. (1997). Letter to Eberhard Bethge, 29 May 1944. In E. Bethge (Ed.), *Letters and papers from prison* (R. H. Fuller, Trans.; pp. 310–312). Touchstone.

Boulton, M. (Ed.). (1976). Social issues [Special issue]. *Transactional Analysis Journal, 6*(1). https://www.tandfonline.com/toc/rtaj20/6/1.

Bove, S., & Rizzi, M. (2009). Listening to intuition: Reflections on unconscious processes in the therapeutic relationship. *Transactional Analysis Journal, 39*(1), 39–45. https://doi.org/10.1177/036215370903900105.

Boyce, M. (1978). Twelve permissions. *Transactional Analysis Journal, 8*(1), 30–32. https://doi.org/10.1177/036215377800800108.

Boyd, H. S. (1976). Therapeutic leverage. *Transactional Analysis Journal, 6*(4), 401–404. https://doi.org/10.1177/036215377600600413

Boyd, H. S., & Cowles-Boyd, L. (1980). Blocking tragic scripts. *Transactional Analysis Journal, 10*(3), 227–229. https://doi.org/10.1177/036215378001000310

Brady, F. N. (1980a). Philosophical links to TA: Hegel and the concept of the Adult ego state. *Transactional Analysis Journal, 10*(3), 255–258. https://doi.org/10.1177/036215378001000317.

Brady, F. N. (1980b). Philosophical links to TA: Kant and the concept of Reason in the Adult ego state. *Transactional Analysis Journal, 10*(3), 252–254 https://doi.org/10.1177/036215378001000316.

British Association for Counselling. (1995). *Code of ethics and practice for supervisors of counsellors*. Author.

British Association for Counselling. (1996). *Code of ethics and practice for trainers*. Author.

British Association for Counselling. (1997). *Code of ethics and practice for counsellors*. Author.

Bronowski, J. (1953). An English philosopher's answer to the question: What is science? [Review of *Scientific explanation* by R. B. Braithwaite]. *Scientific American, 189*(3), 140–142. https://www.jstor.org/stable/10.2307/24944343.

Brook, K. A. (1996). A fresh look at permission. *Transactional Analysis Journal, 26*, 160–166. https://doi.org/10.1177/036215379602600207.

Bryant, J., & Tudor, K. (2022). The lived reality of men who have been violated and violent. In K. Tudor & E. Green (Eds.), *Psyche and academia: Papers from 21 years of the Auckland University of Technology psychotherapy Master's programmes* (pp. 17–30). Tuwhera Open Access Publishing. https://ojs.aut.ac.nz/tuwhera-open-monographs/catalog/book/10.

Bulhan, H. A. (1979). Black psyches in captivity and crises. *Race & Class, 20*(3), 243–261. https://doi.org/10.1177/030639687902000302.

Burrell, G., & Morgan, G. (1979). *Sociological paradigms and organisational analysis*. Heinemann.

Bush, G. W. (2001). President Bush addresses the nation. *The Washington Post*. https://www.washingtonpost.com/wp-srv/nation/specials/attacked/transcripts/bushaddress_092001.html.

Campos, L. (1970). Transactional analysis of witch messages. *Transactional Analysis Bulletin, 9*(34), 51–57.

Campos, L. P. (1988). Empowering children II: Integrating protection into script prevention work. *Transactional Analysis Journal, 18,* 137–140. https://doi.org/10.1177/03621537 8801800209.

Campos, L. P. (2003). Care and maintenance of the tree of transactional analysis. *Transactional Analysis Journal, 33*(2), 115–125. https://doi.org/10.1177/036215370303300204.

Campos, L. (2010). Redecision therapy and social justice. *Transactional Analysis Journal, 40*(2), 85–94. https://doi.org/10.1177/036215371004000202.

Campos, L. P. (2011). Update on transactional analysts for social responsibility. *The Script, 41*(1), 5.

Campos, L. P. (2014). A transactional analytic view of war and peace. *Transactional Analysis Journal, 44*(1), 68–79. https://doi.org/10.1177/0362153714531722.

Campos, L. P. (2015). Cultural scripting for forever wars. *Transactional Analysis Journal, 45*(4), 276–288. https://doi.org/10.1177/0362153715607242.

Carroll, L. (2021). *Through the looking-glass: And what Alice found there.* Duke Classics. (Original work published 1872)

Casement, P. (2002). *Learning from our mistakes: Beyond dogma in psychoanalysis and psychotherapy.* Guilford Press.

Cheney, W. (1971). Eric Berne: Biographical sketch. *Transactional Analysis Journal, 1*(1), 14–22. https://doi.org/10.1177/036215377100100104.

Childs-Gowell E., & Kinnaman P. (1978). *Body-script blockbusting: A transactional approach to body awareness.* Transactional Pubs.

Chinnock, K., & Minikin, K. (2015). Multiple contemporaneous games in psychotherapy. *Transactional Analysis Journal, 45*(2), 141–152. https://doi.org/10.1177/0362153715585096.

Choy, A. (1990). The winner's triangle. *Transactional Analysis Journal, 20*(1), 40–46. https://doi.org/10.1177/036215379002000105.

Christoph-Lemke, C. (1999). The contributions of transactional analysis to integrative psychotherapy. *Transactional Analysis Journal, 29*(3), 198–214. https://doi.org/10.1177/ 036215379902900305.

Clare, S., & Tudor, K. (2023). Ecotherapy: Perceived obstacles and solutions. Ecological transactional analysis (Eco-TA) [Special issue]. *Transactional Analysis Journal, 53*(1), 21–37. https://doi.org/10.1080/03621537.2023.2152547.

Clark, B. D. (1991). Empathic transactions in the deconfusion of child ego states. *Transactional Analysis Journal, 21*(2), 92–98. https://doi.org/10.1177/036215379102 100204.

Clark, F. (1998). [Review of the book *Ego states: Theory and practice*, by J. G. Watkins and H. H. Watkins]. *Transactional Analysis Journal, 28*(2), 175–176. https://doi. org/10.1177/036215379802800213.

Clark, J. V. (1963). Authentic interaction and personal growth in sensitivity training groups. *Journal of Humanistic Psychotherapy, 3*(1), 1–13. https://doi.org/10.1177/002216786 300300101.

Clarkson, B. (2021). Is it God who cures? A transpersonal perspective on script formation, the role of physis, and the "soul work" of the therapeutic process. *Transactional Analysis Journal, 51*(3), 317–330. https://doi.org/10.1080/03621537.2021.1949804.

Clarkson, P. (1987). The bystander role. *Transactional Analysis Journal, 17*(3), 82–87. https://doi.org/10.1177/036215378701700305.

Clarkson, P. (1989). Metanoia: A process of transformation. *ITA News, No. 23,* 5–14.

Clarkson, P. (1990). A multiplicity of psychotherapeutic relationships. *British Journal of Psychotherapy, 7,* 148–163.

Clarkson, P. (1992). *Transactional analysis psychotherapy: An integrated approach.* Routledge.

Clarkson, P. (1993). Bystander games. *Transactional Analysis Journal, 23*(3), 158–172. https://doi.org/10.1177/036215379302300307.

Clarkson, P. (1994). In recognition of dual relationships. *Transactional Analysis Journal, 24*(1), 32–38. https://doi.org/10.1177/036215379402400107.

Clarkson, P. (1995). *The therapeutic relationship.* Whurr.

Clarkson, P., & Fish, S. (1988). Rechilding: Creating a new past in the present as a support for the future. *Transactional Analysis Journal, 18*(1), 51–59. https://doi.org/10.1177/036215378801800109.

Clarkson, P., & Gilbert, M. (1990). Transactional analysis. In W. Dryden (Ed.), *Individual therapy: A handbook* (pp. 199–225). Open University Press.

Clarkson, P., with Gilbert, M. (1988). Berne's original model of ego states: Some theoretical considerations. *Transactional Analysis Journal, 18*(1), 20–29. https://doi.org/10.1177/036215378801800105

Clarkson, P., Gilbert, M., & Tudor, K. (1996). Transactional analysis. In W. Dryden (Ed.), *Handbook of individual therapy* (pp. 219–253). Sage.

Clarkson, P., & Lapworth, P. (1992). The psychology of the self in transactional analysis. In P. Clarkson (Ed.), *Transactional analysis psychotherapy: An integrated approach* (pp. 175–203). Routledge.

Cohen, S. H. (1961). A growth theory of neurotic resistance to therapy. *Journal of Humanistic Psychology, 1*(1), 48–63. https://doi.org/10.1177/002216786100100106

Concannon, J. P. (1971). My introduction to Eric Berne. *Transactional Analysis Journal, 1*(1), 60–61. https://doi.org/10.1177/036215377100100111.

Cook, R. (2022). Connection, hungers, and time structuring: A relational, inclusive, and transpersonal development of autonomy. *Transactional Analysis Journal, 52*(4), 279–294. https://doi.org/10.1080/03621537.2022.2115641.

Cooper, J. (2022). *Oscar Wilde in America.* https://www.oscarwildeinamerica.org/quotations/took-out-a-comma.html.

Cornell, W. F. (1988). Life script theory: A critical review from a developmental perspective. *Transactional Analysis Journal, 18*(4), 270–282. https://doi.org/10.1177/036215378801800402.

Cornell, W. F. (1994). Dual relationships in transactional analysis: Training, supervision and therapy. *Transactional Analysis Journal, 24*(1), 21–29. https://doi.org/10.1177/036215379402400105.

Cornell, W. F. (2000). If Berne met Winnicott: Transactional analysis and relational analysis. *Transactional Analysis Journal, 30*(4), 270–275. https://doi.org/10.1177/036215370003000403.

Cornell, W. F. (2005). In the terrain of the unconscious: The evolution of a transactional analysis therapist. *Transactional Analysis Journal, 35*(2), 119–131. https://doi.org/10.1177/036215370503500203.

Cornell, W. F. (2008). What do you say if you don't say 'unconscious'?: Dilemmas created for transactional analysts by Berne's shift away from the language of unconscious experience. *Transactional Analysis Journal, 38*(2), 93–100. https://doi.org/10.1177/036215370803800202.

Cornell, W. F. (2010). Aspiration or adaptation?: An unresolved tension in Eric Berne's basic beliefs. *Transactional Analysis Journal, 40*(3–4), 243–253. https://doi.org/10.1177/036215371004000309.

Cornell, W. F. (2013). 'Special fields': A brief history of an anxious dilemma and its linger-
ing consequences for transactional analysis. *Transactional Analysis Journal*, *43*(1), 7–13.
https://doi.org/10.1177/0362153713483274.

Cornell, W. F. (2015). Ego states in the social realm. *Transactional Analysis Journal*, *45*(3),
191–199. https://doi.org/10.1177/0362153715597897.

Cornell, W. F. (2020). Transactional analysis and psychoanalysis: Overcoming the narcissism of small differences in the shadow of Eric Berne. *Transactional Analysis Journal*,
50(3), 164–178. https://doi.org/10.1080/03621537.2020.1771020.

Cornell, W. F. (2022). Schiffian reparenting theory reexamined through contemporary
lenses: Comprehending the meanings of psychotic experience. *Transactional Analysis
Journal*, *52*(1), 40–58. https://doi.org/10.1080/03621537.2021.2011035.

Cornell, W. F., & Deaconu, D. (Eds.). (2022). Schiffian reparenting theory and practice reexamined [Special issue] *Transactional Analysis Journal*, *52*(1). https://www.tandfonline.
com/toc/rtaj20/52/1.

Cornell, W. F., & Hargaden, H. (Eds.). (2005). *From transactions to relations: The emergence of a relational tradition in transactional analysis*. Haddon Press.

Cornell, W. F. (Ed.), Hargaden, H., Allen, J. R., Erskine, R., Moiso, C., Sills, C., Summers, G.,
& Tudor, K. (2006) Roundtable on the ethics of relational transactional analysis. *Transactional Analysis Journal*, *36*(2), 105–119. https://doi.org/10.1177/036215370603600204.

Cornell, W. F., & Monin, S. (Eds.). (2018). Social responsibility in a vengeful world [Special
issue]. *Transactional Analysis Journal*, *48*(2).

Cornell, W. F., & Shadbolt, C. (2009). Letter from the coeditors. *Transactional Analysis
Journal*, *39*(2), 82–83. https://doi.org/10.1177/036215370903900201.

Cornell, W. F., & Simerly, T. (2004). Letter from the coeditors. *Transactional Analysis Journal*, *34*(2), 106–108. https://doi.org/10.1177/036215370403400201.

Corsover, H. D. (1979). Life scripts of Asklepieion Therapeutic Community residents. *Transactional Analysis Journal*, *9*(2), 136–140. https://doi.org/10.1177/036215377900900219.

Coto, M. (2004). Similitude. In *Star trek: Enterprise* (L. Burton, Director; Series 3, Episode
10). United Paramount Network.

Cowles-Boyd, L, & Boyd, H. S. (1980). Playing with games: The game/play shift. *Transactional Analysis Journal*, *10*(1), 8–11. https://doi.org/10..1177/036215378001000103.

Cox, M. (1997, April). Dual relationships. Presentation at *European Association for Transactional Analysis Training Endorsement Workshop*, Keele, UK.

Cox, M. (2000). The equal relationship in psychotherapy: Roles, rights, and responsibilities.
ITA News, *56*, 17–20.

Cox, M. (2007). On doing supervision, *Transactional Analysis Journal*, *37*(2), 104–114,
https://doi.org/10.1177/036215370703700203.

Cox, R. W. (1996). Towards a posthegemonic conceptualization of world order: Reflections
on the relevancy of Ibn Khaldun. In R. W. Cox with T. J. Sinclair (Eds.), *Approaches to
world order* (pp. 144–173). Cambridge University Press.

Crossman, P. (1966). Permission and protection. *Transactional Analysis Bulletin*, *5*(19),
152–154.

Crossman, P. (2002). Letter to the editor. *The Script*, *32*(6), 5.

Dalal, F. (1998). *Taking the group seriously. Towards a post-Foulkesian group analytic
theory*. Jessica Kingsley.

Dashiell, S. R. (1978). The parent resolution process: Reprogramming psychic incor-
porations in the parent. *Transactional Analysis Journal*, *8*(4), 289–294. https://doi.
org/10.1177/036215377800800403.

Davies, W. H. (1911). *Songs of joy and others*. A. C. Fifield.

Dawes, R. M. (1994). *House of cards: Psychology and psychotherapy built on myth*. Free Press.

Deaconu, D. (2020). The therapist's agency as a subsymbolic working tool in the clinical encounter: On the phenomenology of thinking Martian. *Transactional Analysis Journal, 50*(3), 193–206. https://doi.org/10.1080/03621537.2020.1771024.

Deaconu, D., & Rowland, H. (2021). Normativity, marginality, and deviance [Special issue]. *Transactional Analysis Journal, 51*(1). https://www.tandfonline.com/toc/rtaj20/51/1.

Deaconu, D., & Stuthridge, J. (Eds.). (2015). Games and enactments. [Special issue] *Transactional Analysis Journal, 45*(2). https://www.tandfonline.com/toc/rtaj20/45/2.

de Graaf, A., & Monin, S. (Eds.). (2019). Transactional analysis and existential perspectives: Religion, faith, spirituality, and beyond [Special issue]. *Transactional Analysis Journal, 49*(2).

de Graaf, A., & Rosseau, M. (2015). Transactional analysis and conflict management. *Transactional Analysis Journal, 45*(4), 250–259. https://doi.org/10.1177/0362153715606172.

de Graaf, A., & Tigchelaar, H. (2021a). TSTA at the expense of the environment? A call to action. *The Script, 51*(8), 5–6.

de Graaf, A., & Tigchelaar, H. (2021b). The world is our oyster: Opening up TA training for everyone everywhere? *The Script, 51*(4), 8–9.

de Saint-Pierre, C. (2004). The contract for change: An original model. *Transactional Analysis Journal, 34*(1), 46–51. https://doi.org/10.1177/036215370403400106.

Dewey, J. (1963). *Reconstruction in philosophy*. Holt & Co. (Original work published 1920)

Dhananjaya, D. (2022). We are the oppressor and the oppressed: The interplay between intrapsychic, interpersonal, and societal intersectionality. *Transactional Analysis Journal, 52*(3), 244–258. https://doi.org/10.1080/03621537.2022.2082031.

Dijkman, B., & Geuze, J. (Eds.). (2021). Schools in TA [Special issue]. *TA Magazine, 1* [English edition]. http://www.professioneelbegeleiden.nl/public/files/TA-2020-05-99.pdf.

Dillon, G. (2020). The road to registration: the New Zealand Association for Psychotherapy and its long search for identity and recognition through legislation. In K. Tudor (Ed.), *Pluralism in psychotherapy: Critical reflections from a post-regulation landscape*. Tuwhera Open Access Books. https://ojs.aut.ac.nz/tuwhera-open-monographs/catalog/book/1. (Original work published 2011)

Douglas, M., & Tudor, K. (2007). Child protection. In K. Tudor (Ed.), *The Adult is parent to the child: Transactional analysis with children and young people* (pp. 48–65). Russell House.

Drego, P. (1994a). *Happy family: Parenting through family rituals*. Alfreruby.

Drego, P. (1994b). *Talk to me mum and dad: Permissions for young people*. Alfreruby.

Drego, P. (2006). Freedom and responsibility: Social empowerment and the altruistic model of ego states. *Transactional Analysis Journal, 36*(2), 90–104. https://doi.org/10.1177/036215370603600203.

Drego, P. (2009). Bonding the ethnic child with the universal parent: Strategies and ethos of a transactional analysis ecocommunity activist. *Transactional Analysis Journal, 39*(3), 193–206. https://doi.org/10.1177/036215370903900303.

Drummond, H. (1904). *The Ascent of Man*. James Pott & Co.

Dryden, J. (1990). *The hind and the panther*. Macmillan. (Original work published 1687)

Drye, B. (1980). Psychoanalytic definitions of cure: Beyond contract completion. *Transactional Analysis Journal, 10*(2), 124–130. https://doi.org/10.1177/036215378001000210.

Dusay, J. M. (1966). Response. *Transactional Analysis Bulletin, 5*(18), 136–137.

Dylan, B. (1964). The times they are a-changin'. On *The times they are a-changin'* [Album]. Columbia.

Education Act 1989 [New Zealand]

Embleton Tudor, L. (1997). The contract boundary. In C. Sills (Ed.), *Contracts in counselling* (pp. 125–141). Sage.

Embleton Tudor, L. (2020). The neuroscience and politics of regulation. In K. Tudor (Ed.), *Pluralism in psychotherapy: Critical reflections from a post-regulation landscape*. Tuwhera Open Access Books. https://ojs.aut.ac.nz/tuwhera-open-monographs/catalog/book/1. (Original work published 2011)

Emde, R. N. (1988a). Development terminable and interminable: I. Innate and motivational factors from infancy. *International Journal of Psychoanalysis, 69*(1), 23–42.

Emde, R. N. (1988b). Development terminable and interminable: II. Recent psychoanalytic theory and therapeutic considerations. *International Journal of Psychoanalysis, 69*(2), 283–296.

Enari, D., Freeth, R., Hutchinson, R., Marshall, H., Matapo, J., O'Neil, G., & Stawiarski, B. (2023). Reflections and responses. In D. Key & K. Tudor, *Ecotherapy: A field guide* (pp. 79–112). Karnac.

English, F. (1972). Rackets and real feelings: Part II. *Transactional Analysis Journal, 2*(1), 23–25. https://doi.org/10.1177/036215377200200108.

English, F. (1975a). The fifth position: I'm OK—you're OK (adult). *Transactional Analysis Journal, 5*(4), 416–419. https://doi.org/10.1177/036215377500500423.

English, F. (1975b). Shame and social control. *Transactional Analysis Journal, 5*(1), 24–28. https://doi.org/10.1177/036215377500500105.

English, F. (1975c). The three-cornered contract. *Transactional Analysis Journal, 5*(4), 383–384. https://doi.org/10.1177/036215377500500413.

English, F. (1977). Let's not claim it's script when it ain't. *Transactional Analysis Journal, 7*(2), 130–138. https://doi.org/10.1177/036215377700700203.

English, F. (1978). Potency as a female therapist. *Transactional Analysis Journal, 8*(4), 297–299. https://doi.org/10.1177/036215377800800406.

English, F. (1979). Talk by Fanita English on receiving the Eric Berne Memorial Scientific Award for the concept of rackets as substitute feelings. *Transactional Analysis Journal, 9*(2), 90–97. https://doi.org/10.1177/036215377900900201.

English, F. (1994). Shame and social control revisited. *Transactional Analysis Journal, 24*(2), 109–120. https://doi.org/10.1177/036215379402400206.

English, F. (1995). Commentary. *Transactional Analysis Journal, 25*(3), 239–240. https://doi.org/10.1177/036215379502500308.

English, F. (1998). Ego-state controversy continues [Letter to the editor]. *The Script, 28*(6), 8, 7.

English, F. (2005). How did you become a transactional analyst? *Transactional Analysis Journal, 35*(1), 78–88. https://doi.org/10.1177/036215370503500110.

Erikson, E. H. (1950). *Childhood and society* (2nd ed.). W. W. Norton & Co.

Erikson, E. H. (1958). *Young man Luther: A study in psychoanalysis and history*. W. W. Norton & Co.

Erikson, E. (1965). *Childhood and society*. Norton. (Original work published 1951)

Erikson, E. (1968). *Identity, youth and crisis*. Norton.

Ernst, F. H. (1971a). Editor's note, *Transactional Analysis Journal, 1*(4), 257.

Ernst, F. H., Jr. (1971b). The OK corral: The grid for get-on-with. *Transactional Analysis Journal, 1*(4), 33–42. https://doi.org/10.1177/036215377100100409.

Ernst, K. (1972). *Games students play (and what to do about them)*. Celestial Arts.

Erskine, R. G. (1980). Script cure: Behavioral, intrapsychic and physiological. *Transactional Analysis Journal, 10*(2), 102–106. https://doi.org/10.1177/036215378001000205.

Erskine, R. G. (1988). Ego structure, intrapsychic function, and defense mechanisms: A commentary on Eric Berne's original theoretical concepts. *Transactional Analysis Journal, 18*(1), 15–19. https://doi.org/10.1177/036215378801800104.

Erskine, R. G. (1991). Transference and transactions: Critiques from an intrapsychic and integrative perspective. *Transactional Analysis Journal, 21*(2), 63–76. https://doi.org/10.1177/036215379102100202.

Erskine, R. G. (1993). Inquiry, attunement, and involvement in the psychotherapy of dissociation. *Transactional Analysis Journal, 23*(4), 184–190. https://doi.org/10.1177/036215379302300402.

Erskine, R. G. (1995). Commentary: Taxonomies, theories, and therapeutic relationships. *Transactional Analysis Journal, 25*(3), 236–239. https://doi.org/10.1177/036215379502500308.

Erskine, R. G. (1998). The therapeutic relationship: Integrating motivation and personality theories. *Transactional Analysis Journal, 28*(2), 132–141. https://doi.org/10.1177/036215379802800206.

Erskine, R. G. (2010). *Life scripts: A transactional analysis of unconscious relational patterns*. Routledge.

Erskine, R. G., Clarkson, P., Goulding, R. L., Groder, M. G., & Moiso, C. (1988). Ego state theory: Definitions, descriptions, and points of view. *Transactional Analysis Journal, 18*(1), 6–14. https://doi.org/10.1177/036215378801800103.

Erskine, R. G., & Moursund, J. P. (1988). *Integrative psychotherapy in action*. Sage.

Erskine, R. G., Moursund, J. P., & Trautmann, R. L. (1999). Beyond empathy: A therapy of contact-in-relationship. Brunner/Mazel.

Erskine, R. G. (Ed.), Tosi, M. T., O'Reilly-Knapp, M., Napper, R., English, F., & Stuthridge, J. (2011). Lifescripts: Definitions and points of view. *Transactional Analysis Journal, 41*(3), 255–264. https://doi.org/10.1177/036215371104100307.

Erskine, R. G., & Trautmann, R. L. (1997). The process of integrative psychotherapy. In R. G. Erskine, *Theories and methods of an integrative transactional analysis: A volume of selected articles* (pp. 79–95). TA Press. (Original work published 1993)

Erskine, R. G., & Zalcman, M. J. (1979). The racket system: A model for racket analysis. *Transactional Analysis Journal, 9*(1), 51–59. https://doi.org/10.1177/036215377900900112.

European Association of Transactional Analysis Professional Training and Standards Committee. (2022) *Training and examinations handbook*. https://eatanews.org/eata-training-and-examination-handbook/.

Eusden, S. (2011). Minding the gap: Ethical considerations for therapeutic engagement. *Transactional Analysis Journal, 41*(2), 101–113. https://doi.org/10.1177/036215371104100202.

Eusden, S., & Pierini, A. (2015). Exploring contemporary views on therapeutic relating in transactional analysis game theory. *Transactional Analysis Journal, 45*(2), 128–140. https://doi.org/10.1177/0362153715588300.

Eze, M. O. (2010). *Intellectual history in contemporary South Africa*. Palgrave Macmillan.

Faiman, P. (Director). (1986). *Crocodile Dundee* [Film]. Rimfire Films.

Fairbairn, W. R. D. (1954). *An object-relations theory of the personality*. Basic Books.

Fay, J. (2011). Birth of an independence movement: The organisation of Independently Registered Psychotherapy Practitioners. In K. Tudor (Ed.), *The turning tide: Pluralism and partnership in psychotherapy in Aotearoa New Zealand* (pp. 199–214). LC Publications.

Federn, P. (1928). Narcissism in the structure of the ego. *International Journal of Psycho-Analysis, IX*, 401–419.

Federn, P. (1932). Ego feeling in dreams. *Psychoanalytic Quarterly, I*, 511–542.

Federn, P. (1934). The awakening of the ego in dreams: I Orthriogenesis, II. Postulates to serve as a basis for an ego psychology. *International Journal of Psycho-Analysis, XV*, 296–301.

Federn, P. (1938). The undirected function in the central nervous system. *International Journal of Psycho-Analysis, 19*(2), 1–26.

Federn, P. (1949). Mental hygiene of the ego. *American Journal of Psychotherapy, III*, 290–291.

Federn, P. (1952a). The awakening of the ego in dreams. In *Ego psychology and the psychoses* (E. Weiss, Ed.) (pp. 90–96). Basic Books. (Original work published 1934)

Federn, P. (1952b). The ego as subject and object in narcissism. In *Ego psychology and the psychoses* (E. Weiss, Ed.) (pp. 283–322). Basic Books. (Original work published 1929)

Federn, P. (1952c). Ego psychological aspect of schizophrenia. In *Ego psychology and the psychoses* (E. Weiss, Ed.). (pp. 210–226). Basic Books.

Federn, P. (1952d). *Ego psychology and the psychoses* (E. Weiss, Ed.). Basic Books.

Federn, P. (1952e). On the distinction between healthy and pathological narcissism. In *Ego psychology and the psychoses* (E. Weiss, Ed.) (pp. 323–364). Basic Books. (Original work published 1936)

Fischer, G. P. (1993). The changing organizational parent. *Transactional Analysis Journal, 23*(2), 70–76. https://doi.org/10.1177/036215379302300204.

Fontana, D. C. (1973). Yesteryear. In *Star trek: The animated series* (H. Sutherland, Director; Series 1, Episode 2). Filmation.

Ford, L. B. (1987). The potent permissions of role-modeling. *Transactional Analysis Journal, 17*(3), 105–106. https://doi.org/10.1177/036215378701700310.

Fornaro, A. (2016). Rethinking ego states in an intersubjective context. *Transactional Analysis Journal, 46*(3), 209–221. https://doi.org/10.1177/0362153716650653.

Foulkes, S. H. (1975). *Group analytic psychotherapy: Method and principles*. Gordon & Breech, Science Publishers.

Fowlie, H., & Sills, C. (2011). *Relational transactional analysis: Principles in practice*. Karnac.

Fox, M. A. (2007, July/August). A new look at personal identity. *Philosophy Now, 62*. https://philosophynow.org/issues/62/A_New_Look_At_Personal_Identity.

Frankl, V. (1963). *Man's search for meaning*. Pocket Books.

Freud, A. (1937). *The ego and the mechanisms of defence* (C. Baines, Trans.). Hogarth. (Original work published 1936)

Freud, A. (1966). Links between Hartmann's ego psychology and the child analyst's thinking. In R. M. Loewenstein, L. M. Newman, M. Schur, & A. J. Solnit (Eds.), *Psychoanalysis—A general psychology: Essays in honor of Heinz Hartmann* (pp. 16–27). International Universities Press.

Freud, S. (1924). Recommendations to physicians practising psycho-analysis. In *The standard edition of the complete works of Sigmund Freud* (Vol. 12; J. Riviere, Trans.; pp. 109–120). Psychoanalytic Electronic Publishing. (Original work published 1912)

Freud, S. (1959). The question of lay analysis: Conversations with an impartial person. In *The standard edition of the complete psychological works of Sigmund Freud* (Vol. 20; J. Strachey, Ed. & Trans.; pp. 177–250). The Hogarth Press/The Institute of Psycho-Analysis. (Original work published 1926)

Freud, S. (1964). Analysis terminable and interminable. In *The standard edition of the complete psychological works of Sigmund Freud* (Vol. 23; J. Strachey Ed. & Trans.; pp. 216–253). Hogarth Press/The Institute of Psycho-Analysis. (Original work published 1937)

Freud, S. (1977). Three essays on the theory of sexuality. In *The Pelican Freud library* (Vol. 7; J. Strachey, Trans.; A. Richards, Ed.; pp. 45–169). Penguin. (Original work published 1905)

Freud, S. (1979). Inhibitions, symptoms, and anxiety. In *The Pelican Freud library* (Vol. 10; J. Strachey, Trans.; A. Richards, Ed.; pp. 229–339). Penguin. (Original work published 1925)

Freud, S. (1984a). The ego and the id. In *The Pelican Freud library* (Vol. 11; J. Strachey, Trans.; A. Richards, Ed.; pp. 339–407). Penguin. (Original work published 1923)

Freud, S. (1984b). Mourning and melancholia. In *The Pelican Freud library* (Vol. 11; J. Strachey, Trans.; A. Richards, Ed.; pp. 245–268). Penguin. (Original work published 1915)

Frick, W. B. (1990). The symbolic growth experience: A chronicle of heuristic inquiry and a quest for synthesis. *Journal of Humanistic Psychology, 30*(1), 64–80. https://doi.org/10.1177/0022167890301004.

Friedlander, M. G. (Ed.). (1987). Power [Theme issue]. *Transactional Analysis Journal, 17*(3).

Friedlander, M. G. (1988). Script [Theme issue]. *Transactional Analysis Journal, 18*(4).

Friedman, M. S. (1992). *Dialogue and the human image: Beyond humanistic psychology.* Sage.

Fritzche, K. (2013). *Praxis der ego-state-therapie* [The practice of ego-state therapy]. Carl Auer.

Fromkin, V., & Rodman, R. (1983). *An introduction to language.* Holt-Saunders.

Gardiner, H. (1983). *Frames of mind: The theory of multiple intelligences.* Basic Books.

Gellert, S D., & Wilson, G. (1978). Contracts. *Transactional Analysis Journal, 8*(1), 10–15. https://doi.org/10.1177/036215377800800103.

Gelso, C. J., & Carter, J. A. (1985). The relationship in counseling and psychotherapy: Components, consequences and theoretical antecedents. *The Counseling Psychologist, 13*(2), 115–243. https://doi.org/10.1177/0011000085132001.

Gendlin, E. T. (1981). *Focusing.* Bantam.

Gendlin, E. T. (1991). Thinking beyond patterns: body, language and situations. In B. den Ouden & M. Moen (Eds.), *The presence of feeling in thought* (pp. 25–151). Peter Lang.

Gentelet, B., & Widdowson, M. (2016). Paradoxical alliances in transactional analysis psychotherapy for anxiety. *Transactional Analysis Journal, 46*(3), 182–195. https://doi.org/10.1177/0362153716650657.

George, V., & Wilding, P. (1976). *Ideology and social welfare.* Routledge and Kegan Paul.

Giusti, M. A. (2002). Therapeutic stages and intervention plans. *Transactional Analysis Journal, 32*(2), 92–106. https://doi.org/10.1177/036215370203200204.

Ghan, L. (1977). The monkey puzzle tree. *Transactional Analysis Journal, 7*(3), 228–230. https://doi.org/10.1177/036215377700700310.

Gheorghe, N., Brunke, M., Deaconu, D., Gheorghe, A., & Ionas, L. (2022). A therapeutic stance addressing destructiveness: What we can learn from looking back at the experience with Schiffian reparenting. *Transactional Analysis Journal, 52*(1), 59–73. https://doi.org/10.1080/03621537.2021.2011037.

Gjurković, T., & Tudor, K. (2018). Treatment stages for working with children: An approach rooted in transactional analysis and play therapy. *Transactional Analysis Journal, 48*(3). 242–257. https://doi.org/10.1080/03621537.2018.1471291.

Glover, E. (1955). *The technique of psycho-analysis.* International Universities Press.

Glover, E. (1956a). The concept of dissociation. *On the early development of mind: Selected papers on psycho-analysis* (Vol. 1, pp. 307–323). Imago. (Original work published 1943)

Glover, E. (1956b). A psycho-analytic approach to the classification of mental disorders. *On the early development of mind: Selected papers on psycho-analysis.* (Vol. 1, pp. 161–186). Imago. (Original work published 1932)

Gobes, L. (1990). Ego states—Metaphor or reality? *Transactional Analysis Journal, 20*(3), 163–165. https://doi.org/10.1177/036215379002000304.

Goldstein, K. (1995). *The organism.* Zone Books. (Original work published 1934)

Goodman, M. (2007). Focusing on the 'bodily felt sense': A tool for transactional analysts. *Transactional Analysis Journal, 37*(4), 278–285. https://doi.org/10.1177/03621 5370703700405.

Goulding, M. (1978). To my clients. In R. L Goulding & M. M. Goulding, *The power is in the patient* (p. 15). TA Press. (Original work published 1975)

Goulding, M. M., & Goulding, R. (1979). *Changing lives through redecision therapy.* Grove Press.

Goulding, R. (1972). New directions in transactional analysis: Creating an environment for redecision and change. In C. J. Sager & H. S. Kaplan (Eds.), *Progress in group and family therapy* (pp. 105–134). Brunner/Mazel.

Goulding, R. L. (1976). Four models of transactional analysis. *International Journal of Group Psychotherapy, 26*(3), 385–392. https://doi.org/10.1080/00207284.1976.11491957.

Goulding, R., & Goulding M. (1976). Injunctions, decisions, and redecisions. *Transactional Analysis Journal, 6*(1), 41–48. https://doi.org/10.1177/036215377600600110.

Goulding, R. L., & Goulding, M. M. (1978). *The power is in the patient: A TA/gestalt approach to psychotherapy.* TA Press. (Original work published 1975)

Graff, R. H. (1976). A game transactional analysts play. *Transactional Analysis Bulletin, 6*(3), 263–267. https://doi.org/10.1177/036215377600600306.

Grant, J. (2004). How the philosophical assumptions of transactional analysis complement the theory of adult education. *Transactional Analysis Journal, 34*(3), 272–276. https://doi.org/10.1177/036215370403400312.

Greenberg, J., & Aron, L. (2018). The emergence of the relational tradition. In L. Aron, S. Grand, & J. Slochower (Eds.), *De-idealizing relational theory: A critique from within.* Routledge.

Greenson, R. R. (1967). *The technique and practice of psychoanalysis* (Vol. 1). International Universities Press.

Grégoire, J. (2007). *Les Orientations Récentes de L'analyse Transactionnelle* [The recent orientations of transactional analysis]. Les Éditions d'Analyse Transactionnelle.

Gregory, J. (2000). Human science research: A matter of quality. *Transactional Analysis Journal, 30*(2), 150–158. https://doi.org/10.1177/036215370003000208.

Groder, M. G. (1971). Kiud. *Transactional Analysis Bulletin, 1*(2), 19–20. https://doi.org/10.1177/036215377100100207.

Groder, M. G. (1972). *Asklepieion: An effective treatment method for incarcerated character disorders.* Unpublished manuscript.

Groder, M. (1977a). Asklepieion: An integration of psychotherapies. In G. Barnes (Ed.), *Transactional analysis after Eric Berne: Teachings and practices of three TA schools* (pp. 134–137). Harper's College Press.

Groder, M. (1977b). Groder's 5 OK diagrams. In G. Barnes (Ed.), *Transactional analysis after Eric Berne: Teachings and practices of three TA schools* (pp. 161–168). Harper's College Press.

Gross, S. J. (1978). The myth of professional licensing. *American Psychologist, 33*(11), 1009–1016. https://doi.org/10.1037/0003-066X.33.11.1009.

Guggenbühl-Craig, A. (1996). *Power in the helping professions.* Spring Publications. (Original work published 1971)

Guglielmotti, R. L. (2008). The quality of the therapeutic relationship as a factor in helping to change the client's protocol or implicit memory. *Transactional Analysis Journal, 38*(2), 101–109. https://doi.org/10.1177/036215370803800203.

Gurowitz, E. M. (1975). Group boundaries and leadership potency. *Transactional Analysis Journal, 5*(2), 183–185. https://doi.org/10.1177/036215377500500224.

Haiberg, G., Sefness, W. R., & Berne, E. (1963). Destiny and script choices. *Transactional Analysis Bulletin, 2*(6), 59–60.

Haimowitz, N. (1975). Protection. *Transactional Analysis Journal, 5*(1), 51–54. https://doi.org/10.1177/036215377500500110.

Hargaden, H. (2005). Letter from the guest editor: All that jazz… *Transactional Analysis Journal, 35*(2), 106–109. https://doi.org/10.1177/036215370503500201.

Hargaden, H. (2016). The role of the imagination in an analysis of unconscious relatedness. *Transactional Analysis Journal, 46*(4), 311–321. https://doi.org/10.1177/036215 3716662624.

Hargaden, H., & Sills, C. (1999). The Child ego state – An integrative view: An exploration of the deconfusion process. *ITA News*, No. *55*, 22–24.

Hargaden, H., & Sills, C. (2001). Deconfusion of the Child ego state. *Transactional Analysis Journal, 31*(1), 55–70. https://doi.org/10.1177/03621537010310010.

Hargaden, H., & Sills, C. (2002). *Transactional analysis: A relational perspective.* Routledge.

Harley, B. (2019). Confronting the crisis of confidence in management studies: Why senior scholars need to stop setting a bad example. *Academy of Management Learning & Education, 18*(2), 286–297. https://doi.org/10.5465/amle.2018.0107.

Harley, K. (2006). A lost connection: Existential positions and Melanie Klein's infant development. *Transactional Analysis Journal, 36*(4), 252–269. https://doi.org/10.1177/036215370603600402.

Harris, A., & Harris, T. (1986). *Staying OK.* Pan Books. (Original work published 1985)

Harris, T. (1967). *I'm OK—you're OK: A practical guide to transactional analysis.* Avon Books.

Harris, T., & Dusay, J. (1967). What is OK? *Transactional Analysis Bulletin, 6*(24), 94–96.

Hartmann, H. (1942). Psycho-analysis and the concept of health. *International Journal of Psycho-Analysis, 20*, 308–321.

Hartmann, H. (1958). *Ego psychology and the problem of adaptation.* Imago. (Original work published 1939)

Hawkes, L. (2007). The permission wheel. *Transactional Analysis Journal, 37*(3), 210–217. https://doi.org/10.1177/036215370703700305.

Haynes, E. (2023). The maternal: An integral part of eco-TA. *Transactional Analysis Journal, 53*(1), 67–79. https://doi.org/10.1080/03621537.2023.2152549.

Health Practitioners Competence Assurance Act 2003. [New Zealand] https://www.legislation.govt.nz/act/public/2003/0048/latest/DLM203312.html.

Heath, J. (2022). The impact of a model of nonmaterial consciousness on the concept of mind in action. *Transactional Analysis Journal, 52*(4), 295–310. https://doi.org/10.1080/03621537.2022.2115647.

Heathcote, A. (2010). Eric Berne's development of ego state theory: Where did it all begin and who influenced him? *Transactional Analysis Journal, 40*(3–4), 254–260. https://doi.org/10.1177/036215371004000310.

Heiller, B., & Sills. C. (2010). Life scripts: An existential perspective. In R. G. Erskine (Ed.), *Life scripts: A transactional analysis of unconscious relational patterns* (pp. 239–267). Karnac.

Herlihy, B., & Corey, G. (Eds.). (1992). *Dual relationships in counseling*. American Association for Counseling and Development.

Hilgard, E. R. (1973). Dissociation revisited. In M. Henle, J. Jaynes, & J. Sullivan (Eds.), *Historical conceptions of psychology*. Springer.

Hillman, J., & Ventura, M. (1992). *We've had a hundred years of psychotherapy and the world's getting worse*. Harper.

Hine, J. (1990). The bilateral and ongoing nature of games. *Transactional Analysis Journal, 20*(1), 28–39. https://doi.org/10.1177/036215379002000104.

Hine, J. (1995). Commentary. *Transactional Analysis Journal, 25*(3), 240–241. https://doi.org/10.1177/036215379502500308.

Hine, M. (1993). On reading the Stamford papers on constructivism: A physicist's reactions. *Transactional Analysis Journal, 23*(1), 45–47. https://doi.org/10.1177/036215379302300106.

Hinshelwood, R. (1991). Psychodynamic formulation in assessment for psychotherapy. *British Journal of Psychotherapy, 8*(2), 166–174. https://doi.org/10.1111/j.1752-0118.1991.tb01173.x.

Hiremath, M. (1995). Race and culture in the context of impasse theory. *ITA News, No. 41*, pp. 22–24.

Hogan, D. B. (1979). *The regulation of psychotherapists* (4 Vols.). Ballinger.

Holloway, R. R., & Holloway, W. H. (1973). *The monograph series: Numbers I–X*. Midwest Institute for Human Understanding.

Holloway, W. (1973). Shut the escape hatch: Monograph IV, in R. R. Holloway and W. H. Holloway, *The monograph series: Numbers I–X*. Midwest Institute for Human Understanding.

Holloway, W. H. (1974). Beyond permission. *Transactional Analysis Journal, 4*(2), 15–17. https://doi.org/10.1177/036215377400400205.

Holloway, W. H. (1976). President's Page. *Transactional Analysis Bulletin, 6*(2), 126–126. https://doi.org/10.1177/036215377600600201.

Holmes, J. (2002). *The search for the secure base: attachment theory and psychotherapy*. London, UK: Routledge.

Holt, R. R. (1975). The past and future of ego psychology. *The Psychoanalytic Quarterly, 44*(4), 550–576. https://doi.org/10.1080/21674086.1975.11926731.

Horney, K. (1999). *Our inner conflicts: A constructive theory of neurosis*. Routledge. (Original work published 1945)

Hostie, R. (1982). Eric Berne, the Martian. *Transactional Analysis Journal, 12*(2), 168–170. https://doi.org/10.1177/036215378201200215.

House, R., & Totton, N. (Eds.). (1997). *Implausible professions: Arguments for pluralism and autonomy in psychotherapy and counselling*. PCCS Books.

Hunt, P. (2022). Discovering John Macmurray. *The John Macmurray Fellowship*. http://johnmacmurray.org/further-reading/discovering-john-macmurray/. (Original work published 1988)

Ingram, R. (1980). Programming for permission (PFP), a game. *Transactional Analysis Journal, 10*(1), 16. https://doi.org/10.1177/036215378001000106.

Institute of Transactional Analysis. (1995). *Transactional analysis: A humanistic psychotherapy. Information sheet*. London, UK: Author.

International Energy Agency. (2021). *World energy outlook 2021*. https://iea.blob.core.windows.net/assets/4ed140c1-c3f3-4fd9-acae-789a4e14a23c/WorldEnergyOutlook2021.pdf.

International Transactional Analysis Association. (1995). *Transactional analysis counseling. Definition*. San Francisco, CA: Training and Certification Council of Transactional Analysts, Training Standards Committee, Counseling Task Force.

International Transactional Analysis Association. (2014). *Code of ethical conduct.* http:// itaaworld.org/sites/default/files/itaa-pdfs/govadmin-docs/12-514%20Revised%20 Ethics_0.pdf.

International Transactional Analysis Association. (2020). *Anti-racism statement.* https://www.itaaworld.org/sites/default/files/itaa-pdfs/gov-admin-docs/ITAA-Anti-Racism-Statement.pdf.

International Transactional Analysis Association. (2023). *Key concepts in transactional analysis: A brief overview.* Author. https://www.itaaworld.org/key-concepts-transactional-analysis.

International Transactional Analysis Association Bilbao Conference Organising Committee. (2011). Welcome letters. In A. M. Etxabe (Co-ordinator) *Conference handbook* (pp. 3–4).

International Transactional Analysis Association. International Board of Certification. (2022). *Certification and examinations handbook.* https://www.itaaworld.org/ iboc-certification-examinations-handbook.

Jackson, P. Z., & Summers, G. (2010). Constructive games people play: e-Organisations and people. *Association for Management Education and Development, 17*(1), 41–45.

Jacobs, A. (1987). Autocratic power. *Transactional Analysis Journal, 17*(3), 59–71. https:// doi.org/10.1177/036215378701700303.

Jacobs, A. (1990). Nationalism. *Transactional Analysis Journal, 20*(4), 221–228. https://doi. org/10.1177/036215379002000403.

Jacobs, A. (1991). Autocracy: Groups, organizations, nations, and players. *Transactional Analysis Journal, 21*(4), 199–206. https://doi.org/10.1177/036215379102100402.

Jacobs, A. (1994). Theory as ideology: Reparenting and thought reform. *Transactional Analysis Journal, 24*(1), 39–55. https://doi.org/10.1177/036215379402400108.

Jacobs, A. (1997a). Berne's life positions: Science and morality. *Transactional Analysis Journal, 27*(3), 197–206. https://doi.org/10.1177/036215379702700309.

Jacobs, A. (2000). Psychic organs, ego states, and visual metaphors: Speculation on Berne's integration of ego states. *Transactional Analysis Journal, 30*(1), 10–22. https://doi. org/10.1177/036215370003000103.

Jacobson, E. (1954). The self and the object world. *The Psychoanalytic Study of the Child, 9,* 75–127.

Jacobson, E. (1964). *The self and the object world.* International Universities Press.

James, J. (1973). The game plan. *Transactional Analysis Journal, 3*(4), 194–197. http://doi. org/10.1177/036215377300300406.

James, J. (1977). Family therapy with TA. In M. James & Contributors, *Techniques in transactional analysis for psychotherapists and counselors* (pp. 351–371). Addison-Wesley.

James, J. (1983a). Cultural consciousness: The challenge to TA. *Transactional Analysis Journal, 13*(4), 207–216. https://doi.org/10.1177/036215378301300402.

James, J. (Ed.). (1983b). Cultural scripts [Special issue]. *Transactional Analysis Journal, 13*(4). https://www.tandfonline.com/toc/rtaj20/13/4.

James, M. M. (1971). Curing impotency with transactional analysis. *Transactional Analysis Journal, 1*(1), 88–94. https://doi.org/10.1177/036215377100100116.

James, M. (1973). *Born to love: Transactional analysis in the church.* Addison-Wesley.

James, M. (1974). Self-reparenting: Theory and process. *Transactional Analysis Journal, 4*(3), 32–39. https://doi.org/10.1177/036215377400400307.

James, M. (1977). TA therapists: As persons and professionals. In M. James & Contributors, Techniques in transactional analysis for psychotherapists and counselors (pp. 33–47). Addison-Wesley.

James, M. (1981a). *Breaking free: Self-reparenting for a new life*. Addison-Wesley.

James, M. (1981b). TA in the 80s: The inner core and the human spirit. *Transactional Analysis Journal, 11*(1), 54–65. https://doi.org/10.1177/036215378101100112.

James, M., & Goulding, M. (1988). Self-reparenting and redecision. *Transactional Analysis Journal, 28*(1), 16–19. https://doi.org/10.1177/036215379802800106.

James, M., & Jongeward, D. (1971). *Born to win: Transactional analysis with gestalt experiments*. Addison-Wesley.

James, M., & Savary, L. M. (1977). *A new self: Self-therapy with transactional analysis*. Addison-Wesley.

James, W. (1981). *Principles of psychology* (Vol. 1). Harvard University Press. (Original work published 1890)

Janet, P. (1907). *The major symptoms of hysteria*. Macmillan Publishing.

Janssens, A. (1984). Treatment of pre-orgasmic women. In E. Stern (Ed.), *TA: The state of the art. A European contribution* (pp. 219–224). Foris Publications.

Jaoui, G. (1988, 1–2 March). *Les permissions en AT* [Permissions in TA]. Workshop presented by G. Jaoui, Paris, France.

Jenkins, B., Morrison, E., & Schwebel, R. (2020). Radical therapy: From the first decade onwards. In K. Tudor (Ed.), *Claude Steiner, emotional activist: The life and work of Claude Michel Steiner* (pp. 116–130). Routledge.

Jenkins, P. (1997). *Counselling, psychotherapy and the law*. Sage.

Joines, V. (2006). The role and function of psychotherapy in the future. *The Script, 36*(9), 1–3.

Joseph, M. R. (2012). Therapeutic operations can be educational operations too. *Transactional Analysis Journal, 42*(2), 110–117. https://doi.org/10.1177/036215371204200204.

Jorgensen, E. W., & Jorgensen, H. I. (1984). *Eric Berne: Master gamesman. A transactional biography*. Grove Press.

Kahler, T. (1979). Existential and behavioral life positions. *Bulletin of the Eric Berne Seminar, 1*(3), 16–17.

Kahler, T, I. (2008). Letter to the Editors. *Transactional Analysis Journal, 38*(3), 258–259.

Kahler, T., with Capers, H. (1974). The miniscript. *Transactional Analysis Bulletin, 4*(1), 26–42. https://doi.org/10.1177/036215377400400110.

Kahn, E., & Cohen, L. H. (1936). The way of experiencing as a psychiatric concept. *Psychological Monographs, 47*(2), 381–389. https://doi.org/10.1037/h0093424.

Karpman, S. (1968). Fairy tales and script drama analysis. *Transactional Analysis Bulletin*, 1–9, 51–56.

Karpman, S. (1971). Options. *Transactional Analysis Journal, 1*(1), 79–87. https://doi.org/10.1177/036215377100100115.

Karpman, S. B. (1975). The bias box for competing psychotherapies. *Transactional Analysis Journal, 5*(2), 107–116. https://doi.org/10.1177/036215377500500204.

Karpman, S. B. (1981). The politics of theory. *Transactional Analysis Journal, 11*(1), 68–76. https://doi.org/10.1177/036215378101100114.

Karpman, S. (2008). Letter to the Editors. *Transactional Analysis Journal, 38*(3), 259.

Karpman, S. (2019). 'Don't say anything you can't diagram': The creative brainstorming of Eric Berne. *International Journal of Transactional Analysis Research, 10*(1), 4–20. https://doi.org/10.29044/v10i1p4.

Karpman, S. B., & Callaghan, V. L. (1985). Protection and nutritional nervosa. *Transactional Analysis Journal, 15*(2), 168–172. https://doi.org/10.1177/036215378501500210.

Kaufman, G. (1993). *The psychology of shame*. Routledge.

Keats, J. (2011). Letter to George and Thomas Keats, 22 December 1817. In S. Colvin (Ed.), *Letters of John Keats to his family and friends*. Project Gutenberg. https://www.gutenberg.org/files/35698/35698-h/35698-h.htm. (Original work published 1817)

Keepers, T. D., & Babcock, D. E. (1986). *Raising kids OK: Human growth and development throughout the life span*. Menalto Press.

Kellet, P. (2004). Queer constructions: The making of gay men and the role of the homoerotic in therapy. *Transactional Analysis Journal, 34*(2), 180–190. https://doi.org/10.1177/036215370403400208.

Kenny, V. (1997). Constructivism—Everybody has won and all must have prizes! *Transactional Analysis Journal*, 27(2), 110–117. https://doi.org/10.1177/036215379702700206.

Kernberg, O. (1975). *Borderland conditions and pathological narcissism*. Aronson.

Kernberg, O. F. (1982). Self, ego, affects, and drives. *Journal of the American Psychoanalytic Association, 30*(4), 893–917. https://doi.org/10.1177/000306518203000404.

Key, D., & Tudor, K. (2023). *Ecotherapy: A field guide*. Karnac.

King, L., & Moutsou, C. (2010). *Rethinking audit cultures: A critical look at evidence-based practice in psychotherapy and beyond*. PCCS Books.

King, P., & Temple, S. (2018). Transactional analysis and the ludic third (TALT): A model of functionally fluent reflective play practice. *Transactional Analysis Journal, 48*(3), 258–271. https://doi.org/10.1080/03621537.2018.1471292.

Kirshner, L. A. (1991). The concept of the self in psychoanalytic theory and its philosophical foundations. *Journal of the American Psychoanalytic Association, 39*(1), 157–182. https://doi.org/10.1177/000306519103900108.

Klein, G. S. (1976). *Psychoanalytic theory: An exploration of essentials*. International Universities Press.

Klein, M. (1949). Preface to the third edition. In M. Klein, *The psycho-analysis of children* (3rd Ed.; pp. xiii–xiv). Hogarth Press and the Institute of Psycho-Analysis. (Original work published 1936)

Klein, M. (1980). *Lives people live: A textbook of transactional analysis*. Wiley.

Kobrin, N. (2013). Freud's concept of autonomy and Strachey's translation: A piece of the puzzle of the Freudian self. *The Annual of Psychoanalysis, 5*(21), 201–223.

Kohut, H. (1971). *The analysis of the self: A systematic approach to the psychoanalytic treatment of narcissistic personality disorders*. University of Chicago Press.

Koopmans, L. (2020). A fruitless attempt to cultivate physis. *Transactional Analysis Journal, 50*(1), 81–92. https://doi.org/10.1080/03621537.2019.1690247.

Kovel, J. (1976). *A complete guide to therapy: From psychoanalysis to behavior modification*. Pantheon.

Kramer, R. (1995). The birth of client-centered therapy: Carl Rogers, Otto Rank, and 'the beyond'. *Journal of Humanistic Psychology, 35*(4), 54–110. https://doi.org/10.1177/00221678950354005.

Krausz, R. (1993). Organizational scripts. *Transactional Analysis Journal, 23*, 77–86.

Krausz, R. (2005). Transactional executive coaching. *Transactional Analysis Journal, 35*(4), 367–373. https://doi.org/10.1177/036215370503500414.

Kreyenberg, J. (2005). Transactional analysis in organizations as a systemic constructivist approach. *Transactional Analysis Journal, 35*(4), 300–310. https://doi.org/10.1177/036215370503500402.

Kritzman, L. (1988). Power and sex [A discussion with B-H Lévy]. In L. D. Kritzman (Ed.), *Michel Foucault: Politics, philosophy, culture: Interviews and other writings, 1977–1984* (pp. 110–124) (D. J. Parent, Trans.). Routledge.

Künkel, F. (1984). *Fritz Künkel: Selected writings* (J. A. Sanford, Ed.). Paulist Press.

Lambert, J. J. (1992). Psychotherapy outcome research: Implications for integrative and eclectic therapists. In J. Norcross & M. R. Goldfried (Eds.), *Handbook of Psychotherapy Integration* (pp. 94–129). Basic.

Langguth, J. (1966, 17 July). Dr. Berne plays the celebrity game; The Celebrity Game, *The New York Times Magazine*, pp. 10–11, 41–43.

Lankton, S. R., Lankton, C. H., & Brown, M. (1981). Psychological level communication in transactional analysis. *Transactional Analysis Journal, 11*(4), 287–299. https://doi.org/10.1177/036215378101100402.

Lapworth, P., Sills, C., & Fish, S. (1993). *Transactional analysis counselling*. Winslow Press.

Lasch, C. (1979). *Culture of narcissism: American life in an age of diminishing expectations.* Warner Books.

Leck, K. (2016). Insider knowledge: Going by the book. In A. Tuck (Ed.), *Singapore* (pp. 85–86). Gestalten.

Lee, A. (1997). Process contracts. In C. Sills (Ed.), *Contracts in counselling* (pp. 94–112). Sage.

Lee, A. (2001). *Schools of change* [handout]. Privately circulated manuscript.

Lee, D. (1963). Autonomous motivation. *Journal of Humanistic Psychology, 1*(2), 12–22. https://doi.org/10.1177/002216786100100203.

Leutner, S., & Piedfort-Marin, O. (2021). The concept of ego state: From historical background to future perspectives. *European Journal of Trauma & Dissociation, 5*(4), 100184. https://doi.org/10.1016/j.ejtd.2020.100184.

Leuzinger-Bohleber, M., & Fischmann, T. (2006). What is conceptual research in psychoanalysis? *The International Journal of Psychoanalysis, 87*(5), 1355–1386. https://doi.org/10.1516/73MU-E53N-D1EE-1Q8L.

Levaggi, J. A., Callaghan, V. L., & Berger, C. (1971). A living Euhemerus never dies. *Transactional Analysis Journal, 1*(1), 64–70. https://doi.org/10.1177/036215377100100113.

Levin, P. (1974). *Becoming the way we are: A transactional analysis guide to personal development.* Transactional Publications.

Levin, P. (1977). Women's oppression. *Transactional Analysis Journal, 7*(1), 87–91.

Levin, P. (1985). *Becoming the way we are: A transactional guide to personal development* (2nd ed.). Directed Media.

Levin, P., & Fryer, R. (1980). Coming together: The evolution of women in ITAA. *The Script, 10*(9), 1–2.

Levinas, E. (1969) *Totality and infinity: An essay on exteriority* (A. Lingis, Trans.) Duquesne Studies. Philosophical Series. Vol 24. Duquesne University Press. (Original work published 1961)

Levinas, E. (1985). Ethics and infinity (R. A. Cohen, Trans.) Duquesne University Press. (Original work published 1982)

Levin-Landheer, P. (1982). The cycle of development. *Transactional Analysis Journal, 12*(2), 129–139. https://doi.org/10.1177/036215378201200207.

Lewin, K. (1952). *Field theory in social science*. Harper & Row.

Little, A. (2022, July 29). *More counsellors to boost mental health workforce* [Press release]. New Zealand government. https://www.beehive.govt.nz/release/more-counsellors-boost-mental-health-workforce.

Little, R. (2005). Integrating psychoanalytic understandings in the deconfusion of primitive child ego states. *Transactional Analysis Journal, 35*(2), 132–146. https://doi.org/10.1177/036215370503500204.

Lloyd, A. P. (1992). Dual relationship problems in counselor education. In B. Herlihy & G. Corey (Eds.), *Dual relationships in counseling* (pp. 71–76). American Association for Counseling and Development.

Loewald, H. (1980). *Papers on psychoanalysis.* Yale University Press.

Lomas, P. (2001). *The limits of interpretation.* Jason Aronson. (Original work published 1987)

Loomis, M. (1982). Contracting for change. *Transactional Analysis Journal, 12*(1), 51–54. https://doi.org/10.1177/036215378201200107.

Loria, B. R. (1990). Epistemology and reification of metaphor in transactional analysis. *Transactional Analysis Journal, 20*(3), 152–162. https://doi.org/10.1177/036215379002000303.

Macmurray, J. (1969). *The self as agent.* Faber & Faber. (Original work published 1957)

Macmurray, J. (1991). *Persons in relation.* Faber & Faber. (Original work published 1961)

Mahler, M. (1968). *On human symbiosis and the vicissitudes of individuation.* International Universities Press.

Marcus, E. R. (1999). Modern ego psychology. *Journal of the American Psychoanalytic Association, 47*(3), 843–871. https://doi.org/10.1177/00030651990470031501.

Marshall, H. (2013/2014, Winter). Greening the adult ego state. *The Transactional Analyst, 4*(1), 37–38.

Marshall, H. (2021a). *Ecological transactional analysis: Allowing the leopards into the temple.* Keynote speech to the Conference of the United Kingdom Association of Transactional Analysis, UK.

Marshall, H. (2021b). Ecological transactional analysis: Allowing the leopards into the temple. *The Transactional Analyst, 11*(2), 31.

Marshall, H. (2023). A place for the ecological third: Eco-TA in therapeutic practice. *Transactional Analysis Journal, 53*(1), 93–108. https://doi.org/10.1080/03621537.2023.2152567.

Marshall, J. (2000). The boundaries of belief: Territories of encounter between indigenous peoples and western philosophies. *Educational Philosophy and Theory, 32*(1), 15–24. https://doi.org/10.1111/j.1469-5812.2000.tb00429.x.

Mart, L., Nichols, T., & Cantrell, M. (1975). Parent shrinkers revisited. *Transactional Analysis Journal, 5*(3), 259–263. https://doi.org/10.1177/03621537750050031.

Maslow, A. H. (1954). *Motivation and personality.* Harpers.

Massey, R. F. (1985). TA as a family systems therapy. *Transactional Analysis Journal, 15*(2), 120–141. https://doi.org/10.1177/036215378501500203.

Massey, R. F. (1986). Paradox, double binding, and counterparadox: A transactional analysis perspective (A response to Price). *Transactional Analysis Journal, 16*(1), 24–46, https://doi.org/10.1177/036215378601600105.

Massey, R. (1987). Transactional analysis and the social psychology of power. Reflections evoked by Jacobs' 'Autocratic power'. *Transactional Analysis Journal, 17*(3), 107–120. https://doi.org/10.1177/036215378701700311.

Massey, R. (1989). Script theory synthesized systematically. *Transactional Analysis Journal, 19*(1), 14–25.

Massey, R. F. (1996). Transactional analysis as a social psychology. *Transactional Analysis Journal, 26*(1), 91–99. https://doi.org/10.1177/036215379602600114.

Massey, R. F. (2007). Reexamining social psychiatry as a foundational framework for transactional analysis: Considering a social-psychological perspective. *Transactional Analysis Journal, 37*(1), 51–79. https://doi.org/10.1177/036215370703700109.

McLean, B., & Cornell, W. (Eds.). (2017). Gender, sexuality, and identity [Special issue]. *Transactional Analysis Journal, 47*(4). https://www.tandfonline.com/toc/rtaj20/47/4.

McLeod, J. (2003). *Doing counselling research* (2nd ed.). Sage.

McNeel, J. R. (1976). The parent interview. *Transactional Analysis Journal, 6*(1), 61–68. https://doi.org/10.1177/036215377600600114.

Mead, G. H. (1934). *Mind, self and society* (C. W. Morris, Ed.). University of Chicago Press.

Mearns, D. (1994). *Developing person-centred counselling*. Sage.

Mellor, K. (1980). Impasses: A developmental and structural understanding. *Transactional Analysis Journal, 10*(3), 213–220. https://doi.org/10.1177/036215378001000307.

Mellor, K. & Schiff, E. (1975). Discounting. *Transactional Analysis Journal, 5*(3), 295–302. https://doi.org/10.1177/036215377500500321.

Micholt, N. (1992). Psychological distance and group interventions. *Transactional Analysis Journal, 22*(4), 228–233. https://doi.org/10.1177/036215379202200406.

Milner, M. (1952). Aspects of symbolism and comprehension of the not-self. *International Journal of Psycho-analysis, 33*, 181–185.

Milnes, P. (2019). 'Written on my heart in burning letters': Putting soul and spirit into a transcendent physis. *Transactional Analysis Journal, 49*(2), 144–157. https://doi.org/10.1080/03621537.2019.1577338.

Minikin, K. (2018). Radical relational psychiatry: Toward a democracy of mind and people. *Transactional Analysis Journal, 48*(2), 111–125. https://doi.org/10.1080/03621537.2018.1429287.

Minikin, K. (2023). *Radical-relational perspectives in transactional analysis psychotherapy*. Routledge.

Minikin, K., & Rowland, H. (2022). Letter from the coeditors. *Transactional Analysis Journal, 52*(3), 175–177. https://doi.org/10.1080/03621537.2022.2080263.

Minikin, K., & Tudor, K. (2016). Gender psychopolitics: Men being, becoming, and belonging. In R. Erskine (Ed.), *Transactional analysis in contemporary psychotherapy* (pp. 255–273). Karnac.

Ministry of Health. (2003, May). *Health Practitioners Competence Assurance Bill. Treaty of Waitangi—The Health Practitioners Competence Assurance Bill and the New Zealand Public Health and Disability Act*. Committee Report No. 11.

Ministry of Health. (2010a). *Health Practitioners Competence Assurance Act 2003*. http://www.moh.govt.nz/hpca.

Ministry of Health. (2010b). *How do we determine if statutory regulation is the most appropriate way to regulate health professions? Discussion document*. http://www.moh.govt.nz/moh.nsf/pagesmh/9894/$File/statutory-regulation-health-professions-discussion-document-jan10.pdf.

Ministry of Health. (2018). *Health Practitioners Competence Assurance Act*. https://www.health.govt.nz/our-work/regulation-health-and-disability-system/health-practitioners-competence-assurance-act. (Original work published 2010)

Ministry of Health. (2021). *Allied Health Business Plan 2021–2023*. https://www.health.govt.nz/publication/allied-health-business-plan-2021-2023.

Mitchell, S. A. (1988). *Relational concepts in psychoanalysis: An integration*. Harvard University Press.

Moiso, C. (1976). The contract card. *Transactional Analysis Journal, 6*(3), 298–299. https://doi.org/10.1177/036215377600600320.

Moiso, C. (1985). Ego states and transference. *Transactional Analysis Journal, 15*(3), 194–201. https://doi.org/10.1177/036215378501500302.

Moiso, C. (1995). The commitments. *Transactional Analysis Journal, 25*(1), 75–76. https://doi.org/10.1177/036215379502500118.

Moiso, C. (1998). Being and belonging. An appreciation and application of Berne's social psychiatry. *The Script, 28*(9), 1,7.

Moiso, C., & Novellino, M. (2000). An overview of the psychodynamic school of transactional analysis and its epistemological foundations. *Transactional Analysis Journal, 30*(3), 182–187. https://doi.org/10.1177/036215370003000302.

Money, M. (1997). Defining mental health—What do we think we're doing? In M. Money & L. Buckley (Eds.), *Positive mental health and its promotion*. Institute for Health, John Moores University.

Monin, S., & Cornell, W. F. (2015). Conflict: Intrapsychic, interpersonal, and societal [Special issue]. *Transactional Analysis Journal, 45*(4).

Morena, S. (2019). Therapeutic transactions in clinical work with children. *Transactional Analysis Journal, 49*(3), 195–210. https://doi.org/10.1080/03621537.2019.1602404.

Morgan, S. (1988). Public agencies, minority clients. In B. Roy & C. Steiner (Eds.), *Radical psychiatry: The second decade* (pp. 189–193). Privately circulated manuscript.

Morgan, S. (2004). Strengths-based practice. *OpenMind, 126*, 16–17.

Morgan, S., & Juriansz, D. (2002). Practice-based evidence. *OpenMind, 114*, 12–13.

Morrison, A. P. (1994). The breadth and boundaries of a self-psychological immersion in shame a one-and-a-half-person perspective. *Psychoanalytic Dialogues, 4*(1), 19–35. https://doi.org/10.1080/10481889409539003.

Mountain, C. (2022). Schiffian reparenting: A critical evaluation. *Transactional Analysis Journal, 52*(1), 74–88. https://doi.org/10.1080/03621537.2021.2011041.

Moustakas, C. E. (1990). *Heuristic research: Design, methodology, and applications.* Sage.

Mowbray, R. (1995). *The case against psychotherapy registration: A conservation issue for the human potential movement*. Trans Marginal Press.

Mowbray, R. (1997). A case to answer. In R. House & N. Totton (Eds.), *Implausible professions: Arguments for pluralism and autonomy in psychotherapy and counselling* (pp. 71–85). PCCS Books.

Müller, U. (2000). Old roots revisited: Reassessing the architecture of transactional analysis. *Transactional Analysis Journal, 30*(1), 41–51. https://doi.org/10.1177/036215370003000105.

Müller, U. (2002). What Eric Berne meant by 'unconscious': Aspects of depth psychology in transactional analysis. *Transactional Analysis Journal, 32*(2), 107–115. https://doi.org/10.1177/036215370203200205.

Murray, G. (1915). *The stoic philosophy*. Appeal Publishing Co.

Napper, R. (2009). Positive psychology and transactional analysis. *Transactional Analysis Journal, 39*(1), 61–74. https://doi.org/10.1177/036215370903900107.

Nathanson, D. L. (1994). Shame transactions. *Transactional Analysis Journal, 24*(2), 121–129. https://doi.org/10.1177/036215379402400207.

Naughton, M., & Tudor, K. (2006). Being white. *Transactional Analysis Journal, 36*(2), 159–171. https://doi.org/10.1177/036215370603600208.

Neville, B. (2018, 11th July). *Taking Rogers seriously* [Keynote speech]. PCE2018 – the Conference of the World Association for Person-Centered & Experiential Psychotherapy & Counseling, Vienna, Austria.

Neville, B., & Tudor, K. (2024). *Eco-centred therapy: Revisioning person-centred psychology for a living world*. Routledge.

New Zealand Association of Counsellors. (2016a). *Self-regulation vs HPCA registration history*. https://nzac.org.nz/publications/other-publications/.

New Zealand Association of Counsellors. (2020). *Code of ethics*. https://nzac.org.nz/ethics/code-of-ethics/.

New Zealand Association of Counsellors. (2022). *Statement of practice for counselling in health settings*. Author. https://www.nzac.org.nz/document/7227/Questions_and_Answers-Te_Whatu_Ora_Accreditation.pdf.

Newton, T., & Wong, G. (2003). A chance to thrive: Enabling change in a nursery school. *Transactional Analysis Journal, 33*(1), 79–88. https://doi.org/10.1177/036215370303300112.

Nietzsche, F. (2022). *Thus spake Zarathustra* (M. Hulse, Trans.). New York Review Books. (Original work published 1883–1892)

Noel, J. R., & DeChenne, T. K. (1974). Three dimensions of psychotherapy: I–we–thou. In D. A. Wexler & L. N. Rice (Eds.), *Innovations in client-centered therapy* (pp. 247–257). Wiley.

Novak, E. T. (2015). Are games, enactments, and reenactments similar? No, yes, it depends. *Transactional Analysis Journal, 45*(2), 117–127. https://doi.org/10.1177/0362153715578840.

Novellino, M. (1984). Self-analysis of countertransference in integrative transactional analysis. *Transactional Analysis Journal, 14*(1), 63–67. https://doi.org/10.1177/036215378401400110.

Novellino, M. (1987). Redecision analysis of transference: The unconscious dimension. *Transactional Analysis Journal, 17*(1), 271–276. https://doi.org/10.1177/036215378701700103.

Novellino, M. (1990). Unconscious communication and interpretation in transactional analysis. *Transactional Analysis Journal, 20*(3), 168–172. https://doi.org/10.1177/036215379002000306.

Novellino, M. (2000). The Pinocchio syndrome. *Transactional Analysis Journal, 30*(4), 292–298. https://doi.org/10.1177/036215370003000406.

Novellino, M. (2003). Transactional psychoanalysis. *Transactional Analysis Journal, 33*(3), 223–230. https://doi.org/10.1177/036215370303300304.

Novellino, M. (2005). Transactional psychoanalysis: Epistemological foundations. *Transactional Analysis Journal, 35*(2), 157–172. https://doi.org/10.1177/036215370503500206.

Novellino, M. (2008). A transactional psychoanalysis of Frodo: The conflict of the male adolescent in becoming a man. *Transactional Analysis Journal, 38*(3), 233–237. https://doi.org/10.1177/036215370803800305.

Novellino, M. (2010). The demon and sloppiness: From Berne to transactional psychoanalysis. *Transactional Analysis Journal, 40*(3–4), 288–294. https://doi.org/10.1177/036215371004000313.

Novellino, M. (2011). Six steps for the first interview: Establishing the frame and work environment in transactional psychoanalysis. *Transactional Analysis Journal, 41*(4), 284–290. https://doi.org/10.1177/036215371104100402.

Novellino, M. (2012). The shadow and the demon: The psychodynamics of nightmares. *Transactional Analysis Journal, 42*(4), 277–284. https://doi.org/10.1177/036215371204200406.

Novellino, M., & Moiso, C. (1990). The psychodynamic approach to transactional analysis. *Transactional Analysis Journal, 20*(3), 187–192. https://doi.org/10.1177/036215379002000308.

Novey, T. (Ed.). (1996). Integrative psychotherapy [Special Issue]. *Transactional Analysis Journal, 26*(4). https://www.tandfonline.com/toc/rtaj20/26/4.

Novey, T. (1998). A proposal for an integrated self [Letter to the editor]. *The Script, 28*(7), 6.

Novey, T. B., Porter-Steele, N., Gobes, L., & Massey, R. F. (1993). Ego states and the self-concept: A panel presentation and discussion. *Transactional Analysis Journal, 23*(3), 123–138. https://doi.org/10.1177/036215379302300303.

Nuttall, J. (2006). The existential phenomenology of transactional analysis. *Transactional Analysis Journal, 36*(3), 214–227. https://doi.org/10.1177/036215370603600305.

O'Hara, M. (1999). Moments of eternity: Carl Rogers and the contemporary demand for brief therapy. In I. Fairhurst (Ed.), *Women writing in the person-centred approach* (pp. 63–77). PCCS Books.

O'Hearne, J. J. (1977). Pilgrim's progress. In G. Barnes (Ed.), *Transactional analysis after Eric Berne: Teachings and practices of three TA schools* (pp. 458–484). Harper's College Press.

O'Reilly-Knapp, M. (Ed.). (1994). Shame [Special issue]. *Transactional Analysis Journal, 24*(2). https://www.tandfonline.com/toc/rtaj20/24/2.

Oden, T. C. (1974). *Game free: The meaning of intimacy. An exploration in and beyond transactional analysis.* Harper & Row.

Oller-Vallejo, J. (1997). Integrative analysis of ego state models. *Transactional Analysis Journal, 27*(4), 290–294. https://doi.org/10.1177/036215379702700408.

Oller-Vallejo, J. (2003). Three basic ego states: The primary model. *Transactional Analysis Journal, 33*(2), 162–167. https://doi.org/10.1177/036215370303300207.

Onions, C. T. (Ed.). (1973). *The shorter Oxford English dictionary* (3rd ed.). Clarendon Press. (Original work published 1933)

Orange. D. (2018). Endorsement. In K. Tudor. *Psychotherapy: A critical examination.* PCCS Books.

Osnes, R. E. (1974). Spot reparenting. *Transactional Analysis Journal, 4*(3), 40–46. https://doi.org/10.1177/036215377400400308.

Oxford English Dictionary. (2023a). *Method.* https://www.oed.com.

Oxford English Dictionary. (2023b). *Methodology.* https://www.oed.com.

Palmer, G. (1974). *The currency wheel of life.* Sacramento.

Panksepp, J. (1998). *Affective neuroscience: The foundations of human and animal emotions.* Oxford University Press.

Park, S. N. (1971). The waiting game. *Transactional Analysis Bulletin, 1*(4), 54–57. https://doi.org/10.1177/036215377100100412.

Parker, I., & Revelli, S. (Eds.). (2008). *Psychoanalytic practice and state regulation.* Karnac.

Parkin, F. (2002). Expanding permissions: New perspectives on working with transactional analysis and sexual difficulties. *Transactional Analysis Journal, 32*(1), 56–61. https://doi.org/10.1177/036215370203200108.

Parr, J. (2008). Letter to the Editors. *Transactional Analysis Journal, 38*(3), 259–260.

Paul, L. (1970). A game analysis of Albee's 'Who's afraid of Virginia Woolf?': The core of grief. *Transactional Analysis Bulletin, 9*(36), 122–127.

Penfield, W. (1952). Memory mechanisms. *Archives of Neurology and Psychiatry, 67*, 178–198. https://doi.org/10.1001/archneurpsyc.1952.02320140046005.

Perls, F. S. (1969). *Ego, hunger and aggression.* Vintage. (Original work published 1947)

Perrett, R. W., & Patterson, J. (1991). Virtue ethics and Maori ethics. *Philosophy East and West, 41*(2), 185–202. https://www.jstor.org/stable/1399769.

Pfaffenberger, A. H. (2005). Optimal adult development: An inquiry into the dynamics of growth. *Journal of Humanistic Psychology, 45*(3), 279–301. https://doi.org/10.1177/0022 167804274359.

Piaget, J. (1950). *The psychology of intelligence.* Routledge and Kegan Paul.

Piccinino, G. (2018). Reflections on physis, happiness, and human motivation. *Transactional Analysis Journal, 48*(3), 272–285. https://doi.org/10.1080/03621537.2018. 1471293.

Pine, F. (1990). *Drive, ego, object, and self: A synthesis for clinical work.* Basic Books.

Pirnie, C. (1976). A permission/protection score card. *Transactional Analysis Journal, 6*(1), 88–89. https://doi.org/10.1177/036215377600600122.

Pohatu, T. W. (2004). Āta: Growing respectful relationships. Wellington, Aotearoa New Zealand: Massey University.

Pohatu, T. W. (2013). Āta: Growing respectful relationships. *Ata: Journal of Psychotherapy Aotearoa New Zealand, 17*(1), 13–26. https://doi.org/10.9791/ajpanz.2013.02.

Polanyi, M. (1962). *Personal knowledge: Towards a post-critical philosophy.* Routledge.

Polanyi, M. (1964). *Science, faith and society.* University of Chicago Press.

Polanyi, M. (1966). *The tacit dimension.* Doubleday.

Polanyi, M. (1969). *Knowing and being.* Routledge & Kegan Paul.

Porter-Steele, N. (1990). Response to 'Over the Border': The nonreification of 'Self'. *Transactional Analysis Journal, 20*(1), 56–59. https://doi.org/10.1177/036215379002 000107.

Postle, D. (2007). *Regulating the psychological therapies—From taxonomy to taxidermy.* PCCS Books.

Postle, D., & House, R. (Eds.). (2009). *Compliance? Ambivalence? Rejection? Nine papers challenging the Health Professions Council proposals for the state regulation of the psychological therapies.* Wentworth Learning Resources/eIpnosis.

Price, D. A. (1978). Social-psychological roots of transactional analysis: Exchange as symbolic interaction. *Transactional Analysis Journal, 8*(3), 212–215. https://doi.org/10.1177/036215377800800306.

Proctor, G. (2002). *The dynamics of power in counselling and psychotherapy: Ethics, politics and practice.* PCCS Books.

Psychoanalytic Electronic Publishing. (2024). *Library* [Database]. https://pep-web.org/

Psychotherapists Board of Aotearoa New Zealand. (2008, 4 September). Notice of scopes of practice and related qualifications prescribed by The Psychotherapists Board of Aotearoa New Zealand. *New Zealand Gazette, 136*, 3647.

Psychotherapists Board of Aotearoa New Zealand. (2013). *Psychotherapist standards of ethical conduct.*

Psychotherapists Board of Aotearoa New Zealand. (2019). *Ngā āheitanga ahurea mā ngā kaihanumanu hinengaro Psychotherapist cultural competencies.* https://www.pbanz.org.nz/common/Uploaded%20files/Standards/Psychotherapist%20Cultural%20Competencies%20July%202019.pdf.

Psychotherapists Board of Aotearoa New Zealand. (2021). *Accreditation standards | Ngā paerewa whakamanatanga.* https://pbanz.org.nz/Public/Rauemia-Ipurangi-Online-resources/Accreditation%20Standards.aspx.

The Radical Therapist Collective. (1971). *The radical therapist* [J. Agel, Producer]. Ballantine Books.

Rangell, L. (1965). The scope of Heinz Hartmann—Some selected comments on his essays on ego psychology an appreciative survey on the occasion of his 70th birthday. *The International journal of Psychoanalysis, 46,* 5–30.

Rangell, L. (1985). On the theory of theory in psychoanalysis and the relation of theory to psychoanalytic therapy. *Journal of the American Psychoanalytic Association, 33,* 59–92.

Rapaport, D. (1967). *The collected papers of David Rapaport* (M. M. Gill, Ed.). Basic Books.

Rath, I. (1993). Developing a coherent map of transactional analysis theories. *Transactional Analysis Journal, 23*(4), 201–215. https://doi.org/10.1177/036215379302300405.

Rawls, J. (1971). *A theory of justice.* Belknap Press.

Reddemann, L. (2011). *Psychodynamisch-imaginative Traumatherapie, PITT. Das Manual. 3. erw. Auflage* [Psychodynamic imaginative traumatherapy, PITT. The manual]. Klett-Cotta.

Riebel, L. (1996). Self-sealing doctrines, the misuse of power, and recovered memory. *Transactional Analysis Journal, 26*(1), 40–45. https://doi.org/10.1177/036215379602600108.

Rinzler, D. (1984). Human disconnection and the murder of the earth. *Transactional Analysis Journal, 14*(4), 231–236. https://doi.org/10.1177/036215378401400406.

Ritchie, H., Roser, M., & Rosado, P. (2022). *Energy.* https://ourworldindata.org/energy.

Roberts, D. L. (1975). Treatment of cultural scripts. *Transactional Analysis Journal, 5*(1), 29–35. https://doi.org/10.1177/036215377500500106.

Roberts. J. P. (1982). Foulkes' concept of the matrix. *Group Analysis, 15,* 111–126. https://doi.org/10.1177/053331648201500203.

Robertson, C. (1993). Dysfunction in training organisations. *Self & Society, 21*(4), 31–35. https://doi.org/10.1080/03060497.1993.11085357.

Robinson, J. (1998). Reparenting in a therapeutic community. *Transactional Analysis Journal, 28*(1), 88–94. https://doi.org/10.1177/036215379802800117.

Robinson, J. (2003). Groups and group dynamics in a therapeutic community. *Transactional Analysis Journal, 33*(4), 315–320. https://doi.org/10.1177/036215370303300406.

Robinson, P. (2020). Cocreative transformational learning as a way to break out of script. *Transactional Analysis Journal, 50*(1), 41–55. https://doi.org/10.1080/03621537.2019.1690237.

Rodgers, B., & Tudor, K. (2020). Person-centred therapy: A radical paradigm in a new world. *New Zealand Journal of Counselling, 40*(2), 21–35. https://www.nzac.org.nz/assets/Journals/Vol-40-No-2/Chapter_2_Person-centred_therapy.pdf.

Rogers, C. R. (1942). *Counseling and psychotherapy: Newer concepts in practice.* Houghton Mifflin.

Rogers, C. R. (1951). *Client-centered therapy.* Constable.

Rogers, C. R. (1957a). The necessary and sufficient conditions of therapeutic personality change. *Journal of Consulting Psychology, 21,* 95–103.

Rogers, C. R. (1957b). A note on the 'nature of man.' *Journal of Counseling Psychology, 4*(3), 199–203. https://doi.org/10.1037/h0048308.

Rogers, C. R. (1959). A theory of therapy, personality and interpersonal relationships, as developed in the client-centered framework. In S. Koch (Ed.), *Psychology: A study of science, Vol. 3: Formulation of the person and the social context* (pp. 184–256). McGraw-Hill.

Rogers, C. R. (1963). The actualizing tendency in relation to "motive" and to consciousness. In M. Jones (Ed.), *Nebraska symposium on motivation 1963* (pp. 1–24). University of Nebraska Press.

Rogers, C. R. (1967a). *On becoming a person: A therapist's view of psychotherapy*. Constable. (Original work published 1961)

Rogers, C. R. (1967b). A process conception of psychotherapy. In C. R. Rogers, *On becoming a person: A therapist's view of psychotherapy* (pp. 125–159). Constable. (Original work published 1958)

Rogers, C. R. (1967c) Some hypotheses regarding the facilitation of personal growth. In *On becoming a person* (pp. 31–38). Constable. (Original work published in 1954)

Rogers, C. R. (1980). Empathic: An unappreciated way of being. In *A way of being* (pp. 137–163). Houghton Mifflin. (Original work published 1975).

Rogers, C. R., & Russell, D. E. (2002). *Carl Rogers: The quiet revolutionary: An oral history*. Penmarin Books.

Rossi, E. L. (1967). Game and growth: Two dimensions of our psychotherapeutic zeitgeist. *Journal of Humanistic Psychology, 7*(2), 139–154. https://doi.org/10.1177/00221 6786700700203.

Rossi, E. L. (1971). Growth, change and transformation in dreams. *Journal of Humanistic Psychology, 11*(2), 147–169. https://doi.org/10.1177/002216787101100205.

Rotondo, A. (2020). Rethinking contracts: The heart of Eric Berne's transactional analysis. *Transactional Analysis Journal, 50*(3), 236–250. https://doi.org/10.1080/03621537.2020. 1771032.

The Rough Times Staff. (1973). *Rough times* [J. Agel, Producer]. Ballantine Books.

Rovics, H. (1981). Contract grading in the college classroom. *Transactional Analysis Journal, 11*(3), 254–255. https://doi.org/10.1177/036215378101100313.

Rowland, H. (2016). On vulnerability. *Transactional Analysis Journal, 46*(4), 277–287. https://doi.org/10.1177/0362153716662874.

Roy, B. (1988). Loss of power – Alienation. In B. Roy & C. Steiner (Eds.), *Radical psychiatry: The second decade* (pp. 3–13). Unpublished manuscript.

Roy, B., & Steiner, C. M. (Eds.) (1988). *Radical psychiatry: The second decade*. Unpublished manuscript. https://www.radicaltherapy.org/resources.

Royal Commission on Social Policy. (1988). *The April report*, Volumes I to IV. https:// gg.govt.nz/sites/default/files/2021-06/RC%20140%20Social%20Policy_Part1.pdf.

Salters, D. (2006). Simunye—sibaningi: We are one—we are many. *Transactional Analysis Journal, 36*(2), 152–158. https://doi.org/10.1177/036215370603600207.

Salters, D. (2021). Eco TA focus group. *The Script, 51*(10), 7.

Samuels, S. D. (1971). Games therapists play. *Transactional Analysis Journal, 1*(1), 95–99. https://doi.org/10.1177/036215377100100117.

Saner, R. (1989). Culture bias of gestalt therapy: Made-in-USA. *The Gestalt Journal, 12*(2), 57–73.

Sayers, J. (1976). A woman's work, *Social Work Today, 8*(12), 12–13.

Schaeffer, B. (1981). *Corrective parenting chart* [Handout; self-published].

Schafer, R. (1968). *Aspects of internalization*. International Universities Press.

Schiff, A. W., & Schiff, J. L. (1971). Passivity. *Transactional Analysis Journal, 1*(1), 71–78. https://doi.org/10.1177/036215377100100114.

Schiff, J. (1969). Reparented schizophrenics. *Transactional Analysis Bulletin, 8*(31), 47–63.

Schiff, J. (1975). Editorial. Social action [Special issue]. *Transactional Analysis Journal, 5*(1), 6. https://doi.org/10.1177/036215377500500102.

Schiff, J. L. (1977). *All my children*. Jove.

Schiff, J. L., Schiff, A. W., Mellor, K., Schiff, E., Schiff, S., Richman, D., Fishman, J., Wolz, L., Fishman, C., & Momb, D. (1975). *Cathexis reader: Transactional analysis treatment of psychosis*. Harper & Row.

Schmid, P. (1999). 'Face to face'—The art of encounter. In B. Thorne & E. Lambers (Eds.), *Person-centred therapy: A European perspective* (pp. 74–90). Sage.

Schmid, P. (2006). The challenge of the other: Towards dialogical person-centered psychotherapy. *Person-Centered & Experiential Psychotherapies*, 5(4), 240–254. https://doi.org/10.1080/14779757.2006.9688416.

Schneider, P. (1967). The squire of Gothos. In *Star Trek* (D. McDougall, Director; Series 1, Episode 17). Desilu Productions.

Schwebel, B. (1974). Trashing the stroke economy. *Issues in Radical Therapy*, 3(3), 13–15.

Sedgwick, J. (2021). *Contextual transactional analysis: The inseparability of self and world*. Routledge.

Seidler, V. J. (1989). *Rediscovering masculinity*. Routledge.

Shakespeare, W. (1985). *Hamlet*. The New Cambridge Shakespeare. (Original work published 1602)

Shakespeare, W. (2018). *The Merchant of Venice*. The New Cambridge Shakespeare. (Original work published 1597)

Shakespeare, W. (2019). *Hamlet*. The New Cambridge Shakespeare. (Original work published 1603)

Shaw, S., & Tudor, K. (2022). The Emperors' new clothes: The socialisation and regulation of health professions. *Journal of Interprofessional Education and Practice*, 28. https://doi.org/10.1016/j.xjep.2022.100519.

Sherrard, E. (2011). Once was a psychotherapist. In K. Tudor (Ed.), *The turning tide: Pluralism and partnership in psychotherapy in Aotearoa New Zealand* (pp. 119–125). LC Publications.

Sherrard, E. M. (2020). Once was a psychotherapist. In K. Tudor (Ed.), *Pluralism in psychotherapy: Critical reflections from a post-regulation landscape*. Tuwhera Open Access Books. https://ojs.aut.ac.nz/tuwhera-open-monographs/catalog/book/1. (Original work published 2017)

Sherwood, V. (2019). *Haunted: the death mother archetype*. Chiron Publications.

Shivanath S., & Hiremath M. (2003). The psycho-dynamics of race and culture. In H. Hargaden & C. Sills (Eds.), *Ego states* (Key concepts in transactional analysis: Contemporary views) (pp. 169–185). Worth Publishing.

Shmukler, D. (2001). Reflections on transactional analysis in the context of contemporary relational approaches. *Transactional Analysis Journal*, 31(2), 94–102. https://doi.org/10.1177/036215370103100204.

Shohet, R. (Ed.). (2007). *Passionate supervision*. Jessica Kingsley.

Siddique, S. (2017). Ellipses. *Transactional Analysis Journal*, 47(2), 152–166. https://doi.org/10.1177/0362153717695071.

Siegler, M., & Osmond, H. (1974). The three medical models. *Journal of Orthomolecular Psychiatry*, 3(2), 96–108.

Siegler, M., & Osmond, H. (1976). *Models of madness, models of medicine*. Macmillan.

Sills, C. (2006). *Contracts in counselling and psychotherapy*. Sage.

Sills C., & Salters D. (1991). The comparative script system. *ITA News*, No. 31, 1–15.

Sills, C., & Tudor, K. (2017). Transactional analysis. In C. Feltham, T. Hanley, & L. A. Winter (Eds.), *The Sage handbook of counselling and psychotherapy* (4th ed.; pp. 355–360). London, UK: Sage.

Sills, C., & Tudor, K. (2023). Transactional analysis. In T. Hanley & L. A. Winter (Eds.), *The Sage handbook of counselling and psychotherapy* (5th Ed.; pp. 503–509). Sage.

Singer, M. (1996). Therapy, thought reform, and cults. *Transactional Analysis Journal*, *26*(1), 15–22. https://doi.org/10.1177/036215379602600105.

Smith, G. T. (1977). *Kaupapa Māori as transformative praxis* [Unpublished doctoral thesis]. University of Auckland, Auckland, Aotearoa New Zealand.

Smith, J. B. (2011). Licensing of psychotherapists in the United States: Evidence of societal regression? *Transactional Analysis Journal*, *41*(2), 139–146. https://doi.org/10.1177/036215371104100209.

Smith K., & Tudor, K. (2015). To be registered, or not to be registered—is that the question? *Asia Pacific Journal of Counselling and Psychotherapy*, 6(1–2), 3–16. https://doi.org/10.1080/21507686.2015.1091020.

Social Workers Registration Act 2003. [New Zealand] https://www.legislation.govt.nz/act/public/2003/0017/42.0/DLM189915.html.

Solms, M. (1999). Controversies in Freud translation. *Psychoanalysis and History*, *1*(1), 28–43.

Solomon, C. (1986). Treatment of eating disorders. *Transactional Analysis Journal*, *16*(4), 224–228. https://doi.org/10.1177/036215378601600403.

Speierer, G-W. (1990). Toward a specific illness concept of client-centered therapy. In G. Lietaer, J. Rombauts, & R. Van Balen (Eds.), *Client-centered and experiential psychotherapy in the nineties* (pp. 337–359). Leuven University Press.

Spinrad, N. (1967). The doomsday machine. In *Star Trek* (M. Daniels, Director; Series 2, Episode 6). Desilu Productions.

Spitz, R. A. (1944). Psychosomatic principles and methods and their clinical application. *Medical Clinics of North America*, *28*(3), 553–564. https://doi.org/10.1016/S0025-7125(16)36374-X.

Sprietsma, L. C. (1982). Adult ego state analysis with apologies to 'Mr Spock'. *Transactional Analysis Journal*, *12*(3), 227–231. https://doi.org/10.1177/036215378201200314.

Stapleton, R. J., & Stapleton, D. C. (1998). Teaching business using the case method and transactional analysis: A constructivist approach. *Transactional Analysis Journal*, *28*(2), 157–167. https://doi.org/10.1177/036215379802800209.

Stark, M. (1999). *Modes of therapeutic action: Enhancement of knowledge, provision of experience, and engagement in relationship*. Jason Aronson.

Stark, M. (2004). *A primer on working with resistance*. Rowman & Littlefield Publishers.

Stark, M. (2016). *How does psychotherapy work?* International Psychotherapy Institute. www.FreePsychotherapyBooks.org.

Stark, M. (2017). *Relentless hope: The refusal to grieve*. International Psychotherapy Institute. www.FreePsychotherapyBooks.org.

Stark, M. (2021). *Understanding life backward but living life forward: Analysing to understand but envisioning possibilities to incentivize action*. International Psychotherapy Institute. www.FreePsychotherapyBooks.org.

Steele, C. A., & Porter-Steele, N. (2003). OKness-based groups. *Transactional Analysis Journal*, *33*(4), 276–281. https://doi.org/10.1177/036215370303300402.

Steinberg, H. (2004). Die Errichtung des ersten psychiatrischen Lehrstuhls: Johann Christian August Heinroth in Leipzig. [Creation of the first university chair in psychiatry: Johann Christian August Heinroth in Leipzig] *Der Nervenartz*, *73*, 303–307. https://doi.org/10.1007/s00115-003-1605-3.

Steinberg, H., & Himmerich, H. (2012). Johann Christian August Heinroth (1773–1843): The first professor of psychiatry as a psychotherapist. *Journal of Religion & Health*, *51*(2), 256–258. https://doi.org/10.1007/s10943-011-9562-9.

Steiner, C. (1966). Script and counterscript. *Transactional Analysis Bulletin*, *5*(18), 133–135.

Steiner, C. (1967). The treatment of alcoholism. *Transactional Analysis Bulletin*, *6*(23), 69–71.

Steiner, C. (1968). Transactional analysis as a treatment philosophy. *Transactional Analysis Bulletin*, *7*(27), 61–64.

Steiner, C. (1971a). *Games alcoholics play: The analysis of life scripts*. Grove Press.

Steiner, C. M. (1971b). Radical psychiatry: Principles. In The Radical Therapist Collective (Ed.), *The radical therapist* (J. Agel, Producer; pp. 3–7). Ballantine Books

Steiner, C. (1971c). The stroke economy. *Transactional Analysis Journal*, *1*(3), 9–15. https://doi.org/10.1177/036215377100100305.

Steiner, C. M. (1971d). *TA: Transactional analysis made simple: Ego states, games, scripts*. TA Press.

Steiner, C. (1974). *Scripts people live: Transactional analysis of life scripts*. Grove Press.

Steiner, C. (1975a). Radical psychiatry: Principles. In C. Steiner (Ed.), *Readings in radical psychiatry* (pp. 9–16). Grove Press.

Steiner, C. (Ed.). (1975b). *Readings in radical psychiatry*. Grove Press.

Steiner, C. (1976). Working cooperatively. *Issues in Radical Therapy*, *3*(4), 22–25.

Steiner, C. M. (1978). The Pig Parent. *Issues in Radical Therapy*, *23*, 5–11.

Steiner, C. M. (1979). *Healing alcoholism*. Grove Press.

Steiner, C. (1981). *The other side of power*. Grove Press.

Steiner, C. (1988). The pig parent. In B. Roy & C. Steiner (Eds.), *Radical psychiatry: The second decade* (pp. 36–54). Unpublished manuscript. Retrieved from www.emotional-literacy.com/rp0.htm.

Steiner, C. (2000). Radical psychiatry. In R. J. Corsini (Ed.), *Handbook of innovative therapy* (pp. 578–586). Chichester, UK: Wiley.

Steiner, C. (Ed.). (2003). Core concepts [Special issue]. *Transactional Analysis Journal*, *33*(2). https://www.tandfonline.com/toc/rtaj20/33/2.

Steiner, C. (2006). Quo vadis transactional analysis? Change and trust. *The Script*, *36*(9), 1, 6–7.

Steiner, C. (2008). *Confessions of a psychomechanic*. Unpublished manuscript.

Steiner, C. M. (2010). Eric Berne's politics: 'The great pyramid'. *Transactional Analysis Journal*, *40*(3–4), 212–216. https://doi.org/10.1177/036215371004000306.

Steiner, C. M. (2020). Confessions of a psychomechanic—Excerpts on power. In K. Tudor (Ed.), *Emotional activist: The work and life of Claude Michel Steiner* (pp. 147–154). Routledge.

Steiner, C., & Cassidy, W. (1969). Therapeutic contracts in group treatment. *Transactional Analysis Bulletin*, *8*(30), 29–31.

Steiner, C., Campos, L., Drego, P., Joines, V., Ligabue, S., Noriega, G., Roberts, D. & Said, E. (2003). A compilation of core concepts. *Transactional Analysis Journal*, *33*(2), 182–191. https://doi.org/10.1177/036215370303300210.

Steiner, C., & Roy, B. (1988). Cooperation. In B. Roy & C. Steiner (Eds.), *Radical psychiatry: The second decade* (pp. 29–35). Unpublished manuscript.

Steiner, C., & Tudor, K. (2014, 7 August). *Still radical after all these years: TA and politics* [Workshop]. International Transactional Analysis Association World Conference, San Francisco, USA. https://www.youtube.com/watch?v=0m5zzQyAe_M.

Steiner, C., & Wyckoff, H. (1975). Alienation. In C. Steiner (Ed.), *Readings in radical psychiatry* (pp. 17–27). Grove Press.

Steiner, C., Wyckoff, H., Golstine, D., Lariviere, P., Schwebel, R., Marcus, J., & Members of the Radical Psychiatry Center. (1975). *Readings in radical psychiatry*. Grove Press.

Steinfeld, G. J. (1998). Personal responsibility in human relationships: A cognitive-constructivist approach. *Transactional Analysis Journal*, *28*(3), 188–201. https://doi.org/10.1177/036215379802800302.

Stern, D. (1985). *The interpersonal world of the infant*. Basic Books.

Stern, D. N. (1998). *The interpersonal world of the infant: A view from psychoanalysis and developmental psychology* (Rev. Ed.). Basic Books.

Stern, D. N. (2004). *The present moment in psychotherapy and everyday life*. Norton.

Stewart, I. (1989). *Transactional analysis counselling in action*. Sage.

Stewart, I. (1992). *Eric Berne*. Sage.

Stewart, I. (1996). *Developing transactional analysis counselling*. Sage.

Stewart, I. (2001). Ego states and the theory of theory: The strange case of the little professor. *Transactional Analysis Journal*, *31*(2), 133–147. https://doi.org/10.1177/036215370103100209.

Stewart, I., & Joines, V. (1987). *TA today: A new introduction to transactional analysis*. Lifespace Publishing.

Stewart-Harawira, M. (2005). *The new world order: Indigenous responses to globalization*. Huia.

Stummer, G. (2002). An update on the use of contracting. *Transactional Analysis Journal*, *32*(2), 121–123. https://doi.org/10.1177/036215370203200207.

Stuntz, E. C. (1971). *Transactional game analysis: A review of TA literature 1962 through 1970*. Privately circulated manuscript.

Stuthridge, J. (2012). Traversing the fault lines: Trauma and enactment. *Transactional Analysis Journal*, *42*(4), 238–251. https://doi.org/10.1177/036215371204200402.

Stuthridge, J. (2015). All the world's a stage. *Transactional Analysis Journal*, *45*(2), 104–116. https://doi.org/10.1177/0362153715581174.

Summers, G. (2014). Introduction. In Tudor, K. & Summers, G. *Co-creative transactional analysis: Papers, dialogues, responses, and developments* (pp. xxxi–xxxviii). Karnac Books.

Summers, G., & Tudor, K. (2000). Cocreative transactional analysis. *Transactional Analysis Journal*, *30*(1), 23–40. https://doi.org/10.1177/036215370003000104.

Summers, G., & Tudor, K. (2008). Introducing transactional analysis. In K. Tudor (Ed.), *The Adult is Parent to the Child: Transactional analysis with children and young people* (pp. 1–11). Russell House.

Summers, G., & K. Tudor. (2014). Response to 'Co-creative contributions'. In Tudor, K. & Summers, G. *Co-creative transactional analysis: Papers, dialogues, responses, and developments* (pp. 183–200). Karnac Books.

Summers, G., & Tudor, K. (2021). Reflections on co-creative transactional analysis: Acceptance speech for the 2020 Eric Berne Memorial Award. *Transactional Analysis Journal*, *51*(1), 7–18. https://doi.org/10.1080/03621537.2020.1853345.

Summerton, O. (1979). RANI: A new approach to relationship analysis. *Transactional Analysis Journal*, *9*(2), 115–118. https://doi.org/10.1177/036215377900900213.

Summerton, O. (1985). The game pentagon. *Tasi Darshan*, *5*(4), 39–51.

Summerton, O. (1992). Game analysis in two planes. *Transactional Analysis Journal*, *22*(4), 210–215. https://doi.org/10.1177/036215379202200403.

Summerton, O. (1993). Games in organizations. *Transactional Analysis Journal*, *23*(2), 87–103. https://doi.org/10.1177/036215379302300206.

Suriyaprakash, C. (2011). Ethics in organizations: My Eastern philosophical perspective. *Transactional Analysis Journal*, *41*(2), 133–135. https://doi.org/10.1177/03621 5371104100207.

Sutich, A. (1967). The growth-experience and the growth-centered attitude. *Journal of Humanistic Psychology*, *7*(2), 155–162. https://doi.org/10.1177/002216786700700204.

Symor, N. K. (1977). The dependency cycle: Implications for theory, therapy and social action. *Transactional Analysis Journal*, *7*(1), 37–43. https://doi.org/10.1177/0362153777 00700110.

Taft, J. (1973). *The dynamics of therapy in a controlled relationship.* Macmillan. (Original work published 1933)

Tangolo, A. E. (2015). Group imago and dreamwork in group therapy. *Transactional Analysis Journal*, *45*(3), 179–190. https://doi.org/10.1177/0362153715597722.

Temple, S. (1999). Functional fluency for educational transactional analysts. *Transactional Analysis Journal*, *29*(3), 164–174. https://doi.org/10.1177/036215379902900302.

Thandeka. (1999). White racial induction and Christian shame theology: A primer. *Gender and Psychoanalysis*, *4*(4), 455–495.

Thatcher, M. (2022). Interview for *Woman's Own* ('No such thing as society'). In *Speeches, interviews and other statements.* Margaret Thatcher Foundation. https://www.margaretthatcher.org/document/106689 (Original work published 1987)

Tolle, E. (1997). *The power of now: A guide to spiritual enlightenment.* New World Library.

Tosi, M. T. (2008). The many faces of the unconscious: A new unconscious for a phenomenological transactional analysis. *Transactional Analysis Journal*, *38*(2), 119–127. https://www.tandfonline.com/doi/abs/10.1177/036215370803800205.

Tosi, M. T. (2018). Personal identity and moral discourse in psychotherapy. *Transactional Analysis Journal*, *48*(2), 139–151. https://doi.org/10.1080/03621537.2018.1429295.

Totton, N. (1999). The baby and the bathwater: 'Professionalisation' in psychotherapy and counselling. *British Journal of Guidance and Counselling*, *27*(3), 313–324.

Totton, N. (2011). *Wild therapy: Undomesticating inner and outer worlds.* PCCS Books.

Traue, J. E. (1990). *Ancestors of the mind: A pakeha whakapapa.* Gondwanaland Press.

Trautmann, R. (Ed.). (1984). Nuclear disarmament [Special issue]. *Transactional Analysis Journal*, *14*(4). https://www.tandfonline.com/toc/rtaj20/14/4.

Trautmann, R. L., & Erskine, R. G. (1981). Ego state analysis: A comparative view. *Transactional Analysis Journal*, *11*(2), 178–185. https://doi.org/10.1177/036215378101100218.

Trautmann, R. L., & Erskine, R. G. (1999). A matrix of relationships: Acceptance speech for the 1998 Eric Berne memorial award. *Transactional Analysis Journal*, *29*(1), 14–17. https://doi.org/10.1177/036215379902900106.

Tudor, K. (1990). Using TA to understand organisations. *ITA News*, No. *28*, 8–10.

Tudor, K. (1990/1991). One step back, two steps forward: Community care and mental health. *Critical Social Policy*, *30*, 5–22.

Tudor, K. (1991). Children's groups: Integrating TA and gestalt perspectives. *Transactional Analysis Journal*, *21*(1), 12–20. https://doi.org/10.1177/036215379102100103.

Tudor, K. (1995a). Shame, shaming and 'shame': A transactional analysis. *ITA News*, No. *41*, 25–31.

Tudor, K. (1995b). What do you say about saying good-bye?: Ending psychotherapy. *Transactional Analysis Journal*, *25*(3), 228–234. https://doi.org/10.1177/036215379502500307.

Tudor, K. (1996b). Transactional analysis *intra*gration: A metatheoretical analysis for practice. *Transactional Analysis Journal, 26*(4), 329–340. https://doi.org/10.1177/0362 15379602600411.

Tudor, K. (1997a). Being at dis-ease with ourselves: Alienation and psychotherapy. *Changes, 22*(2), 143–150.

Tudor, K. (1997b). A complexity of contracts. In C. Sills (Ed.), *Contracts in counselling* (pp. 157–172). London, UK: Sage.

Tudor, K. (1997c). Counselling and psychotherapy: An issue of orientation. *ITA News*, No. *46*, 40–42.

Tudor, K. (1997d). Social contracts: Contracting for social change. In C. Sills (Ed.), *Contracts in counselling* (pp. 207–215). Sage.

Tudor, K. (1998). Value for money: Issues of fees in counselling and psychotherapy. *British Journal of Guidance and Counselling, 26*(4), 477–493. https://doi.org/10.1080/03069889808253858.

Tudor, K. (1999a). *Group counselling.* Sage.

Tudor, K. (1999b). "I'm OK, You're OK—and They're OK": Therapeutic relationships in transactional analysis. In C. Feltham (Ed.), *Understanding the counselling relationship* (pp. 90–119). Sage.

Tudor, K. (2000b). Transactional analysis. In C. Feltham & I. Horton (Eds.), *Handbook of counselling and psychotherapy* (pp. 363–369). Sage.

Tudor, K. (2001a). Change, time, place and community. In P. Lapworth, C. Sills, & S. Fish (Eds.), *Integration in counselling and psychotherapy* (pp. 142–151). Sage.

Tudor, K. (2001b). 'Forever Young' or Mr Zimmerman's 60th birthday blues. *TA UK, 61*, 25–28.

Tudor, K. (2002a). Introduction. In K. Tudor (Ed.), *Transactional approaches to brief therapy or what do you say between saying hello and goodbye?* (pp. 1–18). London, UK: Sage.

Tudor, K. (2002b). Transactional analysis supervision or supervision analyzed transactionally? *Transactional Analysis Journal, 32*(1), 39–55. https://doi.org/10.1177/03621 5370203200107.

Tudor, K. (Ed.). (2002c). *Transactional approaches to brief therapy or what do you say between saying hello and goodbye?* Sage.

Tudor, K. (2003a, 25 October). *Creativity and co-creativity* [Paper presentation]. Thinking in Practice Seminar, Oxford, UK.

Tudor, K. (2003b). The neopsyche: The integrating adult ego state. In C. Sills & H. Hargaden (Eds.), *Ego states* (Vol. 1, Key concepts in transactional analysis: Contemporary views) (pp. 201–231). Worth Publishing.

Tudor, K. (2006). Contracts, complexity and challenge. In C. Sills (Ed.), *Contracts in counselling and psychotherapy* (2nd ed.; pp. 119–136). Sage.

Tudor, K. (2007a, December). Making changes. *ITA News, 34*, 1, 3–7. [Also published in *TA Times* (2008, April), 1–8.]

Tudor, K. (2007b, April 13). *On dogma* [Paper presentation]. Institute of Transactional Analysis Annual Conference, York, UK.

Tudor, K. (Ed.). (2008a). *The Adult is parent to the child: Transactional analysis with children and young people.* Russell House.

Tudor, K. (2008b). L'analisi transazionale o è radicale o non è analisi transazionale [Transactional analysis is radical or it is not transactional analysis]. *Neopsiche, 6*, 8–20.

Tudor, K. (2008c). 'Take it': A sixth driver. *Transactional Analysis Journal, 38*(1), 43–57. https://doi.org/10.1177/036215370803800107.

Tudor, K. (2008d). Therapy is a verb. *Therapy Today, 19*(1), 35–37.

Tudor, K. (Ed.) (2008e). Time, limits, and person-centred therapies. In K Tudor (Ed.), *Brief person-centred therapies* (pp. 13–28). Sage. https://doi.org/10.4135/9781446 221297.

Tudor, K. (2008f). Verbal being: From being human to human being. In B. E. Levitt (Ed.), *Reflections on human potential: Bridging the person-centered approach and positive psychology* (pp. 68–83). PCCS Books.

Tudor, K. (2009a). L'analisi transazionale o è radicale o non è analisi transazionale [TA is radical or it is not TA], *Neopsiche, 6*, 8–20.

Tudor, K. (2009b). "In the manner of": Transactional analysis teaching of transactional analysts. *Transactional Analysis Journal, 39*(4), 276–292. https://doi.org/10.1177/0362 15370903900403.

Tudor, K. (2010a). Alpha und Omega, oder: Umfasst die Aktualisierung den Tod? [Alpha and omega, or, Does actualisation encompass death?]. *Person: The International Journal for Person-Centered and Experiential Psychotherapy and Counselling, 14*(2).

Tudor, K. (2010b). Regulation and registration: Protection or protectionism? A plea for pluralism. *The TAttler*, 4–10.

Tudor, K. (2010c). The state of the ego: Then and now. *Transactional Analysis Journal, 40*(3–4), 261–277. https://doi.org/10.1177/036215371004000311.

Tudor, K. (2010d). Transactional analysis: A little liberal, a little conservative, and a little radical. *The Psychotherapist, 46*, 17–20.

Tudor, K. (2011a, July 8). *Challenges of growth* [Keynote speech]. ITAA World Congress, Bilbao, Spain.

Tudor, K. (2011b). Empathy: A cocreative perspective. *Transactional Analysis Journal, 41*(4), 322–335. https://doi.org/10.1177/036215371104100409.

Tudor, K. (2011c). The law is an Act: The *Health Practitioners Competence Assurance Act 2003*. In K. Tudor (Ed.), *The turning tide: Pluralism and partnership in psychotherapy in Aotearoa New Zealand* (pp. 39–68). LC Publications.

Tudor, K. (2011d). Rogers' therapeutic conditions: A relational conceptualization. *Person-Centered & Experiential Psychotherapies, 10*(3), 165–180. https://doi.org/10.1080/1477 9757.2011.599513.

Tudor, K. (2011e). There ain't no license that protects: Bowen theory and the regulation of psychotherapy. *Transactional Analysis Journal, 41*(2), 154–161. https://doi.org/10.1177/ 036215371104100212.

Tudor, K. (Ed.). (2011f). *The turning tide: Pluralism and partnership in psychotherapy in Aotearoa New Zealand*. LC Publications.

Tudor, K. (2011g). Understanding empathy. *Transactional Analysis Journal, 41*(1), 39–57. https://doi.org/10.1177/036215371104100107.

Tudor, K. (2012). Southern psychotherapies. *Psychotherapy and Politics International, 10*(2), 116–129. https://doi.org/10.1002/ppi.1265.

Tudor, K. (2013a). Group imago and group development. *Transactional Analysis Journal, 43*(4), 321–333. https://doi.org/10.1177/0362153713516297.

Tudor, K. (2013b, March). Transactional analysis works: Getting excited about research. *The TAttler*, 8–15.

Tudor, K. (2014a, Summer). The creativity in co-creativity. *The Transactional Analyst, 4*(3), 9–13.

Tudor, K. (2014b). Introduction. In K. Tudor & G. Summers (Eds.), *Co-creative transactional analysis: Papers, responses, dialogues, and developments* (pp. xix–xxix). Karnac Books.

Tudor, K. (2015, 10ᵗʰ April). *The critical Adult: A critical concept for 'interesting times'.* Keynote speech to the Annual Conference of the United Kingdom Association for Transactional Analysis, Edinburgh, Scotland.

Tudor, K. (2016a, 23 August). *The argumentative therapist: Philosophy, psychotherapy, and culture.* Public inaugural professorial lecture given at Auckland University of Technology, Auckland, Aotearoa New Zealand.

Tudor, K. (2016b). Permission, protection, and potency: The three Ps reconsidered. *Transactional Analysis Journal, 46*(1), 50–62. https://doi.org/10.1177/0362153715617475.

Tudor, K. (2016c). Politics in psychotherapy: Meeting 'Meeting the enemy' [L'angolo del discussant (Discussant's corner)]. *AIT Journal, 2*(2), 95–99.

Tudor, K. (2016d). Seeing the world in an individual. *Transactional Analysis Journal, 46*(2), 121–127. https://doi.org/10.1177/0362153716628867.

Tudor, K. (2016e). 'We are': The fundamental life position. *Transactional Analysis Journal, 46*(2), 164–176. https://doi.org/10.1177/0362153716637064.

Tudor, K. (2017a). *Conscience and critic: The selected works of Keith Tudor.* Routledge.

Tudor, K. (Ed.). (2017b). *Pluralism in psychotherapy: Critical reflections from a post-regulation landscape* (revised and extended edition of The turning tide). Resource Books.

Tudor, K. (2017c). The relational, the vertical, and the horizontal: A critique of 'relational depth'. In K. Tudor *Conscience and critic: The selected works of Keith Tudor* (pp. 191–201). Routledge. (Original work published 2014)

Tudor, K. (2017d). 'Take it': A sixth driver (2008). In K. Tudor *Conscience and critic: The selected works of Keith Tudor* (pp. 107–124). London, UK: Routledge. (Original work published 2008)

Tudor, K. (2018a). *Navigating professional identity through strength and vulnerability: A conversation with Keith Tudor* (D. Deaconu, Interviewer, B. Petrascu, Ed.). www. conversationsinta.com/keith-tudor/.

Tudor, K. (2018b). *Psychotherapy: A critical examination.* PCCS Books.

Tudor, K. (2018c, 23ʳᵈ November). *Transactional analysis: Honouring our traditions.* A keynote speech given to the Singapore Transactional Analysis Association's Conference 'Honouring our Traditions, Securing our Future', Singapore.

Tudor, K. (2019). Religion, faith, spirituality, and the beyond in transactional analysis. *Transactional Analysis Journal, 49*(2), 71–87. https://doi.org/10.1080/03621537.2019. 1577341.

Tudor, K. (2020a). Claude Michel Steiner: Death, life, and legacy. In K. Tudor (Ed.), *Claude Steiner, emotional activist: The life and work of Claude Michel Steiner* (pp. 228–249). Routledge.

Tudor, K. (Ed.) (2020b). *Claude Steiner, emotional activist: The life and work of Claude Michel Steiner.* Routledge.

Tudor, K. (2020c, 27 October). Ego and relationships: Professor of Psychotherapy Keith Tudor. On *Nine to noon* [Interview with Kathryn Ryan]. Radio New Zealand. https://www.rnz.co.nz/national/programmes/ninetonoon/audio/2018770082/ego-and-relationships-professor-of-psychotherapy-keith-tudor.

Tudor, K. (2020d). Introduction. In K. Tudor (Ed.), *Claude Steiner, emotional activist: The life and work of Claude Michel Steiner* (pp. 1–6). Routledge.

Tudor, K. (2020e). The law is an Act! *The Health Practitioners Competence Assurance Act 2003*. In K. Tudor (Ed.), *Pluralism in psychotherapy: Critical reflections from a post-regulation landscape* [E-book edition]. Tuwhera Open Access Books. https://ojs.aut.ac.nz/tuwhera-open-monographs/catalog/book/1. (Original work published 2011)

Tudor, K. (Ed.). (2020f). *Pluralism in psychotherapy: Critical reflections from a post-regulation landscape*. Tuwhera Open Access Books. https://ojs.aut.ac.nz/tuwhera-open-monographs/catalog/book/1. (Original work published 2017)

Tudor, K. (2020g). Transactional analysis and politics: A critical review. Transactional analysis and politics [Special issue]. *Psychotherapy and Politics International, 18*(3). http://dx.doi.org/10.1002/ppi.1555.

Tudor, K. (2021a). Alpha and omega, or, does actualisation encompass death. In *20/20 vision, 2020* (pp. 33–35). [E-book] Tuwhera Open Access Books. https://ojs.aut.ac.nz/tuwhera-open-monographs/catalog/book/6. (Original work published [in German] 2010)

Tudor, K. (2021b). Appendix B The quality assurance of this book. In *20/20 vision, 2020* (pp. 218–219). [E-book] Tuwhera Open Access Books. https://ojs.aut.ac.nz/tuwhera-open-monographs/catalog/book/6.

Tudor, K. (2021c, March). Co-creative transactional analysis. Schools in TA [Special issue]. *TA Magazine* [English edition]. *1*, 26–29. http://www.professioneelbegeleiden.nl/public/files/TA-2020-05-99.pdf.

Tudor, K. (2021b–c–d). He tangata Tiriti tatou. In *20/20 vision, 2020* (pp. 1–9). [E-book] Tuwhera Open Access Books. https://ojs.aut.ac.nz/tuwhera-open-monographs/catalog/book/6.

Tudor, K. (2021d–e). Introduction. In *20/20 vision, 2020* (pp. ix–xiii). [E-book] Tuwhera Open Access Books. https://ojs.aut.ac.nz/tuwhera-open-monographs/catalog/book/6

Tudor, K. (2022a). A coragem de ser – e de pertencer [The courage to be – and to belong]. *Revista Brasiliera de Análise Transacional, 29*. https://portal.unat.org.br/manager/arquivos/4PDvib9T20_06122022-a-coragem.pdf.

Tudor, K. (2022b). There and back again: Re-envisioning 'relationship therapy' as the center of a contemporary, cultural, and contextual person-centered therapy. *Person-Centered & Experiential Psychotherapies, 21*(2), 188–206. https://doi.org/10.1080/14779757.2022.2066562.

Tudor, K. (2023). The courage to be, become – and belong: A person-centred perspective. *Person-Centered & Experiential Psychotherapies*. https://doi.org/10.1080/14779757.2023.2234985.

Tudor, K. (2024/in press). Cambiare il mondo una teoria alla volta [Changing the world one theory at a time]. *Rivista Italiana di Analisi Transazionale e Metodologie Psicoterapeutiche*.

Tudor, K., & Begg, K. (2016). Radical therapy: A critical review. *The Journal of Critical Psychology, Counselling and Psychotherapy, 16*(2), 81–92.

Tudor, K., & Cornell, W. (Eds.). (2020). Transactional analysis and politics [Special issue]. *Psychotherapy and Politics International, 18*(3).

Tudor, K. & Francis, J. (2022). Research and practice: Contributions to the discipline of psychotherapy. *Ata: Journal of Psychotherapy Aotearoa New Zealand, 26*(2), 61–89. https://doi.org/10.9791/ajpanz.2022.10.

Tudor, K., & Gledhill, K. (2022). Notes on notes: Note-taking and record-keeping in psychotherapy. *Ata: Journal of Psychotherapy Aotearoa New Zealand, 26*(2), 123–144. https://doi.org/10.9791/ajpanz.2022.12.

Tudor, K., Green, E., & Brett, E. (2022). Critical whiteness: A transactional analysis of a systemic oppression. *Transactional Analysis Journal*. https://doi.org/10.1080/03621537.2022.2076394.

Tudor, K., & Hargaden, H. (2002). The couch and the ballot box: The contribution and potential of psychotherapy in enhancing citizenship. In C. Feltham (Ed.), *What's the good of counselling and psychotherapy? The benefits explained* (pp. 156–178). Sage.

Tudor, K., & Hobbes, R. (2002). Transactional analysis. In W. Dryden (Ed.), *Handbook of individual therapy* (pp. 239–265). Sage.

Tudor, K., & Hobbes, R. (2007). Transactional analysis. In W. Dryden (Ed.), *The handbook of individual therapy* (5th ed.; pp. 256–286). Sage.

Tudor, K., & House, R. (2019, Summer). From client to professor: A personal and professional journey. *AHPB Magazine, 3*, 1–9. https://ahpb.org/wp/wp-content/uploads/2019/08/nl-2019-t2-n6-keith-t-interview.pdf.

Tudor, K., & Rodgers, B. (2023). Can we be of help? Cultural considerations regarding personal growth, relationships, therapy, and life. *Person-Centered & Experiential Psychotherapies*. https://doi.org/10.1080/14779757.2023.2166576.

Tudor, K., Rodgers, B., & Smith, V. (2022). Tihei mauri ora—Contact, culture, and context. *Person- Centred & Experiential Psychotherapies, 21*(2), 102–111. https://doi.org/10.1080/14779757.2022.2066563.

Tudor, K., & Shaw, S. (2022, June). Expertise and expertise: A commentary on 'Experts, establishments, and learning from struggle' by Brian Martin. *Self & Society, 50*(1&2), 96–102.

Tudor, K., & Sills, C. (2006). Transactional analysis. In C. Feltham & I. Horton (Eds.), *The Sage handbook of psychotherapy and counselling* (2nd ed.) (pp. 310–314). Sage.

Tudor, K., & Sills, C. (2012). Transactional analysis. In C. Feltham & I. Horton (Eds.), *The Sage handbook of psychotherapy and counselling* (3rd ed.; pp. 333–338). Sage.

Tudor, K., & Summers, G. (2014). *Co-creative transactional analysis: Papers, dialogues, responses, and developments.* Karnac Books.

Tudor, K., & Widdowson, M. (2002). Integrating views of TA in time-limited therapy. In K. Tudor (Ed.), *Transactional approaches to brief therapy or what do you say between saying hello and goodbye?* (pp. 114–135). Sage.

Tudor, K., & Widdowson, M. (2008). From client process to therapeutic relating: A critique of the process model and personality adaptations. *Transactional Analysis Journal, 38*(3), 218–232. https://doi.org/10.1177/036215370803800304.

Tudor, K., & Worrall, M. (2006). *Person-centred therapy: A clinical philosophy.* Routledge.

Tudor, K., & Wyatt, J. (2023). *Qualitative research approaches for psychotherapy: Reflexivity, methodology, and criticality.* Routledge.

United Kingdom Council for Psychotherapy. (1996). *National register for psychotherapists.* Author.

United Nations. (1948). *Universal Declaration of Human Rights.* Author.

United States of America Transactional Analysis Association. (2023). *Project TA101.* https://www.usataa.org/circles-of-interest/social-justice-circle/project-ta-101/.

Urban Dictionary. (2023). *Meta.* https://www.urbandictionary.com/define.php?term=meta.

Vago, M., & Knapp, B. W. (1977). Parenting: Protection for growth. *Transactional Analysis Journal, 7*(3), 221–223. https://doi.org/10.1177/036215377700700305.

Vago, M., & Knapp, B. W. (1978). Bartering for protection. *Transactional Analysis Journal, 8*(2), 129–131. https://doi.org/10.1177/036215377800800207.

Vaillant, G. (1993). *The wisdom of the ego.* Harvard University Press.

Valéry, P. (1958). *The art of poetry* (D. Folliot, Trans.). Princeton University Press.

van Beekum, S. (2005). The therapist as a new object. *Transactional Analysis Journal*, *35*(2), 187–191. https://doi.org/10.1177/036215370503500208.

van Beekum, S. (2006). The relational consultant. *Transactional Analysis Journal*, *36*(4), 318–329. https://doi.org/10.1177/036215370603600406.

van Beekum, S. (2009). Siblings, aggression, and sexuality: Adding the lateral. *Transactional Analysis Journal*, *39*(2), 129–135. https://doi.org/10.1177/036215370903900206.

van Beekum, S. (2016). Beyond the concepts. *Transactional Analysis Journal*, *46*(1), 8–12. https://doi.org/10.1177/0362153715611687.

van Beekum, S., & Lammers, W. (1990). Over the border: Script theory and beyond. *Transactional Analysis Journal*, *20*(1), 47–55. https://doi.org/10.1177/036215379002000106.

Van Belle, H. A. (1980). *Basic intent and therapeutic approach of Carl R. Rogers: A study of his view of man in relation to his view of therapy, personality and interpersonal relations.* Wedge Publishing Foundation.

van der Ploeg J. D. (1993). Potatoes and knowledge. In M. Hobart (Ed.), *An anthropological critique of development: The growth of ignorance* (pp. 209–227). Routledge.

van Tol, R. (2017). I love you, and you, and you too. *Transactional Analysis Journal*, *47*(4), 276–293. https://doi.org/10.1177/0362153717720191.

Vygotsky, L. (1962). *Thought and language.* MIT Press.

Wadsworth, D., & DiVincenti, A. (2003). Core concepts of transactional analysis: An opportunity born of struggle. *Transactional Analysis Journal*, *33*(2), 148–161. https://doi.org/10.1177/036215370303300206.

Waitangi Tribunal. (2015). *The treaty of Waitangi.* https://www.waitangitribunal.govt.nz/treaty-of-waitangi/.

Walker, R. (1990). *Ka whawhai tonu matou. Struggle without end.* Penguin.

Wallace, G. W. (1973). Sweet charity. *Transactional Analysis Bulletin*, *3*(1), 47–49. https://doi.org/10.1177/036215377300300112.

Wallerstein, R. S. (2000). The growth and transformation of American ego psychology. *Journal of the American Psychoanalytic Association*, *50*(1), 135–169. https://doi.org/10.1177/00030651020500011401.

Wampold, B. (2001). *The great psychotherapy debate: Models, methods, and findings.* Routledge.

Warner, M. S. (2000). Person-centered psychotherapy: One nation, many tribes. *The Person-Centered Journal*, *7*(1), 28–39. https://www.adpca.org/wp-content/uploads/2020/11/7_1_7.pdf.

Watkins, J. G. (1947). *Hypnotherapy of war neuroses.* The Ronald Press Company.

Watkins, J. G. (1978). *The therapeutic self: Developing resonance—key to effective relationships.* Human Sciences.

Watkins, J. G., & Watkins, H. H. (1988). The management of malevolent ego states in multiple personality disorder. *Dissociation: Progress in the Dissociative Disorders*, *1*(1), 67–72.

Watkins, J. G., & Watkins, H. H. (1997). *Ego states: Theory and therapy.* Norton.

Weinhold, B. K. (1977). A philosophical analysis of various TA treatment styles. *Transactional Analysis Journal*, *7*(3), 235–241. https://doi.org/10.1177/036215377700700314.

Weiss, E. (1942). Psychic defence and the technique of its analysis. *The International Journal of Psycho-Analysis*, *23*, 69–80. (Original work published 1937)

Weiss, E. (1950). *Principles of psychodynamics.* Grune & Stratton.

Weiss, E. (1952). Introduction. In *Ego psychology and the psychoses* (E. Weiss, Ed.; pp. 1–21). Basic Books.

Wells, M. (2012). From fiction to freedom: Our true nature beyond life script. *Transactional Analysis Journal*, 42(2), 143–151. https://doi.org/10.1177/03621537120 4200208.

White, J. D., & White, T. (1975). Cultural scripting. *Transactional Analysis Journal*, 5(1), 12–23. https://doi.org/10.1177/036215377500500104.

White, T. (1994). Life positions. *Transactional Analysis Journal*, 24(4), 269–276. https://doi.org/10.1177/036215379402400406.

White, T. (1995a). 'I'm OK, you're OK': Further considerations. *Transactional Analysis Journal*, 25(3), 234–236. https://doi.org/10.1177/036215379502500308.

White, T. (1995b). Response. *Transactional Analysis Journal*, 25(3), 241–244. https://doi.org/10.1177/036215379502500308.

White, T. (1999). No-psychosis contracts. *Transactional Analysis Journal*, 29(2), 133–138. https://doi.org/10.1177/036215379902900207.

White, T. (2001). The contact contract. *Transactional Analysis Journal*, 31(3), 194–198. https://doi.org/10.1177/036215370103100308.

Widdowson, M. (2010). *Transactional analysis: 100 key points and techniques*. Routledge.

Widdowson, M. (2011). Depression: A literature review on diagnosis, subtypes, patterns of recovery, and psychotherapeutic models. *Transactional Analysis Journal*, 41(4), 351–364. https://doi.org/10.1177/036215371104100411.

Widdowson, M. (2018). The importance of research in transactional analysis for transactional analysts. *Transactional Analysis Journal*, 48(1), 33–42. https://doi.org/10.1080/03621537.2018.1397965.

Wilson, J., & Kalina, I. (1978). The splinter chart. *Transactional Analysis Journal*, 8(3), 200–205. https://doi.org/10.1177/036215377800800303.

Windes, K. L. (1977). The three 'c's' of corrections: Cops–cons–counsellors. In G. Barnes (Ed.), *Transactional analysis after Eric Berne: Teachings and practices of three TA schools* (pp. 138–145). Harper's College Press.

Winnicott, D. W. (1957). Further thoughts on babies as persons. In J. Hardenberg, (Ed.), *The child and the outside world: Studies in developing relationships* (pp. 134–140). Tavistock. (Original work published 1947)

Winnicott, D. W. (1965). The theory of the parent-infant relationship. In, *The maturational processes and the facilitating environment* (pp. 37–55). International Universities Press. (Original work published 1960)

Winnicott, D. W. (1971). Mirror-role of mother and family in child development. In *Playing and reality* (pp. 111–118). Penguin. (Original work published 1967)

Wolf, A., & Schwartz, E. K. (1962). *Psychoanalysis in groups*. Grune & Stratton.

Wood, J. K. (1995). The person-centered approach: Towards an understanding of its implications. *The Person-Centered Journal*, 2(2), 18–35.

Woods, K. (1995). The indirect analysis of manifestations of transference and countertransference. *Transactional Analysis Journal*, 25(3), 245–249. https://doi.org/10.11 77/036215379502500310.

Woods, K. (1996). Projective identification and game analysis. *Transactional Analysis Journal*, 26(3), 228–231. https://doi.org/10.1177/036215379602600306.

Woods, K. (2003). The interface between Berne and Langs: Understanding unconscious communication. *Transactional Analysis Journal*, 33(3), 214–222. https://doi.org/10.1177/036215370303300303.

Woollams, S. J. (1977). From 21 to 43. In G. Barnes (Ed.), *Transactional analysis after Eric Berne: Teachings and practices of three TA schools* (pp. 351–379). Harper's College Press.

Woollams, S., & Brown, M. (1978). *Transactional analysis: A modern and comprehensive text of TA theory and practice*. Huron Valley Institute.

Woollams, S., & Brown, M. (1985). *Analisi transazionale* [*Transactional analysis*]. Cittadella.

Woollams, S., Brown, M., & Huige, K. (1977). What transactional analysts want their clients to know. In G. Barnes (Ed.), *Transactional analysis after Eric Berne: Teachings and practices of three TA schools* (pp. 487–525). Harper's College Press.

Wyckoff, H. (1970). Radical psychiatry and TA in women's groups. *Transactional Analysis Bulletin, 36*, 128–133.

Wyckoff, H. (1971). The stroke economy in women's scripts. *Transactional Analysis Journal, 1*(3), 16–20. https://doi.org/10.1177/036215377100100306

Wyckoff, H. (1976a). Problem-solving groups for women. In H. Wyckoff (Ed.), *Love, therapy and politics* (pp. 3–27). Grove Press.

Wyckoff, H. (Ed.). (1976b). *Love, therapy and politics*. Grove Press.

Yeats, W. B. (1962). A dialogue of self and soul. In *W. B Yeats selected poetry* (A. N. Jeffries, Ed.; pp. 142–145). Macmillian. (Original work published 1933)

Younger, J. (2020). The baby and the bathwater: psychodynamic psychotherapy and regulation. In K. Tudor (Ed.), *Pluralism in psychotherapy: Critical reflections from a post-regulation landscape.* Tuwhera Open Access Books. https://ojs.aut.ac.nz/tuwhera-open-monographs/catalog/book/1. (Original work published 2017)

Zalcman, M. (1990). Game analysis and racket analysis: Overview, critique, and future developments. *Transactional Analysis Journal, 20*(1), 4–19. https://doi.org/10.1177/036215379002000102.

Zechnich, R. (1973) Good games; Therapeutic uses and four new ones. *Transactional Analysis Journal, 3*(1), 52–56. https://doi.org/10.1177/036215377300300114.

Zechnich, R. (1975). Editorial. *Transactional Analysis Journal, 5*(2), 105–106. https://doi.org/10.1177/036215377500500203.

Žvelc, G. (2009). Between self and others: Relational schemas as an integrating construct in psychotherapy. *Transactional Analysis Journal, 39*(1), 22–38. https://doi.org/10.1177/036215370903900104.

Žvelc, G. (2010). Relational schemas theory and transactional analysis. *Transactional Analysis Journal, 40*(1), 8–22. https://doi.org/10.1177/036215371004000103.

Žvelc, G., & Žvelc, M. (2020). *Integrative therapy: A mindfulness- and compassion-based approach*. Routledge.

Žvelc, G., Černetič, M., & Košak, M. (2011). Mindfulness-based transactional analysis. *Transactional Analysis Journal, 41*(3), 241–254. https://doi.org/10.1177/036215371104100306.

Index

Note: **Bold** page numbers refer to tables, *italic* page numbers refer to figures and page numbers followed by "n" refer to end notes.

For Product Safety Concerns and Information please contact our EU
representative GPSR@taylorandfrancis.com
Taylor & Francis Verlag GmbH, Kaufingerstraße 24, 80331 München, Germany

www.ingramcontent.com/pod-product-compliance
Lightning Source LLC
Chambersburg PA
CBHW050335270326
41926CB00016B/3470